LIVING A GOOD LIFE WITH DEMENTIA: A PRACTITIONER'S GUIDE

Other books you may be interested in:

Dilemmas and Decision Making in Social Work
by Abbi Jackson ISBN 9781914171208

Relationship-based Social Work with Adults
Edited by Heidi Dix and Sue Hollinrake ISBN 9781912096275

Safeguarding Adults Together under the Care Act 2014: A multi-agency practice guide
by Barbara Starns ISBN 9781913063252

Self-Neglect: A Practical Approach to Risks and Strengths Assessment
by Shona Britten and Karen Whitby ISBN 9781912096862

Self-Neglect: Learning from Life
by Shona Britten and Karen Whitby ISBN 9781913453572

The Social Worker's Guide to the Care Act 2014
by Pete Feldon ISBN 9781913453053

Working with Family Carers
by Valerie Gant ISBN 9781912096978

www.criticalpublishing.com or contact our distributor Ingram Publisher Services, telephone 01752 202301 or email NBNi.Cservs@ingramcontent.com

LIVING A GOOD LIFE WITH DEMENTIA: A PRACTITIONER'S GUIDE

By Liz Leach Murphy and Jayna Patel

CRITICAL PUBLISHING

First published in 2021 by Critical Publishing Ltd

Illustrations by Mollie Williams

British Library Cataloguing in Publication Data
A CIP record for this book is available from the British Library

ISBN: 9781914171567
This book is also available in the following e-book formats:
EPUB ISBN: 9781914171574
Adobe e-book ISBN: 9781914171581

Cover design by Out of House
Text design by Out of House
Project Management by Deanta Global Publishing Services, Dublin, Ireland
Typeset by Deanta Global Publishing Services, Chennai, India
Printed and bound in Great Britain by 4edge, Essex

Critical Publishing
3 Connaught Road
St Albans AL3 5RX

www.criticalpublishing.com

Contents

Meet the authors

Liz Leach Murphy has worked within health and social care for the past 25 years, and within this time she has been committed to improving the experiences of those accessing the care and support they need, which has involved working alongside people living with dementia and their families. She has been trained in and delivered person-centred planning and support brokerage, both of which are approaches to enable people to direct their own care and support in a manner that is rooted in the community rather than services. Liz's work and passion led her to set up Imagineer Development UK CIC in 2010, a social enterprise based in the north of England with a national reach, which specialises in self-direction.

With a degree in journalism and a love for writing, editing, reviewing and blogging, **Jayna Patel** enjoyed putting her research and inquisitive skills to good use, supporting Liz with finding evidence to underpin her case for more community-based person-centred solutions and tidying up all the references. A keen storyteller, helping her illustrate the book with case studies of real people affected by dementia and making these books a valuable and helpful resource for family carers have been an even more rewarding experience. An account manager at a web design and digital marketing agency, she is a Yorkshire lass whose favourite things to do in her free time are walks in nature, exploring new places and discovering new experiences.

Glossary

BSI British Standards Institution sets standards for many areas of industry. The BSI holds the standard set for dementia-friendly communities.

CCG Clinical commissioning group is the local NHS commissioning group. They are responsible for commissioning health support and interventions in the local area and are responsible for the provision of personal health budgets.

CCM Clinical case manager is an approach that integrates services around the needs of individuals with long-term conditions. A community-based and proactive approach to care that involves assessment, care planning and care coordination.

CM Care manager refers to a set of evidence-based, integrated clinical care activities that are tailored to the individual patient and that ensure each patient has their own coordinated plan of care and services.

DH The Department of Health leads, shapes and funds health and care in England. Their aim is to make sure people have the support, care and treatment they need, with the compassion, respect and dignity they deserve.

DP Direct payment is a method a person can choose to manage their personal budget or personal health budget. The budget is deposited into a bank account that is managed by the individual and/or their representatives.

GP A general practitioner is a doctor based in the community who treats patients with minor or chronic illnesses and refers those with serious conditions to a hospital.

HP A health professional or health care provider is an individual who provides preventive, curative, promotional or rehabilitative health care services in a systematic way to people, families or communities.

IB Indicative budget is presented to an individual as an amount to work with when developing the support plan. As the name suggests, this is only intended as an indication and is open for discussion and negotiation. The actual budget is agreed on completion of the person's care and support plan.

ISF Individual service fund is a mechanism for controlling a person's personal budget or personal health budget within an organisation. It is managed specifically on behalf of the person, and it can be spent flexibly to achieve the best possible outcomes for a person.

MDT Multi-disciplinary team is a group of health care workers who are members of different disciplines, for example psychiatrists or social workers, each providing specific services to a person.

PB Personal budget is allocated to the person by a social work team in a local authority. It can be utilised to meet a person's assessed social care need.

PHB Personal health budget is allocated to the person by a clinical team within a CCG to enable a person to meet their assessed health care needs.

RAP Resource allocation panel is the group of people within a local authority or a CCG who make decisions about the level of budget to allocate to an individual. Often there will be a member of the social work or nursing team on the panel alongside a person to represent commissioning and a person to represent the finance department. They will use the information within a completed assessment document to aid their decision.

RAS Resource allocation system is utilised by a local authority or a clinical commissioning group to calculate the level of budget a person would be entitled to based on the content of their assessment. Generally, the system is either a computer-based programme that calculates the budget based on the information entered into it or a comparative process where the social worker or nurse would identify the services a person would have been offered under a traditional service-led approach. The cost of these services would then represent the budget allocated to an individual.

Introduction

Over the past 20 years I have worked within health and social care, with a broad range of people in a variety of circumstances: living in their own home, supported living, residential care and hospital settings, and attending daytime support and respite provision. I have worked with those with dementia, with Down's syndrome and dementia, with long-term health conditions, at the end of life, with autism and Asperger's, with physical disabilities and under a section order.

In this time I have provided direct care and support, managed teams working in care and support settings, delivered district-wide projects to implement person-centred approaches and personalisation and been involved in the development of national strategy. I have worked alongside individuals who required care and support in their lives, their families and those who work in the provision of health and social care, including direct support workers, care workers, team leaders, managers, social workers, directors of adult social care, clinicians, leaders in the delivery of personal budgets and personal health budgets, commissioners and members of the community.

It is this accumulation of learning and experience that has brought me to writing this book, based on a true belief that the provision of care and support can be positive and can be done in a manner that upholds the person's identified choices and wishes. It is possible as I have been part of making this possible and I have seen it work well.

I hope you enjoy reading the book. It is not meant to be read from cover to cover although, if this is how you would like to digest the information, please go ahead. It begins with an understanding of how developments have made a difference over the past 60 plus years, moves on to where we are now in the delivery of care and support and, finally, gives a strong sense of direction for the future – all supported with some really useful tools and approaches.

This book is absolutely directed at dementia care and support although I am sure you will appreciate that many of the ideas and approaches are relevant to anyone wanting to achieve a good life.

1 Innovation within dementia care

Introduction

There are more than 850,000 people in the UK living with dementia. The condition affects 1 in 6 people over 80 and 42,000 people aged under 65 (Alzheimer's Society, n.d.a). People are living longer, which is increasing the number of people who are diagnosed with dementia. It is estimated that by 2025 the number of people with dementia in the UK will exceed one million (NHS, 2020). It is becoming increasingly important to make sure that the health and social care resources available to support these people are used to achieve the best outcomes, where a person is well supported and able to lead a good life. An approach which embraces personalisation is one way to achieve this.

This chapter covers:

- **Personalisation and the personalisation agenda**
- **Self-directed support**
- **Personalisation within service settings**
- **The dementia care triad**
- **Person-centred care**
- **Dementia care mapping**
- **Person-centred practice**
- **The values of inclusion**
- **Person-centred planning**
- **The VIPs framework**

- **The senses framework**
- **Enriched care planning**
- **Dementia and age-friendly communities.**

Personalisation

Defining personalisation

Personalisation is an approach to adult social care and health services which tailors the care and support provided to the individual. It advocates a shift in focus away from large-scale building and service-based solutions to a particular recognition of the person, promoting their individual identity and preferences with choice and control set as a principle to achieve this.

The personalisation agenda

Personalisation focuses on ensuring that the support and care provided to a person is unique to them and that they, and those close to them, have decided upon the way in which their care and support is provided, so they can exercise full control over their life choices and experience. The personalisation agenda encourages all aspects of health and social care to be delivered in a manner that works well for the individual, taking into consideration the person's choices, dignity and identity.

A report by the Alzheimer's Society in 2011 stated that two-thirds of people with dementia were living within the community (Alzheimer's Society, 2011, p 9). The report also showed that the satisfaction with services received was generally high (Alzheimer's Society, 2011, p 12). However, half of the respondents said: '*the person with dementia is not receiving sufficient support and care to meet their needs*' (Alzheimer's Society, 2011, p 11)

The term *personalisation* first appeared in 2007 within the ministerial concordant 'Putting People First'. It focused on delivering personalised adult social care and was the first driver of system-wide transformation (Policy Navigator, 2007) as described by the Department of Health: '*every person who receives support, whether provided by statutory services or funded by themselves, will have choice and control over the shape of that support in all care settings*' (Department of Health, 2010). In the same year, the Social Care Institute for Excellence (SCIE) stated:

> *Personalisation is not just about personal budgets, but about achieving choice and control in many ways and in different settings, including basic needs such as being able to access public transport if you are disabled.*
>
> *Personalisation is about the dignity and well-being of the individual.*
>
> *Delivering personalised services will mean different things to different people – it's about self-determination and self-directed care.*

> *The relationship between social workers/PAs and service users should be based on respect and a recognition of equality.*
>
> (Social Care Institute for Excellence (SCIE), 2011)

Self-directed support

The term *self-directed support* in practice is used interchangeably with *self-directed care*. It is a complementary term to personalisation and describes a situation when the person is central to making the decisions about how to use the budget available to them to meet their care and support needs and whether the person is self-funding or accessing public monies.

Self-directed support means that the person, and their family, directs the care and support they receive to make sure it works well for them and meets their aspirations and needs. It places the person and their family at the centre of *good outcomes* and provides opportunity for them to think about what *good support* would look like and where that support can be found. It broadens the possible solutions beyond the usual array of service solutions and supports a wider consideration for the person. For instance, rather than attend a day centre provision, a person may prefer to spend their time going out for lunch with a friend while they also enjoy an activity that they both have a shared interest in, such as visiting a museum. Depending on the circumstances, this could also be an opportunity for the person who provides the majority of the care to have a rest or a break while the person retains independence, freedom and choice in a supportive environment.

Personalisation and self-directed support encourage people living with dementia to consider all the options available to them when they are looking at how they wish to be supported or cared for with the aim of helping them to find solutions that work best for them. A good starting point when looking to implement self-directed support and personalisation is to listen to and understand what makes sense to the person, including their aspirations and ideas about how their care and support needs can be met. This helps you to look at the bigger picture of what is possible for the person through their existing relationships, the places they know well, the local and wider community as well as the local community associations and groups that are available. This approach to finding support is complementary to 'The National Dementia Strategy: living well with dementia', published in February 2009 (Department of Health, 2009a).

Personalised services

When services form part of someone's support network, these services need to be oriented around their life and be flexible in their approach to ensure the person can maintain their identity and individuality and exercise choice and control.

A personalised service would structure the way that care and support are provided around the person's preferences. This would include following routines that make sense to them, for example, when they like to get up and how they like to get ready in the morning. A service that is not personalised would follow routines designed to suit the smooth running of the service rather than the preferences of each individual being cared for. For example, in a care home, each resident would be supported to get up at a time that fits into a morning routine that makes sure everyone is ready to have breakfast at the same time.

Achieving a personalised approach can prove to be a challenge for services built on rigid structures. These structures can determine when people are to be supported with personal care, who will be providing this care, when meals are to be served, when each room will be cleaned and bedding changed and when and what activities will be offered. Rigid structures prevent staff from having the freedom to think about *what is possible*' when it comes to the care they provide and ensuring that care makes sense to the individual. Staff can be denied the time and creative space to really get to know those they are caring for. These themes are explored further in Chapter 3.

Person-centred care

Person-centred care is explored further later in this chapter but is introduced here as a model for those providing care and support to people living with dementia. The model was unique from its inception in the sense that *personhood* ran as a central theme within its development. Personhood relates to the qualities and conditions that define us as individual human beings. Person-centred care challenges the Medical Model of care (explored further in Chapter 2), which has a focus on diagnosis, medical treatment, finding ways to fix the person's condition and task-oriented approaches. In contrast, person-centred care is built on the needs of the individual and is conditional on developing a good understanding through healthy interpersonal relationships. It is the dominant approach within dementia care settings and was, and continues to be, largely developed through the innovative and pioneering work of Tom Kitwood and Dawn Brooker. Person-centred care is explained in many reviews and research articles, such as 'The experience of dementia' (Kitwood, 1997), where the psychological needs of people with dementia are explored and an evidence base is built for the *six routes of understanding*, as well as 'What is person centred care in dementia?' (Brooker, 2004), where the aspiration surrounding person-centred approaches is compared with the actual experience of receiving care.

Integrating person-centred care into dementia care and clinical settings has demonstrated the valuable difference the approach has on the experience of receiving care and support for those living with dementia (Kim and Park, 2017). Person-centred care highlights the following as areas of focus when supporting or caring for a person living with dementia:

- well-being;
- personality;
- personhood;
- the subjective experience of people with dementia.

The personalisation of services for people living with dementia complements and develops the principles and purpose of person-centred care. The personalisation agenda has introduced functions within the provision of health and social care which helps people living with dementia and their families to take more control over the care and support they receive and to be fully involved in making decisions about how, when and who provides the care and support they require.

Person-centred care recognises all aspects of the person and enhances their sense of self. This includes respecting the person's culture, faith, religious practices, values and lifestyle choices. It focuses on the provision of care within a care setting, for example, residential care, nursing homes and hospitals. In these settings person-centred care has value; however, it is limited in its implementation (see Chapter 3 for more details).

Personalisation, as an agenda for health and social care, sets the principle of people being fully involved in the planning of their care and support and being informed about the options available to them so as to make choices about how, when and where they receive the support and care they need to live their lives.

Personalisation complements the underpinning principles of assessment, management and support for people living with dementia and their carers, as set out by the National Institute for Health and Social Care Excellence, which assert:

- *the human value of people with dementia (regardless of age or cognitive impairment) and those who care for them;*
- *the individuality of people living with dementia, and how their unique personality and life experiences influence their response to dementia;*
- *the importance of the person's [with dementia] perspective;*
- *the importance of relationships and interactions with others to the person living with dementia, and their potential for promoting wellbeing.*

(National Institute for Health and Care Excellence, 2018)

The national drive

Personalisation has been on the government agenda since 2007 but is yet to be achieved at scale. Some of the key reasons for this are a lack of strong leadership and the complexity of changing systems to accommodate a personalised approach. The guidance provided to date has been broad and open to interpretation, causing inconsistent implementation and practice from area to area. Achieving personalisation requires strong leadership (Think Local Act Personal, 2014) in order to review all the systems that govern the provision of services and to enable greater flexibility and individualised arrangements. Steadfast guidance from the government and authoritative organisations is also required to drive through the significant changes needed to achieve a large-scale personalised approach and to secure a sustainable model of practice into the future.

An international focus

In December 2013, a G8 summit was held in the UK with a specialist focus on dementia. The intention of the summit was to bring about a global incentive to address and build understanding about dementia, focusing on the quality of care and support and encouraging ongoing research. This event was heavily supported by the Alzheimer's Society, which ensured people attending had heard the voices of those with the experience of living with dementia. This was the first opportunity for people living with dementia and their families to talk to an audience of this size about what they had been through and to share their thoughts on the priorities with regard to dementia. The main concern they raised was the negative stigma and how this needed to be addressed.

Following the G8 summit, the Scottish Government convened an international meeting in 2014 to galvanise international relations and to discuss opportunities and priorities for international collaboration.

Government policy and international commitment place an emphasis on developing and improving dementia diagnosis, care and support. The question is how do we translate these ideas into the day-to-day life experiences of people with dementia? How can person-centred approaches, personalisation and self-directed support progress these developments, and how do practitioners, families and individuals embrace these ideas and implement them to make a real difference to people's quality of life?

Dementia care triad

The dementia care triad (Adams and Gardiner, 2005) highlights the importance of the relationship between the person with dementia, informal carers and the health and social care professionals.

It is vital that each member of the triad is included and involved in conversations about what good support would look like and what is meant by *quality of life*, which can be subjective and vary from person to person. The connection between the people who make up the dementia care triad enables key conversations to take place that provide detailed insight into how the person living with dementia wishes to be supported, and it sheds light on the different perspectives regarding what is important and what is needed to improve the quality of the support and care the person receives. Personalisation is about individualising service provision and helping recipients of services maintain their identity, choice and control over the services they receive; therefore, conversations between members of the dementia care triad are crucial in achieving the goal of personalisation.

The emphasis is on the person living with dementia retaining choice and control over their lives through sharing their thoughts, opinions and feelings via conversations with their informal carers and those in the health and social care provision; for this to be possible, the principles of respect, dignity and identity need to be present in equal measure.

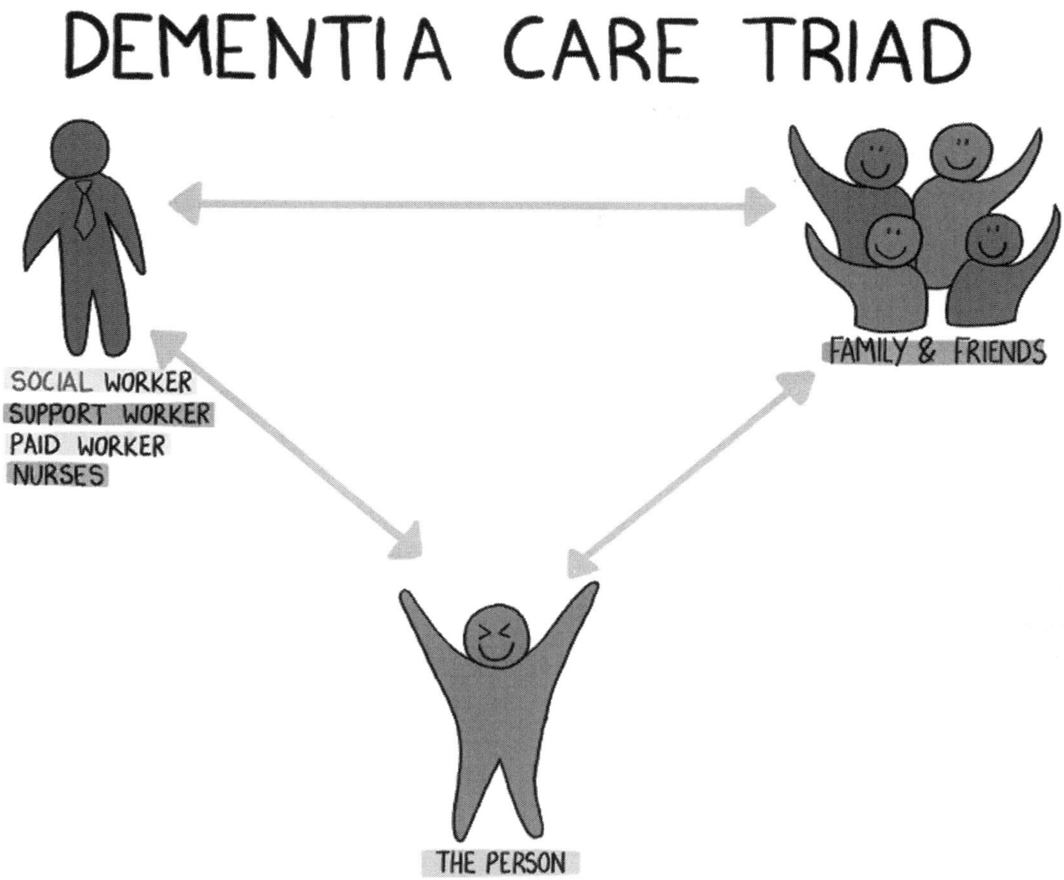

Figure 1.1 *Forms of Positive Person Work (Mitchell and Agnelli, 2015, p 49)*

There is no one individual who is determined as being the responsible person to begin the formation of a dementia care triad; rather it is an approach to building effective relationships with and around the person living with dementia for all involved to recognise. The bringing together of individuals could be instigated by any one person.

Complementary approaches to personalisation

In this section, we will explore person-centred care in greater detail alongside subsequent models of delivering personalised services for those living with dementia in order to understand what personalisation looks like in practice.

Person-centred care

Since this approach was developed by Tom Kitwood in the late 1980s, person-centred care has changed the practice in care homes, and, according to Health Innovation Network

South London (2016), this has given rise to an increased quality of care and a decreased level of agitation and distress in the people cared for in that setting (Plos Medicine, 2018).

The central ideas are:

- the person living with dementia should come first;
- people with dementia have personhood;
- this should be maintained, despite the continuing presence of dementia. Kitwood defines personhood as: '*a standing or status that is bestowed upon one human being, by others, in the context of relationship and social being*' (Kitwood, 1997, p 8). He states that personhood '*implies recognition, respect and trust*' (Kitwood, 1997, p 8). He argues that, unlike biomedical approaches towards people living with dementia, which directly equate changes in the brain to the degree of cognitive and behavioural decline, the extent to which dementia affects a person arises out of biomedical factors and social-psychological factors. Kitwood expresses this relationship by the equation:

Dementia = [physical health + neurological impairment] + [life history + personality + social psychology]

Kitwood and his followers focus on how personhood arises within and through social relationships. Underpinning this thinking is the belief that there is often an emotional gulf that divides paid staff and people living with dementia. While this gulf can protect staff from emotional pain caused by their close proximity to people living with dementia, it also means that people are more likely to be treated as objects and this kind of iteration of care leads to depersonalisation. To address this gulf, Kitwood outlines numerous ways staff can interact with people who have dementia, which allows for better interpersonal engagement to promote personhood as outlined in Figure 1.1.

Celebration – Not just during celebratory occasions, such as birthdays or anniversaries. The person should see their achievements celebrated; for example, the healthcare professional can join the person who is happy and and celebrate with them, irrespective of the reason, by clapping, whistling, singing or smiling.

Collaboration – Partnership between the healthcare professional and the person to carry out an activity or task, for instance having a bath or getting dressed in ways that are comfortable for the person.

Facilitation – Enabling the person to do what otherwise they would be unable to do. This is similar to collaboration, for example, accompanying a person to go for a walk outside of the care setting.

Giving – Accepting whatever kindness the person with dementia gives, such as the person with dementia wanting to give a nurse a flower from the garden.

Holding – Providing a safe psychological space or environment to enable people to truly express themselves, for example, not isolating a person living with dementia if they are experiencing distress but instead staying beside them and validating their experiences without trying to stop or ignore them.

Negotiation – Facilitated through consultation with the person about their preferences in care and their daily lives. Where possible, supporting them in being involved in the decision-making process, serving residents food that they enjoy, for instance.

Creation (creativity) – Encouraging the person to be creative, because this can be therapeutic, for example, spontaneous singing or dancing or horticultural therapy.

Play – The provision of appropriate activity and enablement of self-expression, such as rolling a ball, sharing a joke or playing a game.

Recognition – A person who is recognised by name and acknowledged as a person with unique thoughts, feelings and preferences, greeting a person by their preferred name, for example.

Relaxation – Low level of intensity and recognition that some people may like to relax in solitude, for example, by listening to music or spending time in the garden.

Timealation (Timao – Latin for 'I honour') –A form of interaction, such as aromatherapy, which stimulates the senses.

Validation – Connected to the work of Feil (1993); this is about accepting the reality of another even if it is as a result of hallucinations or misperceptions.

Underlying Kitwood's approach is the idea that people living with dementia can benefit from interpersonal strategies that promote their sense of personhood. To develop this approach, he drew on a range of writers from the biomedical sciences, philosophy, social sciences and counselling, not least Carl Rogers (1959) who highlighted three conditions for effective therapeutic engagement.

- **Genuineness –** also called congruence. This approach within therapy encourages the therapist to be authentic in their relationships with the client. Translated into a care setting, this encourages caregivers to be authentic with the person receiving their care.
- **Unconditional positive regard –** the belief that people need to be valued for being their true selves if they were to grow and fulfil their potential.
- **Empathic understanding –** this is an ability to understand sensitively and accurately a person's feelings and experience without demonstrating sympathy.

Kitwood's focus on personhood and the subjective experience of people with dementia is further developed when he identifies different access routes that staff may use to gain an understanding of people's experience of dementia. These are:

- reading accounts written by people with dementia;
- listening to people with dementia talking about their experience in either one-to-one conversations or group settings;
- listening to what people with dementia say in the course of their life and everyday conversations;
- observing the behaviour and actions of people with dementia;
- consulting people who have gone through conditions or illnesses that are similar to dementia;
- acting out situations in role play.

Kitwood's work within dementia care also covered the effects of malignant social psychology, which raised awareness of the psychological effects of receiving care based on an approach embedded in the Medical Model, as covered in Chapter 2, and how it can be compared with the Enriched Model of Dementia, which recognises all the factors that affect a person's experience of dementia. These factors include neurological impairment, physical health, biography and personality and the person's immediate social environment.

Kitwood's introduction of person-centred care has made a significant and positive difference for people living with dementia who receive care within a care setting (Chenoweth et al, 2009, pp 317–25). It must be recognised that the difference made is largely limited to care settings, although the principles are transferable to any setting such as the family home, community-based support or day centre. Person-centred care fails to consider the experience of living with dementia when the person is still living in their own home in the community or how the principles can be embedded when the person is receiving care and support in shorter time frames from a home care agency.

Person-centred care runs the risk of being driven from a professional perspective, and, as a result, the delivery is done *for* or *to* people living with dementia and in receipt of care rather than an approach that is done *with* or *by* the people living with dementia themselves. It implies that people are not able to manage the aspects of their lives highlighted by the model, for instance when to have time alone, when to be around others, which activities to be involved in and how to self-express. Maintaining the belief that people living with dementia are not able to manage these aspects of their lives can be disempowering and negates agency, the concept of which is discussed in more detail later in this chapter.

Dementia Care Mapping™

Kitwood also developed an important tool for realising person-centred care within care settings called Dementia Care Mapping™ (DCM). This assessment tool has a proven track record of success and is now used internationally.

DCM helps staff observe life through the eyes of a person living with dementia and identifies the extent to which their support enhances their sense of well-being. It is a structured process that involves the following steps.

Preparation and briefing – This would involve providing information about DCM to staff, people living with dementia, family members and visitors. This would build people's understanding of the process that will take place and their role and involvement in that process.

Observation – During the observation period, a trained observer (mapper, often a member of staff in the care setting) records the care experience of up to eight people living with dementia for a length of time determined by the purpose of the observation (map). These can be short focused maps (eg, over mealtime periods), or longer maps to gain a broad picture of the person's day and evening time experience. Once the observer has recorded their findings they make an assessment on the level of relative well or ill-being of the person living with dementia.

Analysis – Analysis of data recorded using the DCM tool provides in-depth detail about how individual and group levels of well-being and ill-being vary across the day. The DCM also identifies how people living with dementia spend their time and how this is linked to relative well-being and pinpoints the staff interactions that promote person-centred care and those that undermine person-centred care and well-being.

Report writing and feedback – Once the data have been analysed, the mapper provides written and verbal feedback to staff teams.

Action plan – Following verbal feedback of the written report, the staff team develops action plans for individuals or groups of individuals. In some instances, this may be facilitated and supported by the mapper.

DCM findings can suggest changes in the way a person is supported to improve their well-being and quality of life. The DCM assesses the quality of support offered by staff and any training needs they may have, and an action plan is implemented to address the changes needed.

The intention is to ensure that the care and support the observed person living with dementia is receiving is person centred and that the outcomes of this support are positive for the individual.

Person-centred planning and practice

Despite its similar name, person-centred planning and practice is a different approach to person-centred care.

Being person centred means having a focus on the individual and gaining a real insight into their perspective of the world including their needs, wishes and aspirations.

Person-centred planning and practice can be of value to a person in a variety of circumstances, whether living at home, in a community setting or in supported living or residential/nursing care. It is a way of relating to people that places the person at the centre of all actions and considerations. It focuses attention on the person experiencing a quality of life that encompasses the things that are important to them, and it places the person very much in the driving seat of the planning and decision-making process. Person-centred practices can be '*used in teams and organisations to ensure that the focus is on what matters to the people receiving support and their families, and pays attention to how to support staff as well. Person-centred approaches ensure that we see people as unique individuals with valuable gifts and contributions*' (National Disability Practitioners (NDP), 2016, p 1). Although they can be utilised by teams and organisations, person-centred practices and the person-centred values that underpin them can be adopted by anyone who is caring for and supporting someone living with dementia. They can also be useful within community settings.

The focus within person-centred practice is to recognise what a good life looks like from the perspective of the person and to develop an appreciation of what can be learnt regarding how a person wishes to be supported or cared for and what they want their day-to-day life to look and feel like.

Delivering person-centred practice requires everyone to relate to each other and work together with the following principles:

- as individuals and equal partners;
- respectfully, irrelevant of the role they play;
- without assumptions;
- as people, not a label or a diagnosis.

Developing and delivering person-centred practice enables those involved to understand:

- what is important to a person, including people, places and routines;
- the person's identity;
- the person's story; the life the person has led;
- how to provide support and care in a meaningful way;
- the person's aspirations and fears for the future;
- how the person communicates and makes decisions;
- what is working well in their life;
- areas of the person's life that are not working well and that are a source of upset and frustration for them.

As well as supporting the current vision for health and social care, person-centred practice has been embraced by individuals, families and communities. The approach has supported many people to experience greater choice and control, which has changed the care and support they have received for the better. It is also an effective approach in changing the culture of the organisations that provide care and support.

Embracing person-centred practice can support personalisation by:

- creating a focus on the person and an opportunity for the person's voice to be heard;
- encouraging the conversations that support people to identify and share what they would like to achieve or change about the way they are supported or cared for;
- introducing tools that the person and the people around them can use to support them to consider how these changes can be achieved.

Person-centred practice supports the person to:

- build understanding about how they communicate;
- have control over their life;
- address the issues they are experiencing;
- identify ways to remain connected to the community;
- draw together a network of support;
- create a picture of what good support and care would look like;
- maintain relationships as they wish to;
- have their voice heard and responded to;
- create a sense of direction for their future.

Person-centred planning

Person-centred planning is a range of methods and approaches that place the person in the driving seat of their lives and at the forefront of any planning about their life. Duffy (2004, pp 7–13) stated that families would like to have more control in the planning and delivery of services. This approach involves the people who are most important to them, which provides a significant shift away from traditional service-based planning involving the person, some family members and the professionals or paid-for people who are involved in the provision of the person's care and support, to an experience of bringing together everyone with whom the person has a meaningful relationship, family, friends, neighbours, members of the community as well as the paid-for professionals with whom the person has a good relationship or who can bring useful knowledge and insight to support the planning process. According to Richie, '*Person Centred Planning is a way of organising around one person to define and create a better future*' (O'Brien and O'Brien, 2002, pp 11–12). The plan could focus on the immediate future so that the person's day-to-day experience improves their quality of life. It can also focus on the long-term plans regarding where the person wants to live and what they would like to achieve.

Person-centred planning was first developed in the 1970s by a group of people who together explored how to achieve a meaningful and community-based life; this included a whole range of people. It was established through drawing on well-tested ideas and approaches to planning for change from community and enterprise development. It was introduced in the early 90s in the UK through small pockets of practice around the country. People learnt about the success stories from these areas of innovation and the improved quality of life people were experiencing, and this started to influence change across the country.

These innovations led the way in demonstrating how people can be in control of their lives and the care and support they receive while remaining active members of their local communities, in turn reducing the level of referrals being made to traditional service provision.

Person-centred planning is built on the principles and values of inclusion.

Values of inclusion

The values of inclusion strengthen communities and create a welcoming place where people are respected and valued for their uniqueness and where everyone's contributions are recognised (Inclusion, 2019).

Everyone belongs within their community:

> Everyone is born into and is part of a community; it is only later that they are removed and placed within a segregated service setting. It should not be assumed that due to a person's diagnosis or disability that they would be better off somewhere other than the community that they are familiar with. Everyone has a need to be a part of society, to be present with other members of the community, and no one is too difficult, too old, too poor or too disabled.

Everyone can communicate:

> Communication is not reliant on the use of words; in fact only 7% of what is communicated is conveyed via words where the rest of communication is dependent on body language, gestures, facial expressions and vocalisations. We work better together when we move away from making sweeping assumptions about someone's ability to communicate on the basis of their use of words and placing the challenge of communicating on the person, 'they have difficulty communicating'. When there is a challenge to understand one another, this is a shared challenge. In these circumstances it is important to make a commitment to learn about how we can get better at communicating. Recognising that communication is the foundation stone in building on person-centred practice and planning, the person needs to be understood first before anything else makes sense.

Everyone has the right to determine their life experience:

Irrelevant of the person's stage in life or their circumstances, they should be able to determine what their day-to-day life experience is like as well as their future.

As a community we are stronger together:

A community functions better if its citizens are all able to be actively involved and contribute. No one present in the community has to meet a certain level or pass a test before they are able to belong. Rather, communities are stronger if people are accepted for who they are, with their unique gifts and qualities they have available to share.

Everyone needs support:

Everyone needs support, a cup of tea made in the morning, someone offering to wash the car, someone helping to set up the internet connection. Sometimes some people need more support than others and the level of support people need may change over time.

Everyone can learn:

As human beings all people grow, change and make mistakes and are all able to learn. This learning does not have to be formal based learning that we find within education systems, but the learning that takes place when people share time and conversations, where people learn about what is happening in their local area or learn something about another person: their culture, experiences or areas of knowledge.

Everyone can contribute:

Contributions to the community do not have to be grand for them to have meaning and value; it could be the person who picks the litter up on the way home or knocks on the neighbours' door to check in on them.

Each person's contributions, including our own, can be recognised and valued.

Everyone can have aspirations and dreams:

It is important to recognise that people can have aspirations and dreams, and often this may form the person's identity, what makes them motivated and enthusiastic. Recognising and listening to a person's dreams leads to identifying opportunities to connect and form meaningful relationships in their community.

People are the most qualified experts in their own lives:

The person is not just the person whom we see today, but they have lived a life with experiences and relationships. Working with a person to plan the care and support they need at this stage in their life without an appreciation of the person's story, their history and their input on what would make sense for them can lead to missing vital insight into what would work best for the person.

Anything is possible:

> A person's ideas should not be led only by what is available but instead should be led by their ideas, including their dreams and aspirations. If the exploration of the person's ideas leads to something that is not currently available within the local service of the support structure or from within the person's community it could be possible, through working together with the person, their family, friends, members of the community and professional input, to find a way to make that unique solution happen.

Never say never:

> No one has the right to say 'no' to a person's ideas, dreams and aspirations. An open dialogue, explorative conversations, involving the right people and having a commitment to the person to find a way to move towards their ideas, dreams and aspirations on the basis of being positive and finding what is possible.

The values of inclusion have informed the development of approaches that place the person at the centre of planning and decision-making and have formed the foundations on which person-centred planning and practice were developed (Pearpoint et al, 1992). They were first written in the early 1980s, and although they have evolved since then, they have largely remained the same. This demonstrates how relevant and important these statements are in underpinning our understanding of inclusion.

Person-centred planning and person-centred practice can be applied in many different scenarios, for instance, when someone is wanting to plan for their future, to help people address their day-to-day routines and to determine what good support looks like for them; supporting a person to maintain or develop connections within the community. This has been proven to achieve real and positive outcomes for individuals and families. Although the implementation hasn't been widespread, it has been successfully utilised in various settings including within supported living settings, supporting people who continue to live in their own home, in day centres and within residential care settings and nursing homes. The emphasis on a community-focused approach, steeped in the principles of inclusion, has to be at the core of any person-centred planning to achieve the intended outcomes.

The strength of this approach resides in the strong emphasis on recognising people's relationships and connections within their community, learning about their history, skills, interests and passions and listening to their ideas of what a good life would look like.

Person-centred planning and practice enables those from within the dementia care triad to learn and understand which relationships and resources are significant to the person and helps to initiate discussions about how to maintain these or develop them further.

As person-centred practice and planning has progressed, a range of practical approaches have been developed to help build a picture of how someone wants to live their day-to-day life, as well as their aspirations for the future. These approaches will be explored further in Chapter 2.

Person-centred planning is based on the Social Model of Disability; this is explored further in Chapter 6, with the intention of working with people to plan for their own lives while recognising and addressing some of the systemic barriers within society: physical, systemic and attitudinal, with the principle that it is these external factors that restrict people from living their life to the fullest, not themselves.

Person-centred planning comprises a range of planning tools and approaches that focus on the individual and their community and network of support; these include PATH, MAP, Essential Lifestyle Planning, Personal Futures Planning; Community Mapping and Relationship Mapping.

When developing a plan, it is important to stay focused on the purpose of the plan, which is the person being in the driving seat of their own plan where they may consider how they want to live their life, what quality of life means to them and what they would like to achieve. The plan is developed at a pace that makes sense to the person. The content of the plan is recorded and communicated in a way the person can engage with: video, big visual records, on a computer or a device.

Here is an explanation of the planning approaches.

PATH stands for Planning Alternative Tomorrows with Hope. This planning approach develops a clear appreciation of a good future for the person and the steps that need to be taken to get there.

MAP stands for Making Action Plans. This planning approach develops an appreciation of the person's life story and the people who are important in their lives and develops an appreciation of what the person would like to see happening in their life and what they would like to avoid.

Essential Lifestyle Planning is a planning approach that develops an understanding of what is important to the person in their day-to-day life and outlines their important routines and preferences.

Community Mapping is a method to capture the resources and connections within a person's community; this may be based on a community of interest, beliefs, culture and spirituality and an area where a person resides. By capturing this information on a map, the connections someone already has within their community can be appreciated and also the potential for new connections and opportunities can be recognised.

Relationship Mapping captures the relationships that a person has in their life; this would include close family and friends. It would also include the relationships the person has within their community and with people who are in their lives in a paid capacity. A Relationship Map helps to recognise the relationships that are important to the person and also the potential to grow and develop new relationships.

These approaches to planning have a clear process to follow to be able to go through the planning process in a logical order to reach the clear outcome of the plan. However, these processes can be facilitated in a manner where the person continues to feel in full control of the planning process.

Person-centred planning allows for creative and imaginative, as well as practical, ways to plan, in which the views and opinions of the person living with dementia can be heard and their choices known.

Person-centred planning encourages people to come together to listen and develop and share in their understanding, experiences and learning. This gathering of people creates a network around the person where the collective resources, skills, knowledge, extended connections and time can be pooled together to support the implementation of the individual's person-centred plan, encouraging those involved to be creative and think about life more than services and what is possible rather than what is available to be able to find solutions.

The VIPS framework

Dawn Brooker, an early student of Tom Kitwood, continues to contribute towards the development and progress of person-centred care and is responsible for developing the VIPS framework, published in 2004. This framework helps staff consider the needs of people living with dementia at an individual and organisational level. The initials 'VIPS' refer to four key elements within person-centred care.

Valuing people with dementia.

Individualised care that treats the person with dementia as a complex person.

Personal perspective of the person with dementia.

Social environment that supports the person's psychological needs.

For each of these key elements there are six key indicators.

V = valuing people

Every person has value regardless of age or cognitive status.

Vision	**Time to share knowledge and understanding**
Identify skills	**Being aware of the environment**
Recognise passions	**Explore personal connections**

I = individualised care

Using an approach that promotes the uniqueness of the individual.

Care planning	**Individual preferences**
Regular reviews	**Life history**
Personal possessions	**Activity and occupation**

P = personal perspectives

Acknowledge and understand life from the perspective of the person with dementia.

Communication with the person	**Physical health**
Empathy and acceptable risk	**Perspectives**
Behaviours of concern as communication	**Advocacy**

S = social environment

Providing a social environment designed to meet the psychological needs of the individual.

Inclusion validation	**Everyday places**
Respect	**Warmth**
Enabling	**Community**

(Brooker, 2004).

At the time of writing the VIPS framework continues to be used in the measurement of the quality of care provision for people living with dementia (Skills for Health and Skills for Care, 2018).

VIPS framework and personalisation

The VIPS framework takes us even closer to achieving personalisation and, in relation to person-centred care, further broadens what is considered important to be understood about the individual. The heading 'Social environment' within the VIPS framework encourages people to consider the importance of community connections and inclusion when measuring the quality of care and support a person is receiving. The rights of the individual are addressed with the recognition of advocacy within the 'Personal perspectives' heading. The importance of personal connections and relationships is highlighted within the 'Valuing people' section of the framework and individual preferences and life history are focused on in the 'Individualised care' section.

Relationship-centred care by Mike Nolan

As person-centred care emphasised the importance of creating positive engagement and interaction between the person working within a dementia care setting and the residents or patients within that setting; relationship-centred care broadens this thinking beyond the immediate relationship between the caregiver and the care receiver and considers the relationships that exist around the person living with dementia. This approach to care states that relationships exist at many levels, including among patients, their families, staff from all disciplines, and the wider community (Nolan et al, 2006).

The quality of the care and support offered to people with dementia depend on the quality of relationships between each of these levels. This is similar to the point raised regarding the dementia care triad, where the quality of support shared between people with dementia, informal carers and health and social care professionals depends on good mutual and reciprocal communication.

The importance of relationship-centred care was emphasised in a report published by the Joseph Rowntree Foundation in 2012, 'My home life: promoting quality of life in care homes'. This report highlighted issues that affect the provision of personalisation in care homes and asserts that relationship-centred care is '*at the heart of best practice and central to quality of life, quality of care and quality of management*' (Owen et al, 2012, p 12) and advocated that to achieve relationship-centred care, it needs to be recognised that people with dementia have a voice and the ability to make choices and decisions for themselves.

Mike Nolan recognises the value of Kitwood's approach and believes that there is the opportunity to further develop person-centred care towards an approach that recognises the input from other people who are offering support to the person living with dementia, such as family members and health and social care professionals.

Nolan highlights a problem with person-centred care: communication is portrayed as a one-way process that occurs *from* the carer *to* the person living with dementia. Communication on this basis could prevent the person living with dementia from expressing their preferences and views, which in turn negatively impacts their level of choice and control. He argues that person-centred care does not go far enough to '*fully capture the interdependencies and reciprocities that underpin caring relationships*' (Nolan et al, 2002, p 203). Consequences of failing to fully capture the interdependencies that underpin caring relationships include the person becoming withdrawn, misunderstood and not respected; staff becoming overwhelmed and overburdened; families becoming concerned and unsupported. Therefore, although person-centred care remains a dominant model within dementia care, it doesn't capture the importance of an open, two-way or multi-way dialogue. This is why progressive models like relationship-centred care make such a positive contribution to the evolution of thinking and approaches within dementia care.

Through the development and implementation of relationship-centred care, it is encouraging that people with dementia are being seen as having agency. *Agency*, as defined by Deacon and Mann (1999, pp 413–35), refers to the ability of people to undertake '*actions, activities, decisions and behaviours that represent some measure of meaningful choice*'.

To achieve relationship-centred care, it is important to address any negative assumptions about a person's ability to demonstrate agency. Goldsmith (1996) called upon staff within care homes to shed preconceived ideas that people living with dementia are not able to express their views and identified that staff members who believed that people living with dementia could not express their views did not effectively engage with people to find out what their views were.

Supporting people with dementia to express their views and display agency should be a key consideration in all their daily interactions, including those regarding their care or support, in order for people living with dementia to experience a better quality of life and to have control, choice and self-determination.

People living with dementia, over time, will experience a diminished cognitive ability. It is, however, possible to capture a person's wishes and preferences to help them inform the provision of care and support through all stages of dementia. In Chapter 6 a range of approaches will be introduced to show how it is possible to support people with dementia to share their views and opinions.

Nolan also suggests that there are '*meaningful triadic relationships based on mutual appreciation of each other's knowledge, recognition of its equal worth, and its sharing in a symbiotic way to enhance and facilitate joint understanding*' (Nolan et al, 2002, p 204). He worked alongside a team at Sheffield Hallam University to develop 'the Senses Framework' (2006), which sees quality care arising out of mutual and reciprocal relationships between those who form the dementia care triad and leads to each party developing subjective *senses* comprising a sense of security, continuity, belonging, purpose, achievement and significance, as can be seen in The Sense Framework below.

The Senses Framework (Nolan et al, 2006)

Sense of security

Feel safe and free from threat, receive complete care and support and to be treated as a competent person who is understood and that their opinions are heard.

For older people: attention to essential psychological needs, to feel safe and free from threat, harm, pain and discomfort. To receive complete and sensitive care. To have the opportunity to share what is important to them and to be reassured when needed.

For staff: to feel free from physical threat, rebuke or censure. To have secure conditions of employment. To have the emotional demands of work recognised. To work within a supportive culture where they have the opportunity to learn about the support people require.

For family carers: to feel confident about their knowledge and ability to provide good care without detriment to their own personal well-being. To have adequate support networks and timely help, when required. To be able to relinquish care when appropriate. To be fully involved in all conversations and to be treated respectfully.

Sense of continuity

To understand the past and how that is reflected in day-to-day life. To have a sense of sustained relationships. To experience positivity in all aspects of the person's life and for everyone to know what is expected.

For older people: recognising the importance of personal biography. To have the opportunity to share what has happened in the past and the meaningful aspects of their history. Skilled use of knowledge of the past to help contextualise the present and future. To recognise what is significant for life now and into the future. Seamless, consistent care delivered within an established relationship by known people.

For staff: positive experience of work with older people from an early stage of their career. Exposure to good role models and environments of care. Expectations and standards of care communicated clearly and consistently. To have the opportunity to hear the person's story and identify how this is significant for the person's life now. To ensure that what is learnt from this reflects in how the support is provided.

For family carers: to maintain shared pleasures/pursuits with the person they care for. To be able to provide competent standards of care, whether delivered by self or others. To ensure that personal standards of care are maintained by others. To have the opportunity to share in the life story and the aspects of the story that are significant to them. To have the opportunity to bring the important aspects of what makes a good life into the person's day-to-day life now.

Sense of belonging

To feel part of the community and to have meaningful relationships within it with valued roles. To not feel alone.

For older people: to have the opportunity to have conversations about the places and the people who are important to them and how they would like to stay involved. Opportunities to maintain and/or create meaningful and reciprocal relationships.

For staff: to feel part of a team where they are recognised and valued for their contribution. To belong to a community of practitioners.

For family carers: to be able to maintain/improve valued relationships. To be able to confide in trusted individuals, to feel that they are 'not in this alone'. To have the opportunity to talk about the people and places that have meaning and how the person wishes to remain involved.

Sense of purpose

To be able to have choice and to take part in purposeful activities, this reflects goals and aspirations. For care to be reciprocal and maintain dignity, integrity, personhood and well-being.

For older people: opportunities to engage in purposeful activity. To be able to identify and pursue goals and challenges. To exercise discretionary choice.

For staff: to have a sense of therapeutic direction, a clear set of goals to aspire to that makes sense to the person they are caring for. To maintain the dignity and integrity, well-being and personhood of the care recipient.

For family carers: to pursue (re)constructive/reciprocal care. Family members share with each other what goals and aspirations each person has for themselves and the family member being cared for. This is an opportunity to notice where people share the similarities and also to discuss differences.

Sense of achievement

To have a sense of progress towards achieving goals and to use abilities and skills to the full while developing new ones. To have a sense that 'we have done our best'.

For older people: opportunities to meet meaningful and valued goals. To feel satisfied with one's efforts and to have the opportunity to celebrate. To make a recognised and valued contribution. To make progress towards personal and therapeutic goals as appropriate.

For staff: to be able to provide good care. To feel satisfied with one's efforts. To make progress towards therapeutic and personal goals as appropriate. To use their skills and abilities to the full. To recognise how each person has played a part in ensuring that achievements and goals are reached and having the chance to share in the celebrations.

For family carers: to feel that they have provided the best possible care. To know they've done their best. To meet challenges successfully. To develop new skills and abilities. Creating the opportunity to talk about the positive things that have happened, for the person and each other. Recognising the difference these achievements make.

Sense of significance

To feel valued and appreciated and that efforts made have a significance.

For older people: to feel recognised and valued as a person of worth, that one's actions and existence are of importance, that they *matter*.

For staff: to feel that working alongside older people is valued and important, that their work and efforts *matter*. Recognising that their function in a person's life has importance in defining their day-to-day experience. Keeping motivated ensures the quality of support provided and that enjoyment of the role can continue to be experienced.

For family carers: to feel that one's caring efforts are valued and appreciated, to experience an enhanced sense of self.

The approach highlights the need to address requirements of those who form the dementia care triad in a manner that had not yet been included in the previous approaches. The Senses Framework addresses how those within the dementia care triad experience the interactions with one another. Each sense can be related to a level on Maslow's *hierarchy of needs*: physiological, safety, love and belonging, esteem and self actualisation (Maslow, 1943).

Enriched care plan

Another important contribution to the development of quality care and support for people living with dementia made by Dawn Brooker, alongside Hazel May and Paul Edwards (2009), is an assessment and planning package titled the *enriched care plan*, which is based on person-centred care. The package provides a practical tool, which is founded on both psychological and biomedical theories, and includes a range of templates that guide professional carers through the assessment process and leads to the completion of an enriched care plan.

An enriched care plan is there to support both people living with dementia and their carers. The following five components look at both the social and psychological aspects of life for the individual at the time the assessment is completed. A completed enriched care plan aims to identify how to meet the person's care and support needs.

1. Life history

Life story – Knowing something about a person's life can help others to know why a person with dementia is behaving or reacting to current events in a particular manner. The enriched care plan package includes a profile relating to *life story*, which gains important information about the person's early years, middle years, post-retirement years and the present time. It also includes information about their lifestyle and future wishes.

Lifestyle – This section of the enriched care plan gathers information about what is important for the person with dementia regarding their lifestyle choices. This includes their preferences regarding food and drink, clothes, daily living activities, work-like activities, relaxing, social activities, personal attachment figures or objects and spirituality.

Future wishes – An enriched care plan captures details about what the person wants in relation to the treatments, health interventions and support they receive, which includes end-of-life and funeral planning.

2. Personality

The person living with dementia will experience their condition in a unique way. The life experience of a person living with dementia will be influenced by a number of factors. This includes their personality, their environment and their interactions with other people around them. When completing an enriched care plan, assessing the personality of the person living with dementia is based on five areas, whether the person is:

sensitive/nervous – a person who sees themselves as more sensitive or nervous is less likely to be emotionally stable, whereas a person who is confident and secure is going to have better control over their emotions;

introvert/extrovert – a person who is extroverted is more likely to be outgoing, active and assertive, whereas a person who is introverted tends to be less sociable and shy;

inventive/curious – those who are inventive are open to new experiences and tend to be more liberal in their outlook. In contrast, people who are *preservers* tend to be more conservative, conventional and prefer familiarity;

friendly/compassionate – this section is linked to the traits of friendliness, which include compassion, caring, warmth and kindness in contrast to competitiveness, jealousy and spitefulness;

efficient/organised – the more conscientious a person the more competent, dutiful, orderly, responsible and thorough they are (McCrae and Costa, 2003). People with this trait are more likely to control their impulses, whereas people who are easy going are more likely to be impulsive.

3. Health

People with dementia may not be able to give a good account of the physical and mental health issues that they have, which may lead to preventable or treatable conditions being missed. The health profile looks at different areas of the person's physical and mental health, including basic details such as weight, height, medication use, diet and fluid intake. Any issues regarding safety, emotional and mental health will also be addressed. It is within this section of the profile that issues regarding memory are discussed and recorded.

4. Neurological impairment

Capacity for doing – While people with dementia are cognitively impaired, they can, to varying degrees, engage with the world, whether engagement comprises higher-level activities, such as driving a car, or lower-level activities, such as watching the events of the day. People with dementia are at particular risk of disengaging from the world, as a person's dependency on other people to initiate engagement increases, or they may begin to lose the skills, coordination and language needed to fulfil activities they have done in the past, which can impair their well-being. The 'capacity for doing' profile allows staff to know what the person with dementia wants to do to remain fully engaged with the world.

5. Life at the moment

This profile assesses the quality of life that is presently experienced by the person living with dementia. The 'life at the moment' profile focuses on the person's psychological needs for comfort, occupation, attachment, identity and inclusion. The quality of life at the moment is profoundly affected by interactions with other people and the *feel* of the social environment in which the person lives and spends time. The profiling process provides a structure that helps reveal and quantify how satisfied the person is with their life at the moment of profiling and the extent to which their psychological needs are being met. This information is fed into the enriched care plan, which then identifies any clear actions that should be taken to improve the quality of life for the person in receipt of care.

Enriched care planning is ongoing and takes place throughout the duration of care provision. It comprises five stages: profiling, identifying needs, documenting needs, implementing the plan and reviewing. This approach builds on the concept of person-centred care; it takes a structured approach to consider a broad range of issues that influence the person's quality of life and day-to-day experience. An enriched care plan helps identify the areas of a person's support and care that need further consideration for improvement and creates an action plan to implement the ideas. The areas covered within an enriched care plan broaden the perspective presented in person-centred care and relationship-centred care to include the direct experience of a person living with dementia.

Evolution in thinking

The development of these six approaches in dementia care demonstrates an evolution of thinking. Earlier approaches and models focused on the delivery of quality of care within a care setting, such as residential care and nursing homes, while, gradually, the focus of approaches has shifted to include a wider perspective of the person's life, including their relationships, life history, interests, personality and preferences. It was once considered that the development of information and planning to enable person-centred care was the responsibility of those paid to work within dementia care provision. Personalisation has begun to significantly shift this emphasis, recognising that often people, alongside their families, friends and those paid to support them, are best working in collaboration to plan, gather and record information, shifting the emphasis of expertise to the person with lived experience.

Developing the concept of the dementia care triad

As the approaches to dementia care have evolved over time, they have come closer to meeting the needs of the three components of the dementia care triad. Relationship-centred care is the latest in these developments, which recognises the need for a reciprocal relationship between the person with dementia, their family and those in a paid role.

To further develop the concept of the dementia care triad would be to propose that the triad is:

- located within communities;
- constructed by the mutual and reciprocal interaction of the members of the triad with members of the local and wider community.

This widens consideration regarding the important relationships in a person's life, and it is possible to suggest that the model of relationship-centred care, as presented by Nolan, may be developed further to consider the importance of relationships among people in the person's immediate and wider community.

By adding a connection to the relationships within a person's community to the dementia care triad, the opportunity for collective agency can develop.

Individual agency

This is where each individual in the dementia care triad has the opportunity for:

- reflection;
- free time to pursue interests and activities;
- active involvement in any decision-making;
- the development of self-awareness;
- seeking support and advice as needed.

Collective agency

This recognises that a group of people can be supportive of one another and work together to support the person living with dementia to live the best life possible and for them to receive health and social care support in a manner that works well for them.

Collectively, people can identify shared interests and goals and support one another to get involved in activities that are suitable for each other on the basis of what they have learnt about one another.

Collective agency can be achieved through the involvement of those within the dementia care triad and can be strengthened further if significant people from the person's community are also invited to take part in important conversations and discussions.

Decision-making can be a complex and difficult process, and mutual support given from a familiar group of people can enable the person to feel better equipped to make decisions. Collective agency needs to be developed and fostered over a period of time, where relationships can grow and meaningful connections and roles can develop. The direction and pace of the collective of people need to go at a speed that makes sense to the group and each individual within it.

Building on the principles of person-centred care and relationship-centred care with complementary approaches, person-centred planning and person-centred practice can ensure an overall approach that achieves the outcomes of personalised practice.

Therefore, personalised practice, as a complement to the dominant model of care for people with dementia (person-centred care), comprises models of care, approaches and interventions that:

- enhance the subjective well-being of the person living with dementia (person-centred care);
- occur within the context of relationships between the person living with dementia, informal carers and those from the health and social care profession (relationship-centred care);
- ensure people living with dementia are fully involved in and at the centre of the planning about their own life, that they make worthwhile choices and stay rooted within their community (person-centred practice and planning).

This may be expressed by the equation:

Personalisation in Dementia Care = Person-Centred Care + Relationship-Centred Care + Person-Centred Practice + Person-Centred Planning

Life in the community

To achieve a good quality of life for people with dementia, consideration must be given to how people can be supported to continue to live in their community if this is what they choose. Thought needs to be given to how to achieve this in a manner that makes sense to the person and their immediate family and friends with an aim to be surrounded by the people and places they know well.

It is important to develop an understanding of the opportunities that exist within the person's community and their existing connections within it.

Communities are vibrant places with a mix of:

- people;
- places;
- events;
- opportunities;
- resources;
- connections.

Exploring what exists within a person's community can lead to identifying untapped potential and solutions for care and support that had not been considered previously.

Communities can have an abundance of strengths and assets that are available to support people with dementia, which can be found after exploration and discovery based on finding what makes sense to the person based on their own interests and aspirations.

The conversations to be held and the connections to be developed can become clearer when seeking the answers to the following question:

'What does the person living with dementia and their family want and need to ensure that they can continue to live the life they choose?'

The assets that exist in communities include the:

- availability of skills;
- time the local people have to share with others;
- local people's passion and commitment to making a difference in their local area;
- knowledge of the local area;
- relationships that exist within the community;
- local services and businesses;
- small community groups and initiatives;
- charities and voluntary organisations;
- statutory provision; police force, education and local MPs.

Developing an understanding about the strengths and assets within the community can lead to a greater scope of ideas and solutions regarding how to achieve the outcomes that are right for the person living with dementia and their family. This could also include solutions to long-standing problems.

An approach that has a focus on the community is supportive of the person maintaining the aspects of their life that mean the most to them. It encourages everyone who is involved, including those from the three aspects of the dementia care triad, to have a focus on what is possible, not just what is currently available through service-based solutions.

Participating in social networks and recognising citizenship

Continuing to be a part of the local community and surrounded by people who are known or connected to the person can help maintain their personhood and their sense of belonging, security, safety, purpose, achievement and significance, as covered by the Senses Framework.

There are two prevailing models for community: dementia-friendly communities and age-friendly communities.

Dementia-friendly communities

Dementia-friendly communities are communities whose residents understand dementia. There those living with dementia continue to be recognised as members of the community, are welcome, are safe and continue to fulfil meaningful roles.

They reflect the diverse range of communities we have in our society such as a local faith group or the services found in a local area. Towns, villages and neighbourhoods have received recognition as dementia-friendly communities, and the dementia friends website keeps an up-to-date list.

Since the publication of the UK National Dementia Declaration (2010), the government has invested in a coordinated approach to community understanding of dementia and greater connectedness through the 'Dementia-Friendly Communities' programme. This programme comprises villages, towns, cities and organisations, such as hospitals and care homes, that are committed to improving the chances of people living with dementia to remain connected in their community.

The idea of dementia-friendly communities was first introduced in the 2010 to 2015 Government Policy: Dementia (Department of Health and Social Care, 2015). The then prime minister, David Cameron, issued a national challenge at the Dementia 2012 conference committing to:

- invest further in dementia research;
- improve the quality of dementia care;
- increase professional and public understanding of dementia;
- implement initiatives to achieve dementia-friendly communities.

> *A dementia friendly community can be defined as: a place or culture in which people with dementia and their carers are empowered, supported and included in society, understand their rights and recognise their full potential.*
>
> (Alzheimer's Disease International, 2016, p 10)

Dementia-friendly communities is an international initiative with a commitment in many countries to engage in the development of a society that understands dementia and supports people living with dementia to continue living an active and full life. A key component to achieving dementia-friendly communities is initiatives like the Dementia Friends Programme, which aims to increase awareness and understanding of dementia across all levels of communities. As of April 2020, there were 67 Dementia Friends Programmes (or national equivalent) launched or in development in 56 countries led by national Alzheimer's associations and other organisations (Alzheimer's Society, n.d.b).

The shape and form dementia-friendly communities take can vary greatly. For example, Banks in the UK have appointed dementia champions who are trained to spot the signs of people living with dementia who may be victims of financial abuse and have implemented recommendations from people living with dementia to make banking easier and more secure, including creating a photo ID bank card and a chip to store information to discreetly indicate to the cashier that the individual may need extra support or a side room to prevent embarrassment. The Northumberland Dementia Forum prompted a dementia awareness training package for local bus drivers, as part of their Certificate of Professional Competency. This means the many older adults living with dementia who use public transport in rural and urban areas across the UK benefit from having a well-trained and sensitive point of contact with their bus drivers. Over in Ireland, Dementia Aware Donegal's Dementia Friendly Community Programme has five project components, each of which covers several key aspects of dementia-friendly communities. These are 'Be a Sport for Dementia', which encourages people living with dementia to continue to participate in local sports clubs; 'Ordinary Man, Extraordinary Memories', a play intended to raise awareness and understanding of dementia; 'You've Got a Friend in Me', a bid to establish dementia champions to recruit and train new dementia friends; 'Hearth and Home', an initiative designed to provide support for those living with dementia in the community; and 'Faith, Hope and Charity', a development of best practices for clergy to better support members of the congregation living with dementia and their families. What all these forward-thinking initiatives have in common is that they all aim to make everyday life as respectful, dignified and inclusive as possible for those living with dementia, regardless of the setting. This demonstrates how dementia-friendly communities transcend one physical place and become a values-based approach practised by and applied in different communities (Alzheimer's Disease International, n.d.).

The principles of dementia-friendly communities

Alzheimer's Disease International asserts that there are four necessary elements needed to achieve a dementia-friendly community: people, communities, organisations and partnerships.

People: the involvement of people living with dementia

Alzheimer's Disease International recommends that dementia-friendly communities be based on a combination of information about the social and economic consequences of dementia, the requirements and thoughts of people living with the condition and contributions from carers. The organisation states: '*Only by ensuring that initiatives are inclusive of people living with dementia at all stages of development, will we succeed in giving them the sense of respect, dignity and purpose they seek*' (Alzheimer's Disease International, 2016, p 10).

Communities: the social environment

According to Alzheimer's Disease International, there is a pressing need to combat the shame and social isolation that are often perceived as being synonymous with dementia. Equally important is the need to empower people living with dementia to engage with and feel included in community activities. Accessible community activities that are suitable for the requirements of people living with dementia and appropriate transport choices need to be readily available. It's important to note that Alzheimer's Disease International views it essential that people living with dementia should be able to participate in community activities that already exist instead of only being able to engage with specialised activities. The importance of people living with dementia being able to stay in their familiar surroundings cannot be underestimated. The organisation says: '*Providing people with dementia with the opportunity to remain in their homes and within their communities should be a guiding principle*' (Alzheimer's Disease International, 2016, p 10), emphasising that dementia or no dementia, we all have the right to expect access to paid or unpaid activities: sporting activities, meeting with friends, attending community activities such as choirs and walking clubs, banking and retail to allow us a chance to remain connected and to socialise.

Communities: the physical environment

It goes without saying that it is crucial that a community that is deemed dementia friendly features a physical environment that supports the needs of people living with dementia. Alzheimer's Disease International views lighting, pathways and clear signage as elements that will need to be carefully considered explaining: [The environment in which the person lives] '*needs to be accessible and easy to navigate*' (Alzheimer's Disease International, 2016, p 10).

Organisations: dementia-friendly organisations

To make it possible for people living with dementia to easily keep engaged with their communities, businesses and organisations need to be on board in the sense that they need to make the effort to show understanding, respect and responsiveness to the needs of people living with dementia who use their services and make use of their business. '*Encouraging organisations to establish dementia friendly approaches and implement strategies that help people with dementia will contribute to a dementia friendly society*' (Alzheimer's Disease International, 2016, p 11).

Partnerships: working together to effect real change

It is no one person or organisation's role to implement the changes required to achieve a dementia-friendly community. Partnership working which brings together cross-cultural and sectoral support is key within this social action initiative. '*The strengths and focus of organisations within a community need to be identified and built into the plan for establishing a dementia friendly society*' (Alzheimer's Disease International, 2016, p 11).

Alzheimer's Disease International has created a clear outline of what a dementia-friendly community would look like to provide a benchmark for any town or local area.

For a list of towns, cities and other areas in the UK that have been recognised as dementia friendly, visit the website of Dementia Friends (Dementia Friends, n.d.) and for information regarding dementia-friendly communities in Scotland, please visit Alzheimer's Scotland (Alzheimer's Scotland, n.d.).

How to become dementia friendly

To have recognition as being a dementia-friendly community in the UK, there is an application process. Once the application has been approved, it is followed by the submission of a six-month report and an annual assessment. The process and accreditation are managed by the Alzheimer's Society and Dementia Action Alliance for England, Wales and Northern Ireland and by Alzheimer's Scotland.

The process of dementia-friendly accreditation is designed to enable communities and organisations to gain public recognition for the work they are doing to be dementia friendly. In England, Northern Ireland and Wales, the process is built on the following criteria developed by the Alzheimer's Society:

> *Make sure you have the right local structure in place to maintain a sustainable dementia friendly community.*
>
> *Identify a person or people to take responsibility for driving forward the work to support your community to become dementia friendly and ensure that individuals, organisations and businesses are meeting their stated commitments.*
>
> *Have a plan to raise awareness about dementia in key organisations and businesses within the community that support people with dementia.*
>
> *Develop a strong voice for people with dementia living in your communities. This will give your plan credibility and will make sure it focuses on areas people with dementia feel are most important.*
>
> *Raise the profile of your work to increase reach and awareness to different groups in the community.*
>
> *Focus your plans on a number of key areas that have been identified locally.*
>
> *Have in place a plan or system to update the progress of your community after six months and one year.*
>
> (Alzheimer's Society, 2014–2015, pp 3–13)

The Alzheimer's Society has also worked with the British Standards Institution to develop a set of standards for dementia-friendly communities. This standard is the PAS 1365:2015 Codes of Practice developed through funding from the Department of Health (BSI Group, n.d.).

The increase in the number of local areas, towns and organisations receiving the dementia-friendly status demonstrates that there is a strong commitment to improving communities for people living with dementia and that those that make up a community are prepared to invest resources to engage with the process.

While the term *dementia-friendly community* is used to describe a village, town or city, it is appropriate to also think of the support and care a person receives as being dementia friendly. Hospitals and care homes can be committed to being dementia friendly as can other service settings. Taking steps towards being dementia friendly can enhance the experience and well-being of people living with dementia. At a time of limited budgets achieving dementia friendliness doesn't have to take a heavy resource. It is about focusing on developing understanding, awareness and interpersonal skills.

When a service is aiming to be dementia friendly, the areas to consider would include the following.

- Are the physical structures and environment accessible and welcoming?
- Is there equipment and resources available to create an accessible and adaptable accommodation?
- Are visits from family and friends encouraged and welcomed?
- Is time allocated to ensure *people time* between the people providing support and those they are supporting?
- Is there active engagement between the organisation/service, the people supported and the local community?
- Does the community around the person living with dementia have an insight into their skills, abilities, interests and passions; is it a place where people are recognised for the life that they have led and the people they are today?
- Is there a good range of activities and opportunities available, and are people living with dementia involved in planning and deciding which activities take place?
- Is it a culture that recognises relationships and associations outside the immediate care/support environment and facilitates the continuation of these?

The concept of dementia-friendly communities improves the experience of living with dementia, and it identifies how to build a stronger community for everyone within it. A community that can work to protect and support people, especially those who are at risk and vulnerable, is a better place for everyone.

Age-friendly communities

An age-friendly community is a place where people of all ages can lead healthy and active lives.

Dementia-friendly communities have, in effect, been a progression of work previously committed to developing age-friendly communities, as supported by the Centre for Ageing Better (Centre for Ageing Better, n.d.a). An age-friendly community is a community that is respectful and enables everyone to actively participate regardless of age or background. It can be argued that an age-friendly approach is a broader, more inclusive approach to develop a community's ability to support the older generation, including those living with dementia.

The communities that are age friendly support people to continue to live in their homes, take part in the activities that are important to them and contribute to their community for as long as possible.

The Centre for Ageing Better is the organisation that supports communities to achieve age-friendly status. There is a growing UK network of age-friendly communities covering Scotland, Northern Ireland, Wales and England. There are currently 40 recognised communities in this network (Centre for Ageing Better, n.d.b).

The World Health Organisation worked with older people to develop the framework for age-friendly communities, and it is built on the evidence of what supports active and healthy ageing in a community. This led to eight domains of an age-friendly community, which can be found on the Centre for Ageing Better website.

Personalisation and dementia/age-friendly communities

The values that underpin dementia-friendly and age-friendly communities, such as inclusiveness, respect and accessibility, are complementary to personalisation, especially in the sense that:

- progress should be shaped around the needs and opinions of older people and people living with dementia, together with input from carers;
- older people and people living with dementia engage in existing community activities, rather than only specialised provision in a service setting;
- older people and people living with dementia can remain in their homes and within their communities.

Therefore it is safe to reach the conclusion that the fourth perspective of the community can be added to accompany the dementia care triad.

The dementia care triad + community

Personalisation in Dementia Care = Person-Centred Care + Relationship-Centred Care + Person-Centred Practice + Person-Centred Planning

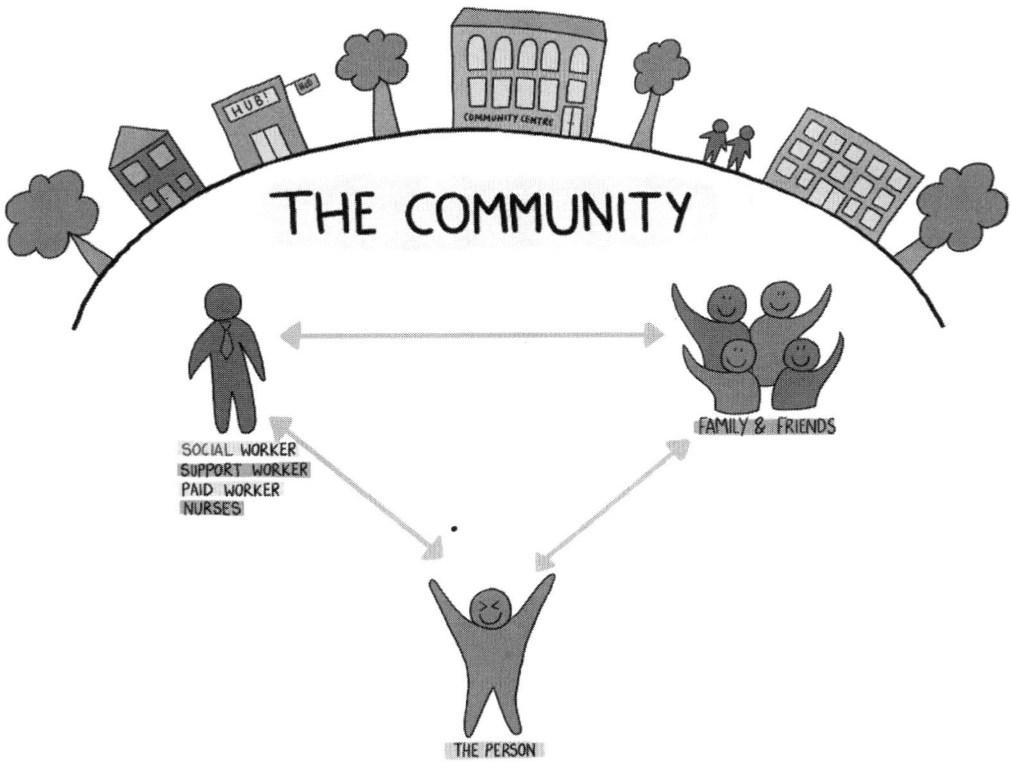

Figure 1.2 *The Dementia Care Triad + 1*

Personalisation and choice

The life of a person with dementia does not have to be determined by the services available to them or by the opinions of others. Personalisation creates the opportunity for the person to explore what is possible to have a voice about what would work best for them. It encourages everyone involved to consider and actively listen to the person and to recognise that some of the best solutions can be found within the person's local community. Any decisions about how to be supported and cared for must, whenever possible, reside with the person living with dementia. They know what works well for them, what they would like to see happen in their life and the connections they already have in place.

The writings of May, Edwards and Brooker on the 'enriched care planning' asserts: '*Delivering Person-Centred Care means providing and supporting an environment in which the person who has dementia is able to live out their drive to engage with the world. All human beings, unless in a coma, are able to engage with their world in some way or other*' (Brooker et al, 2009). This principle supports the idea that people can connect with their own community and make decisions about how they are cared for and supported, which, in turn, is complementary to the principles of personalisation. Considering people's ability and opportunity to make decisions must be done within the context of the principles surrounding capacity, as set out by the Mental Capacity Act (MCA) 2005.

Tom Kitwood (1997) highlights the contribution of socio-political factors, how people within society are functioning and the influence of the political landscape, to people's experience of dementia and, in keeping with this outlook, Bartlett and O'Connor (2010) express the view that there is a need to see people with dementia as having civic rights and participating within society. Bartlett and O'Connor, therefore, not only see personhood as an important focus within support for people living with dementia but also view citizenship as a key focus. The acknowledgement that people with dementia have citizenship opens the idea that people living with dementia have the same rights and should have the same opportunities as those who do not have dementia. This is a positive approach that is a development on the approaches explored in this chapter and a step closer to what is understood to be full personalisation in dementia care.

Personalised approaches

Personalised approaches are significant steps away from the provision of a service that is based on meeting medically or care-assessed needs. Personalisation is a progression towards people leading the life that makes sense to them, while choosing the care and support they want and need to achieve. In this context, the choice of the care and support available moves away from the narrow view of existing service provision to thinking about what is possible in the community.

This requires creative thinking and collectively finding new ideas and initiatives that work well and where the person is in the driving seat of their lives. Organising support in this way is based on the person's preferences, interests, identity and connections. To realise this approach, an alignment and bringing together of the approaches presented in this chapter is required. Personalisation calls for a whole scale change in how care and support are designed, arranged and provided. The tailored approach of personalisation should enable the person to identify the way they wish to be cared for and supported and to have the opportunity to set this up in a practical, local and individualised manner.

Personalisation is possible and often the way to achieve this with people is through very practical and local solutions.

Key lessons learnt

There are now four areas of development that are emerging within dementia care as a result of implementing the models outlined in this chapter. These developments include:

- recognising family and paid-for carers;
- agency;
- citizenship;
- participation in social networks.

Mike Nolan's work on relationship-centred care recognises and includes informal and professional carers within the approach to caring for a person living with dementia and highlights the importance of good relationships between each person. Good relationships of this kind are central to achieving a positive and personalised approach to care and support.

There is some crossover in the different approaches presented in this chapter. These areas of crossover include:

- the person has the right to be central and the lead in all discussions about their life;
- developing an insight into the person's past and their life story;
- understanding how the person wishes to spend their time;
- the relationships that are important to the person;
- how the person wishes to be supported and cared for.

When citizenship, person-centred practices and personalisation are considered in relation to dementia, it is possible to realise that the traditional service-based approach overlooks important aspects in achieving positive outcomes and quality of life.

The integration of person-centred practices and personalisation with the existing approaches would help bridge the gap between person-centred care and the person feeling a sense of control and choice over their life and the care and support they receive.

Personalisation = Person-Centred Care + Person-Centred Practice + Relationship-Centred Care

Questions to aid reflection

1) How do the innovations of Dementia Care Mapping™, the VIPS framework, enriched care planning and relationship-centred care in person-centred care have a positive impact on the experience of living with dementia?

2) If the situation of having dementia applied to you, or a member of your family, what do you think people would need to know to make sure that you, or the person you know well, felt in control and understood?

2 Personalisation

What does it mean for people with dementia?

This chapter covers:

- ***Personalisation* in more depth, building on what we learnt in Chapter 1, with an exploration of the history of the approach**
- **The Social Model and the Medical Model, examining how the two approaches differ**
- **What barriers people living with dementia face, as outlined by the World Health Organisation**
- **How self-directed support and personalisation can help people with dementia overcome barriers**
- **The vision for the future of health and social care and how Personalisation fits into this vision**
- **An exploration of both the Professional Gift Model and the Citizenship Model**
- **Co-production and its impacts**
- **The difference between *outcomes* and *outputs* and what makes quality outcomes for people living with dementia are.**

In Chapter 1 the personalisation in dementia care model and the dementia triad were introduced.

Personalisation in Dementia Care = Person-Centred Care + Relationship Centred Care + Person-Centred Practice + Person-Centred Planning

This chapter further develops these two concepts to introduce *community* as a fourth element.

Based on the principle that remaining connected and developing new connections in the community has the potential to improve a person's quality of life and can lead to positive outcomes for people living with dementia and their families.

Person-Centred Care + Person-Centred Practice + Relationship-Centred Care + Community Connecting = Dementia Care Triad +1

The routes to personalisation

Various strands of thinking and practice have supported the development of personalised approaches.

Normalisation

The principles and practice of *normalisation* stem back to the work of Wolfensberger in the 1970s (Wolfensberger et al, 1972). He was a prolific and often controversial activist in the field of developmental disabilities in the United States. An early organiser and promoter of community organisations for people with disabilities, he worked to liberate those who were ostracised in society and facing barriers and exclusion from the community.

Normalisation was introduced at a time when large psychiatric hospitals were the standard provision for people with disabilities or mental health conditions. In these settings, people became institutionalised as their lives became governed by established routines and practices within the hospital. As a result, people had very little choice, control or self-determination.

The normalisation movement highlighted and addressed the inequalities people experienced in these settings compared to those living in mainstream society and aimed to ensure that everyone received the same life experiences and opportunities. It suggested that every citizen should have the right to experience the patterns and conditions of everyday life, that is, a home, a place to work and a place to share interests. Initially, this concept invoked debates regarding risk: how safe would people be in the community and in everyday places? How safe were people in large psychiatric hospital settings? How would people respond in a less controlled environment? How would members of the community respond?

Although normalisation was initially concerned with the lives of people with developmental disabilities (the term then used), the approach and underpinning values were adopted for a much wider audience, including those affected by institutional practice and thinking. Wolfensberger encouraged people to recognise that having a chance to lead a fulfilling life was preferable to an approach that limits a person's ability to have freedom of choice and self-determination and to experience life as other people do.

Normalisation and personalisation

The principles of normalisation and the outcomes of this approach helped to shape a new vision for how to support and care for people within society during the 1970s. The fundamental changes achieved as a result created a commitment to address the question of how to create a fair society for all. This vision continues to shape the direction of health and social care practice and has led to the current principles that underpin personalisation and self-directed support (Kumar et al, 2015).

Social Model and Medical Model

The Social Model and the Medical Model help illustrate the practices and approaches within the delivery of health and social care, which directly influence the experience of people living with dementia when they access health and social care support. *Medical Model* is the term given by psychiatrist R D Laing in 'The politics of the family and other essays' (1971), for a set of procedures used to assess and treat a condition. Doctors and those in the medical profession are trained in these procedures. The Medical Model is an approach to pathology that aims to find medical treatments for diagnosed diseases and illnesses, and this approach treats the body as a complex mechanism of connected functions.

The Medical Model is professionally led with a focus on a person's condition, diagnosis and corresponding treatment (Figure 2.1). The Royal College of Psychiatrists thus define dementia as a '*global cognitive impairment, which represents a decline from previous level of functioning, and is associated with impairment in functional abilities and, in many cases, behavioural and psychiatric disturbances*' (Commission for National Institute for Health and Clinical Excellence (NICE) and Social Care Institute for Excellence (SCIE), 2007, p

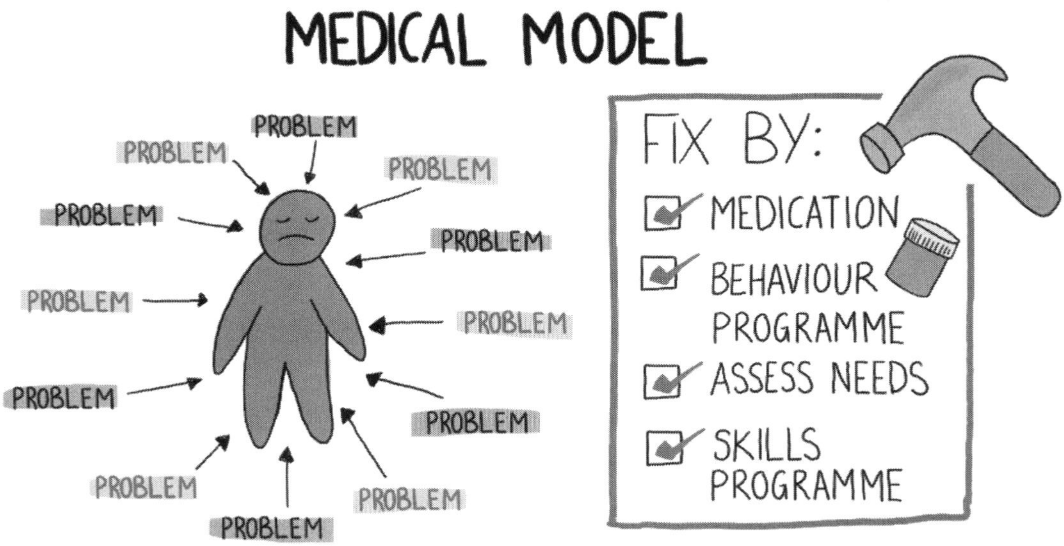

Figure 2.1 *Medical Model.*

67). The Medical Model of dementia focuses on studying the brain disease which leads to dementia, along with the chemical and neurological changes that occur throughout the progression of the condition.

The Medical Model is led by medical professionals and developed through their study of dementia, along with the knowledge and understanding that they accumulate as a consequence of researching the condition. Developments within the medical approach to dementia have led to improvements in the delivery of timely diagnosis and follow-up treatment and care. However, there is the risk that the person becomes defined by their diagnosis of dementia, with the support and care provided having a focus on the treatment and care of the person with dementia rather than the person as a whole.

Malignant social psychology

The impact of an approach underpinned by the Medical Model was studied by Kitwood (1990), who made notes on episodes he observed in care settings. He classified the episodes that were harmful and deeply damaging as malignant social psychology.

Here are some examples.

- **Disempowerment –** a lack of recognition of a person's abilities and opportunities are not given for the person to do what they can do.
- **Objectification –** treating a person as if they were an object rather than as a person.
- **Invalidation –** not recognising the way a person might be feeling in response to what is happening.
- **Infantilisation –** communicating with a person as if they were a young child.

(Dementia Partnership, n.d.)

Questions to aid reflection

1) In your opinion, what kind of environments would you find malignant social psychology?
2) Are people always aware that they are treating another person in this way?
3) What if someone is not aware of how they are treating others and the outcomes of their own interactions; could this be challenged? If so, how and what would happen next?

4) Is this treatment towards an individual determined by the culture within an environment or by the intention of the individual interacting with the person?

5) What would happen to the person who is being cared for in an environment if malignant social psychology was embedded in the culture of that place, and what would need to happen next?

6) If a person has become used to being disempowered, infantilised, objectified or invalidated, would they expect to be treated any differently, and how could this be addressed?

Contrary to the Medical Model, we find the Social Model first introduced in *The Fundamental Principles of Disability* by the Union of the Physically Impaired Against Segregation (UPIAS) in 1975 (Priestley et al, 1997). It stated: '*In our view, it is society which disables physically impaired people. Disability is something imposed on top of our impairments, by the way we are unnecessarily isolated and excluded from full participation in society*' (Union of the Physically Impaired Against Segregation (UPIAS), 1975 cited in Priestley et al, 1997, p 4).

In relation to dementia, the Social Model advocates a holistic approach that considers all aspects of the changes occurring in the person's life including their personal and social capabilities. According to this model, the care and support provided to the person should be in keeping with a holistic outlook, recognising what support would be needed for the person to maintain their independence, choice and control. The changes a person living with dementia experiences only become disabling when the environment and relationships around them do not adapt to accommodate these changes.

The results of the research conducted by Kitwood demonstrate how a purely Medical Model approach has a negative impact on those receiving care and support. The National Institute for Health and Care Excellence, however, advocates that the two models are complementary to one another (Commission for National Institute for Health and Clinical Excellence (NICE) and Social Care Institute for Excellence (SCIE), 2007). This opinion is valid, as the Medical Model is needed to ensure that there is access to dementia expertise and continued learning about the physical condition of dementia, for instance, access to consultants who have the expertise to provide assessments and diagnosis. On the other hand, the Social Model encourages an approach that recognises the whole person and is concerned with the quality of life, aiming to improve the practices and approaches within the provision of care and support for those living with dementia.

The Social Model and personalisation

The Social Model underpins the values that are required to realise personalisation and self-directed support (Commission for Social Care Inspection (CSCI) et al, 2008). It was developed and continues to be led by people with lived experience. This experience

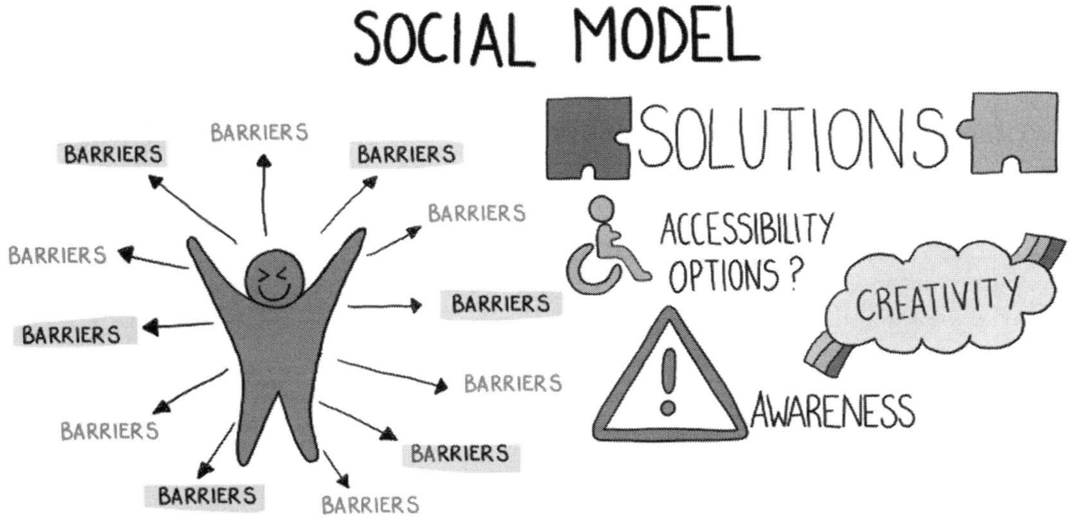

Figure 2.2 *Social Model.*

includes being isolated from full participation in society due to barriers and obstacles within it. It has increased awareness that it is not the diagnosis of dementia that prevents people from living a full life but the barriers that exist in society; this is especially the case during the early stages of dementia.

In August 2014 the Social Model was endorsed by the Government's Equalities Office, which recommended it be used by all government departments when they include and interact with the diverse communities they support (Department for Education, Government Equalities Office and Office for Disability Issues, 2015). In summary, the Social Model asserts:

- the person's condition, for instance, dementia, is a part of who they are and not their whole identity;
- the restrictions and barriers faced by an individual are an issue for society to address and collectively find solutions to;
- medical treatment is required for most conditions, but achieving well-being is much more than a medical issue.

Society is a collective of individuals who have functional differences, whether physical, emotional or sensory. These differences do not lead to disability unless a person's community, or society as a whole, fails to take account of these differences. Society can be enabling and inclusive if:

- the places that make up our community – the buildings, the parks, the local amenities and social gathering spaces – are fully accessible;

- consideration is given to transport and accessibility;
- everyone is treated equally and has the same opportunities available to them;
- people function with each other from a foundation of respect and enable each other to be included and involved.

Tom's story

Read through the excerpt of Tom's story and answer the questions that follow.

Tom is a young man with dementia who talks about his experience of living with the condition and the reactions he has had from other people in his life.

> 'We can follow a conversation but no one gives us a chance to answer and people always ask us closed questions, you know – are you alright? Do you want a cup of tea? You're looking well'. I said that when I'm in a room full of people I know, I feel the loneliest person in the world, because people will talk over me, around me, about me, but never to me. Yet when I'm in a room with strangers, they talk to me, until I say the magic words, 'I've got dementia' and hey presto, I turn invisible. People don't know how to talk to people with dementia; they don't realise we still have our intelligence. You see it with people in wheelchairs; people talk to the chair. With a blind person they speak to the guide dog, but dementia is an invisible illness because we look well.
>
> (Tom Dunne, Young Dementia UK, n.d.)

Reflection

- Can you relate these feelings to disempowerment, invalidation, objectification or infantilisation?
- How could these social situations be improved? What would be a better experience for Tom, one that would improve his quality of life?

Within the Social Model, impairment is defined as a long-term limitation of a person's physical, mental or sensory function. The Social Model of Disability has been internationally accepted within dementia care, with the development of the Social Model of Dementia Care. A variety of articles and publications are available, notably the report 'Dementia, rights, and the social model of disability' published by the Mental Health Foundation in 2015.

The approach to dementia care rooted in the Medical Model remains a challenge to the achievement of personalisation. A report published by the Social Care Institute of Excellence (SCIE) (2012a) stated: '*The way that the Medical Model continues to underpin the approaches of many service providers is seen as a fundamental obstacle to the future development of personalisation'*.

Being aware of both models provides the opportunity to reflect on how a person living with dementia is being supported and cared for. Reflection should also identify how the person is responding to the care and support they are receiving. What is learnt should lead to adapting the approach to ensure that the person faces no unnecessary barriers to prevent them living a full life with meaningful participation in society. To offer a personalised approach, the Social Model must underpin practice and be embraced within the delivery of health and social care as an equal partner to the Medical Model.

Barriers faced by people living with dementia

The World Health Organization (2011) describes barriers as being more than just physical obstacles and recognises that they are created by environmental factors that limit a person's functioning. Often there are multiple barriers which can make it impossible for a person to function. The most common include:

- communication – approaches that do not take into consideration factors affecting communication such as hearing, speaking, reading, writing and/or understanding;
- physical access to facilitates – steps, curbs, narrow doors and over-stimulating environments;
- transportation – a lack of accessible and convenient transport;
- people's attitudes – stereotypes, stigma, assumptions, discrimination and prejudice;
- policy – barriers to accessing the appropriate support and services;
- system shortcomings – inconvenient scheduling of appointments, lack of access to appropriate equipment and short appointment times;
- financial restraints – the level of income available to a person and the additional cost of living with a disability.

Systemic barriers within health and social care are a common issue for people living with dementia. It is important to recognise that people who are not trained within or familiar with such systems may not recognise the terminology which is often nuanced and specific to that area of work and expertise. They may also not be aware of all the options available to them such as a personalised and self-directed approach to their care or support.

It is important for health and social care practitioners to be aware of these barriers, to adopt everyday language and fully explain what specific terminology means.

The information and advice available about personalisation are sometimes sparse, and the range of options available is not fully explored. Practitioners must make sure people are fully informed of the available options, including the support available for them to continue to be included in the community and personal budgets, personal health budgets and direct payments.

The development of direct payments

Direct Payments 1996 onwards

The Community Care (Direct Payments) Act 1996 enabled local authority social care departments to make payments directly to people eligible for support. These payments would be utilised to purchase the support, care and services the person wanted to access to meet their needs/outcomes as identified in their assessment and care plan. When first introduced, the person's assessment was followed by a care plan which documented:

- the person's needs as based on the assessment;
- the services and support available to meet these needs;
- how many hours of support were needed each week;
- what the direct payment could be used for.

During this initial introduction, limits were set regarding how it could be used; to pay for a personal assistant/support worker. The rate of pay offered was determined by the authority.

Direct payments under personal budgets 2005 onwards

Personal budgets

In 2005, the 'Improving the life chances of disabled people final report' emphasised personalised support and direct payments (Prime Minister's Strategy Unit, 2005). Further to this, as well as first acknowledging the term *personalisation*, the 2007 ministerial concordant 'Putting People First' also outlined the then government's commitment to offer personal budgets to those who are eligible and, among other things, to offer direct payments as a mechanism to receive the personal budget to allow recipients to plan and purchase their own care (HM Government, 2007).

A personal budget is intended to meet the care and support needs of people accessing health and social care support in a manner that works best for them.

Once an assessment of needs is completed, the person can develop a support plan, which outlines how they intend to make use of the available budget. The support plan is developed by the person with whoever they choose to help them. This could include family members, friends, support workers, carers, advocates and professionals involved in the person's care and support, such as social workers.

The level of budget available to the person is presented after the completion of the assessment as an indicative budget. With this knowledge, they can develop their support plan which describes:

- who the person is and what is important to them;
- what they wish to change or achieve;
- how they want to be supported;
- how their support will be managed;
- how they will stay in control;
- how they will use the budget available to them;
- contingency plans and risk mitigation plans;
- how the support plan will be put into practice.

The budget section of the support plan clearly shows the level of budget available to the person and how this will be used. The intended use will achieve the best outcomes for the person and meet their needs as identified in their assessment. They may choose to utilise the budget to purchase equipment and adaptations, to purchase specialist support, to support communication, to employ a support/care worker, or to attend sessions that are of interest to them.

Once the support plan is complete, it is sent to the social worker for discussion and is then approved by a member/s of the social work team (depending on the size of the budget and the local arrangements).

A support plan can be developed on person-centred principles and provides the opportunity for the person to consider what would work best for them, placing them in the driving seat. A personal budget can be used flexibly to support the person to achieve the outcomes they have set in their support plan. The only requirements are that:

- the budget is used to meet the needs and outcomes as identified in the person's assessment;
- it is not used to purchase or do anything illegal;
- the planned use will not put the person or anyone close to them at risk;
- it is not used to purchase a service that is usually free at the point of delivery, especially in the case of health care provision.

Within the support plan it is also decided how the person will manage their personal budget. There are a number of options.

- **Individual Service Fund** (ISF) – The budget is managed by an organisation who may or may not also provide support to the individual. It is managed as a restricted fund, which can only be utilised for the purposes of meeting the needs and outcomes of the individual. This can be spent flexibly to achieve the best possible outcomes for the person. There would be clear communication between the individual and the organisation to ensure everything is working well and the budget is being spent appropriately. Changes can be made as to how the budget is spent, which can be discussed and agreed upon between both parties. The authority to make these decisions is passed from the local authority to the person and the organisation with a clear agreement in place on how this will be managed. A percentage of the budget or an overall charge from the budget is utilised by the organisation to cover the cost of administering the budget.
- **Third party managed** – An organisation would manage the budget on behalf of the person; the organisation would provide payroll for those who are employed by the person, and they would arrange for the payments of invoices. This organisation would manage the record keeping for the purposes of the local authority financial audit.
- **Direct payment** – The budget is paid directly into a bank account managed by the person or their representatives/nominees. This has to be a specific account for the sole purpose of the budget. The money is then utilised for the purposes as set out in the support plan. Changes to the use of the budget can still be organised in agreement with the person's social worker or with the local direct payments team. The bank statements, invoices and receipts would need to be kept for the purposes of the financial audit.
- **Local authority/clinical commissioning group (CCG) managed budget** – The person and their family would have developed the support plan but then asked the local authority or the CCG to manage the budget, meaning there is no financial exchange. This can reduce the additional work of setting up an account or finding an organisation to manage this, but it can be restrictive as the person would be expected to choose the services and support they receive from the approved providers list managed by the local authority or CCG, unless the authority is prepared to do a one-off contract with a provider of the person's choosing.
- **Trust fund** – The person being supported asks for their budget to be paid into a trust. This is where the budget is held and managed by a legal trust in the person's name.
- **Mixed package –** It is possible to create a mix of the above-mentioned options; for instance if the person wants to employ their own personal assistant for support at home, they may choose a part of their overall budget as a direct

payment and, then, if they also want to attend the local day centre, they may choose for a local authority–managed budget to cover this aspect of their support.

Overcoming barriers

People with lived experiences are arguably best placed to identify effective ways of overcoming the barriers they personally face to improve their quality of life. Here are some of the ideas that have been put forward by people who have dementia.

- To have more control over the way support and care are provided, with a greater range of choices regarding where to find care and support.
- To be able to utilise the health or social care funding to find solutions within the local community.
- To have access to information that is accurate, easy to understand, accessible and appropriate, with time to be able to discuss this with a knowledgeable person.
- To create greater awareness and understanding among paid professionals; education, benefit application assessors, employers, health and social care professionals as well as the wider community.
- To provide training and raise awareness, delivered by those who experience the barriers.
- To promote positive attitudes where people are treated with greater sensitivity and understanding.

(Copestake et al, 2014)

Hidden barriers

The barriers experienced by people with dementia are often hidden. The Alzheimer's Disease International Report, titled "World Alzheimer Report 2012 – overcoming the stigma of dementia', stated that one in four people with dementia hides their diagnosis, with stigma cited as the main reason. The global survey involved 2500 participants from 50 countries and highlighted that 40% of people with dementia have been avoided, excluded from everyday life or treated differently. The report produced the following recommendations to tackle the stigma surrounding dementia.

- Educate the public.
- Reduce isolation of people with dementia.
- Give people with dementia a voice.
- Recognise the rights of people with dementia and their carers.
- Involve people with dementia in their local communities.

- Support and educate informal and paid carers.
- Improve the quality of care at home and in care homes.
- Improve dementia training of primary healthcare physicians.
- Call on governments to create national Alzheimer's disease plans.
- Increase research into how to address stigma.

(Batsch et al, 2012)

Although these aspirational recommendations are comprehensive and address every level of societal change, from government strategy to local level changes, it would be beneficial to recognise the expertise within paid carers and their experience and knowledge and to create opportunities for them to support and educate other people about what they do and how they do it.

Questions to aid reflection

1) Consider the barriers of day-to-day life and which of the barriers identified are universal.
2) Consider the barriers that would be unique to the individual. What would these be?
3) Barriers are not always physical; they may relate to the person's quality of life in other areas, for instance being able to make fundamental decisions. What other barriers do people with dementia experience?
4) What recommendations would make a real difference in people's lives, and what difference could you make within your own community?

Self-directed support and personalisation

Overcoming barriers involves people with dementia actively choosing how they want to be supported. Self-directed support and personalisation are an approach where people accessing health and social care have more control.

The Adult Social Care Outcomes Framework (ASCOF) England 2018–19 (NHS Digital, 2019a) demonstrated that 90.3% of people aged 65 and over accessing long-term community support were receiving self-directed support, of which 17.6% were receiving a direct payment. This shows a marked increase from the same outcomes framework for 2011–2012, when the proportion for older adults aged 65 or over receiving self-directed support was 45.2%. At this stage there was no measure of the number of people aged 65 and over receiving direct payments (NHS Digital, 2013). We have to note that the measurement methods for the Adult Social Care Outcomes Framework were changed in 2014/15 (NHS Digital, 2015), making it difficult to achieve a completely accurate comparison between the years.

Although the statistical information suggests that more people with dementia are in receipt of self-directed support, it could be argued that this is not reflective of the day-to-day choices made by people with dementia, their experience of care and support or their quality of life. The concern with gathering outcomes regarding the success of self-directed support based on the number of people taking this option is that this does not provide details about the difference this has made for the individual. It is clear that more needs to be done to ensure that the statistical information regarding the uptake of personalisation and self-directed support is presented alongside real stories and the experiences of people with dementia and those in receipt of health and social care support.

When people access social care support, they are largely dependent on the advice regarding their options given to them by those working within social care. When people are provided advice that is weighted with opinion rather than facts, the option of a direct payment can be presented in a negative light. An emphasis on the responsibilities that come with a direct payment such as employer responsibilities and bookkeeping then overshadows the greater sense of control and choice achieved through direct payments. It is through this option that people can be creative and have individualised support and care arrangements.

If a person finds the option of a direct payment appealing, a further conversation is needed to explore the support that person wants to manage responsibilities that come with holding a direct payment. The sources of support available include:

- the employer support line attached to employers' liability insurance;
- the recruitment support available via local independent living association or centres of integrated living;
- a local accountancy firm providing payroll services and bookkeeping;
- the skills and knowledge available through the person's network of family, friends and community associations.

Quality of life itself is multi-dimensional and may reflect a range of elements of importance to the person: family life, friendships, community relationships, work, pursuing hobbies and interests and a sense of achievement, purpose and meaning.

Quality of life is dependent on each individual's perspective and measure of this. Whether a person is assessing their own quality of life, or a practitioner or a family member is doing this on their behalf, it is important to make sure that it is the person's perspective that is used as the measure.

Inevitably, the quality of the care and support a person receives will have a direct influence on the quality of life the person experiences, and this, in turn, depends on the environment in which the person receives their care and support be it within their own home, the community, sheltered living, residential care, nursing homes or a hospital setting.

'Dementia 2015: aiming higher to transform lives', a report published by the Alzheimer's Society in 2015 states: '*32% of people who responded to our survey said that they felt they were not living well with dementia. Half (49%) of people with dementia said they were not getting enough support from the government*' (Kane and Terry, 2015, p 7/v).

Personalisation and self-directed support can make a positive difference, where there is a focus on understanding the person, how they want to live their life and how they want to be supported or cared for, alongside a commitment and intention to reach positive outcomes for the person, their family and the community.

According to Think Local Act Personal's 'The national personal budget survey', the majority (76%) of people reported that personal budgets had made a positive impact on their lives (Hatton et al, 2011, p 2), stating that the freedom and control that is made possible through a personal budget enables people to maximise the resources available to them, often achieving the best outcomes for themselves and their family.

The Department of Health shared stories regarding personal budgets in 'Putting people first: personal budgets for older people – making it happen', which highlighted how personal budgets have made a difference for people living with dementia and their families (Department of Health Putting People First Programme Personalisation, 2010). One story is about a friend (Sarah) who supported a woman (Claire), living with dementia, to return home after an unhappy stay at a care home where Claire had become agitated. Claire no longer had the capacity to manage her personal budget, and Sarah held enduring power of attorney on Claire's behalf. The local authority appointed Sarah to act in the capacity to receive Claire's personal budget. Although initially Sarah was daunted by the additional responsibilities, she eventually found that the task of managing Claire's personal budget had not been a problem in practice and the outcome has been a much-improved quality of life for Claire (Department of Health Putting People First Programme Personalisation, 2010, pp 26–27).

A vision for the future

The vision for the future of health and social care delivery for people with dementia, as set out in the Prime Minister's Challenge on Dementia 2020, recognises the need to provide quality support at the time of diagnosis. The paper states: '*In February 2014 the Secretary of State for Health set out his ambition that everyone diagnosed with dementia should be offered high quality support after receiving a diagnosis of dementia. This may include Personalised information, a dementia advisor, access to support services*' (Department of Health, 2015, p 16). In addition to the areas outlined in the report, the following areas also need to be regarded as necessary in the strive for a better future for those diagnosed with dementia.

- The person living with dementia to be given the time and the support to consider the question 'what is a good life for you?'. Then find the best support arrangement based on their answers to this question, rather than choosing from a range of predetermined services that are currently available in the person's local area.

- A strong focus on the person with dementia when it comes to how their care and support are provided based on their *good life* answers. This applies in any setting: their own home, community, residential care, nursing care and hospitals.
- Led by the person and not their diagnosis, taking into consideration their relationships, interests, community, skills and abilities.
- Avoid a *one-size-fits-all* approach and ensure that a full range of options are available to the person. This would include coproducing unique arrangements that are individualised to meet the best outcomes for that person.
- Access to medical support as required with timely diagnosis. The Medical Model approaches not to dominate the person's experience of care and support but rather a balance between the Medical Model and the Social Model.

The Citizenship Model vs. the Professional Gift Model

The next building block in learning how to provide a good experience of accessing care and support is developing an understanding of the Citizenship Model and the Professional Gift Model, first published by Dr Simon John Duffy in 1991 (Duffy, 2011).

Values, relationships and the infrastructure of the social and health care system form the basis of the models. Firstly, and arguably most importantly, values form the foundation of interaction and behaviour. Therefore, how people experience interaction with others is dependent on the individual's values.

These models created a new perspective on how people who access public services are valued and perceived by:

- employees of public services;
- people within the community;
- professionals who administer public services and funding;
- the person themselves.

> *The Citizenship Model is a new paradigm for public services where support is treated as an entitlement which can be shaped and driven by the citizen, in the context of their community life. It contrasts with the Professional Gift Model, whereby support is defined by professionals and given as a unilateral gift to needy people.*
>
> (Duffy, 2011)

The model recognises and raises awareness of the power dynamics and control embedded within the current system underpinning the delivery of health and social care. This provides the potential to influence practice and decision-making, building a momentum to shift power and control away from the underpinning system and those who have to work within it over to individuals and their families. As a result of this shift of power and control, those accessing health and social care support can continue to have self-determination, identity and community connections.

The Professional Gift Model

The Professional Gift Model is the prevalent model for the delivery of many public services, including education and health and social care. As a starting point it recognises that citizens-paid taxes go to the government (both central and local) and the government works out how to utilise this revenue to take care of local people. The government then transfers that funding to professional bodies including social service departments and the clinical commissioning groups.

Needy people are assessed by professionals to establish what kind of care is appropriate. This is then provided by and paid for, via the funding made available by taxes and the government, from the local authority. The *needy* person then receives this service (Duffy, 2011). The cost of this service is never disclosed or made known; therefore, it appears to be free to the person and is given like a *gift* albeit at times an unwanted one.

People can then experience segregation due to the services they receive, robbing people of their citizenship twice over. This occurs as the services offered are based on what is already available, which tend to be segregated and standardised and the poorest at meeting people's needs, often holding people back from citizenship.

As services continue to be largely commissioned by local authorities and clinical commissioning groups, the principles of best value (Local Government Act 1999) act as a guide in which decisions are made. These principles place an emphasis on the cost element of any contract, which often leads to services demonstrating the lowest cost per person being chosen and awarded the contract. These contracts can be in place for at least three years before any alternative to this arrangement can be considered.

These practices mean that quality and customer experience is a secondary consideration at best. Sitting alongside the best value principles is the Social Value Act (Public Services (Social Value) Act 2012). The Social Value Act clearly states, within a legislative framework, the absolute need to consider the experience of the citizen, the end user of the service and the quality of the provision. '*The first thing to note about the* [Social] *Act is that, where it has been taken up, it has had a positive effect, encouraging a more holistic approach to commissioning which seeks to achieve an optimal combination of quality and best value*' (Cabinet Office, 2015, p 4). One can see then that the two acts, when implemented alongside each other in a complementary fashion, can have a positive impact on citizens. In order to achieve personalisation and self-directed support, cohesion between the two acts needs to be realised in practice.

Improving institutional long-standing services and service infrastructures into something better takes time and demands the energy of the staff within the services. The existing services and infrastructure can naturally resist making such changes and so funding largely remains locked into old-fashioned forms of support and care provision.

Therefore, the professional's *free gift* mostly suits the interests of the giver and is not carefully tailored to suit the individual. Simon Duffy states: '*This may seem too strong: there are many good professionals continually battling to offer people what they really need and to help people take up their rightful place as citizens. But the system is stacked against them, because power and control are in all the wrong places*' (Duffy, 2011). The Professional Gift Model suggests that '*People are not in control of their own lives*' (Duffy, 2011). and can be aligned with the Medical Model of disability. The Professional Gift Model has similar characteristics to the Medical Model, where the individual is:

- treated based on their needs and diagnosis;
- not involved in making decisions about their care and support;
- offered services, care and support based on professional opinion without dialogue regarding what would work best for them;
- dismissed in the sense that the wider context of their life, experiences, skills, relationships and community are not taken into consideration.

The Citizenship Model

In contrast, people as citizens can benefit greatly from exercising real responsibility and power in their own social care affairs as described by the Citizenship Model. Duffy believes this more autonomous approach is possible when the relationships between the person, paid professional groups and the government are equal and balanced, with an open dialogue led by the person focused on what a good life and good support would look like, therefore experiencing a fair say in the support they receive and the life they lead within their community (Duffy, 2011).

Simon Duffy's Professional Gift Model reflects the experience people have when they begin to access support through their local authority. People have reported:

- a lack of control over what was happening in their lives;
- other people are making the important decisions for them;
- they have been told what support they will receive and how/when they will receive it;
- they did not know what to expect when they accessed health and social care, what would happen and when and how much of a say they could have;
- concern in reporting any dissatisfaction regarding the support they receive due to a perception that it would be *taken away* and they would be left with no support at all;

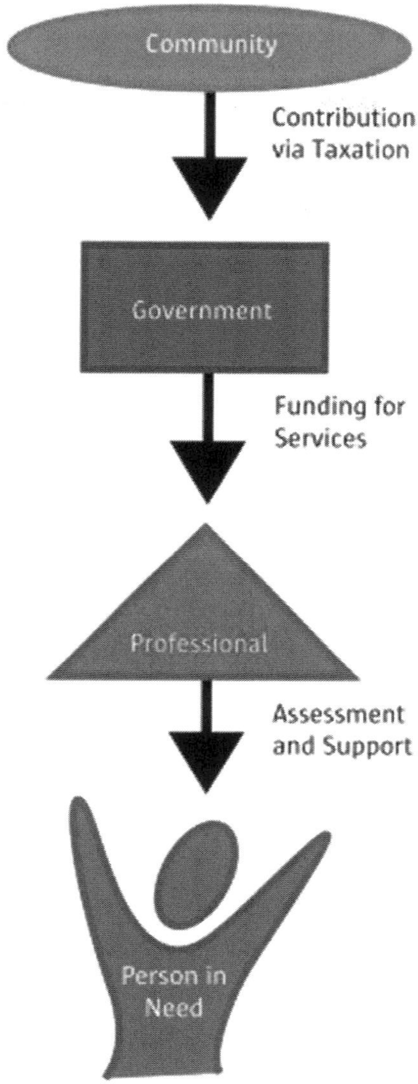

Figure 2.3 *Professional Gift Model (Duffy 2011).*

- a feeling that they had to be thankful for what they were receiving even if it wasn't ideal, as it was free;
- no insight into the monetary value of the support and care they were being provided.

The Citizenship Model aligns with the Social Model and the values that underpin personalisation. The Citizenship Model suggests that:

- a person is recognised as a member of their community and their right to continue to be a valued member of that community is upheld;

- services and support available are a combination of the mutual supports that currently exist, community-based resources, which are free to access, alongside support and services that have a cost associated with them;
- the level of funding available to the individual to meet the health and social care outcomes should be clear at the point of planning care and support;
- to reach or maintain a quality-of-life outcome, the focus should not solely be on the utilisation of the budget available through health and social care but, instead, should be on a wider perspective that recognises all the resources available to the individual;
- the process of accessing health and social care support needs to be open and transparent so people know what to expect, when to expect it and how they will be involved;
- the person, alongside family, friends and their community, can think about how they want to be supported and consider how this can be achieved.

Personalisation is about people experiencing choice and control over their lives. Personalised practice and approaches would therefore be strengthened if there was a strong understanding of the Social Model alongside the Citizenship Model and how this differs from the Medical Model and the Professional Gift Model. Without this understanding,

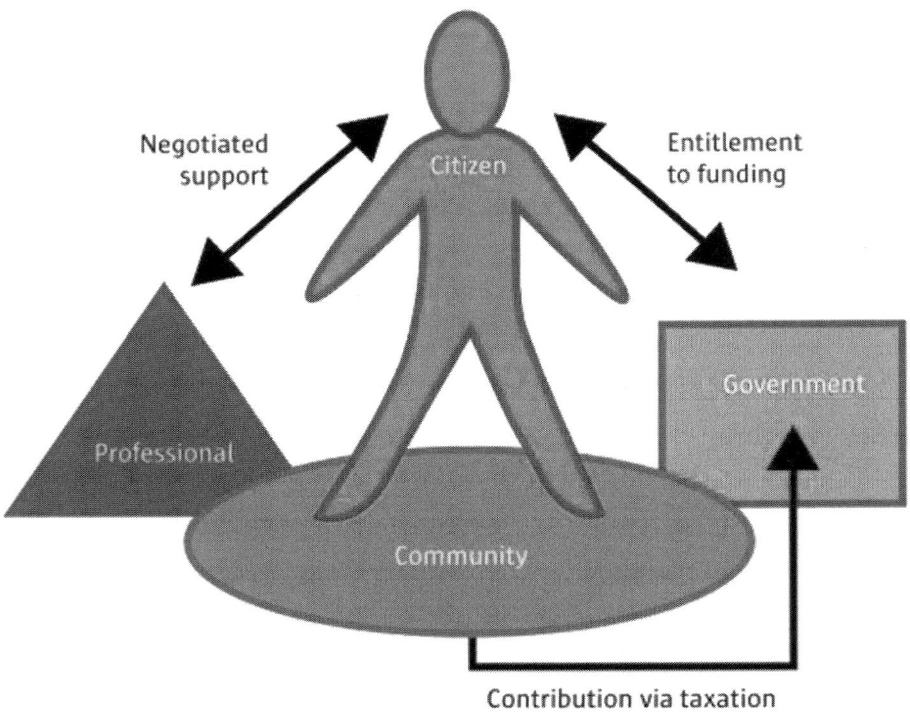

Figure 2.4 *Citizenship Model (Duffy 2011).*

fundamental principles and values would be overlooked, and this could lead to outcomes that are not as aspirational as those intended through personalised practice. It is therefore important that people from all aspects of the dementia care triad + community have an insight into the founding principles of the models.

Putting personalisation into practice

The development of personalisation has spanned decades, and during this time there have been a number of innovative approaches and developments that have resulted in a radical change in people's experience of accessing health and social care. Personalisation and self-directed support have initiated a transformation in the way social care and health care systems function and how personnel within these settings interact with people who are accessing their care and support. These developments have also required people to begin to see themselves differently as:

- experts in their own lives. Moving away from the strong belief that professional people know best and instead recognising that people know what would work best for them. While recognising that professionals are available to share expertise and knowledge to be able to answer any 'how can we make this possible' questions;
- connected to people within their communities and to recognise the resources available to them from the relationships they hold with other members of the community;
- actively engaged in conversations, which enable them to take the lead and state how they would like to be cared for and supported.

The Social Model and Citizenship Model also suggest that the person with dementia should not face any restrictions and limitations due to other people's false assumptions, misunderstanding and prejudices. Instead, they advocate an approach that does not place any limitations or barriers on the person in achieving a good quality of life.

Reflecting and embedding personalisation in practice

- Are there any experiences you could reflect on where you have helped someone talk about how they want to be cared for or supported?
- Looking back on this conversation, what worked well and what didn't work well.
- Was the approach in line with the Social Model and the Citizenship Model?
- What has been learnt through reflecting on this?
- What would you do differently in the future?

The legal framework for self-direction

In Chapter 1, agency and self-direction are presented as integral to personalisation. This idea has been extended further in this chapter to include the Social Model, Citizenship Model and the recognition that people should not simply be passive recipients of services but rather be able to exercise direction and control to achieve the quality of life, and this would include how they are supported or cared for.

The amount a person *self-directs* will, of course, depend on their capability and desire to make decisions and act upon these with those around them. This engagement, with the concept of *self-directing*, could potentially fluctuate over time. The leading principle is that the opportunity to self-direct should not be denied to anyone, regardless of their circumstances.

Memory decline and reduced mental capacity are attributed to dementia, both of which can fluctuate over time. Many people living with dementia do not experience either of these fully until the later stages.

People in the early to middle stages of dementia may still experience full mental capacity and can have a strong voice about their own lives and their plans for the future, including expressing their wishes for when they reach the later stages of dementia and end-of-life care.

This principle is strengthened by the MCA and in legislation via the Care Act 2014.

> *The Government wants the new law to focus on the person and their needs, their choices and what they want to achieve. It should put them in control of their lives and the care and support they receive. The Care and Support Planning process is the way of making this happen. It will provide people who use services, and carers, with clear legal rights to a Care and Support Plan.*
>
> (Department of Health, 2013, p 2)

The Care Act demonstrates progress within the legislature in recognising people's right to self-direction, control and choice, but what holds back the realisation of this in practice is the complex and bureaucratic infrastructure of the health and social care systems (The King's Fund, 2018, p 25). There is a general acknowledgement that systems and structures need to change, but, as already discussed, the process of changing them can be complex and overly time consuming (The King's Fund, 2018, p 1).

Mental Capacity Act

The Mental Capacity Act is an act of parliament of the United Kingdom (Mental Capacity Act 2005) and is especially relevant to those involved in the care, treatment and support of people aged 16 and over living in England and Wales. The Scottish equivalent is the Adults with Incapacity Act 2000 (Adults with Incapacity (Scotland) Act 2000). Meanwhile, the equivalent legislation for Northern Ireland is the Mental Capacity Act (Northern Ireland) 2016 (Mental Capacity Act (Northern Ireland) 2016).

The acts are designed to protect and restore power to people who have been assessed as lacking the capacity to make a decision at a particular time in their life.

The Mental Capacity Act sets out five core principles.

1. A person is assumed to have mental capacity until it is proven otherwise.
2. All practical steps must be taken to help the person understand the decision they are making and the options available to them to support them wherever possible to make the decision for themselves.
3. People with mental capacity have the right to make *unwise* decisions.
4. When it is assessed that the person does not have the capacity to make a decision, these decisions will then be made in the person's *best interests*.
5. Any decision or action must be done in a way that is the *least restrictive* of the person's rights and freedoms.

(*Mental Capacity Act 2005*. s.1.(1)(1–6))

One of the first considerations when assessing the capacity to make decisions is whether the person has an impairment or disturbance of the mind. The elements of the MCA which provide guidance on supporting a person to make a decision only apply to people who meet this descriptor.

If there is concern that the person lacks the capacity to make a decision, then a capacity assessment is completed. Anyone caring for or supporting the person, either in a paid or unpaid capacity, can be involved in this assessment. The completed capacity assessment will have to demonstrate that the person's preferred communication approach has been adopted, while supporting the person to make their own decisions and maintain choice and control.

The Mental Capacity Act states someone who is deemed as lacking capacity cannot do one or more of the following four things.

- Understand the information given to them.
- Retain that information long enough to be able to make a decision.
- Weigh up the information available to make a decision.
- Communicate their decision.

(Mental Capacity Act 2005. s.1(3)(1))

When a capacity assessment is completed it is only:

- for the decision to be made at that time;
- relevant at the time of completion.

Therefore, if a completed capacity assessment concludes that the person does not have the capacity, this is only relevant to the decision to be made at that time. It cannot be assumed that the person doesn't have the capacity for any other decision they need to make. It also cannot be assumed that the person will lack capacity from that point onwards as a person's capacity can fluctuate over time.

If the capacity assessment concludes the person does not have capacity. the following will be considered.

Best interest

A best interest meeting would be needed where an adult has been assessed as lacking mental capacity to make significant decisions for themselves and therefore needs to involve other people to make those decisions on the person's behalf (West and Glover, 2014, p 3).

West and Glover stated that a best interest meeting may be needed to make decisions about:

- where a person wants to live;
- what care services and support the person is to receive at home;
- what care services and or support should the person receive away from the home.

A best interest meeting could also be held to make a decision about serious medical treatment, although some serious medical treatments can only be granted by the Court of Protection (West and Glover, 2014, p 7). During the meeting the person would remain central to the decision-making process, and the significant people involved in the person's life would take part. The meeting would need to be clear, accessible and structured, with record keeping that can hold up to any scrutiny at a later date, including information regarding risk analysis and benefits.

Power of attorney

Anybody over the age of 18 and who is able to make decisions for themselves can select a person to have power of attorney over their affairs to cover the circumstances where they lose capacity. The person who holds power of attorney for an individual would then be able to make decisions on their behalf, following the best interest principles.

There are two types of lasting powers of attorney.

1. Personal welfare – this applies when decisions need to be made regarding medical interventions.
2. Property and affairs – this applies when decisions are to be made regarding property, assets and financial affairs.

When establishing a power of attorney, a person can be specific regarding the areas of decision-making they would like it to hold, for example, dietary considerations or the clothes the person wishes to wear.

Deprivation of liberty

Deprivation of liberty was included in the Mental Capacity Act after an amendment was made in 2007. This aspect of the act ensures that a person's liberty is not compromised. This will soon be replaced by a new approach called Liberty Protection Safeguards, which will provide protection to people of the age of 16 or above who need to be deprived of their liberty to enable their care and treatment but lack the capacity to consent to this. To support understanding around the Mental Capacity Act in relation to dementia, Alzheimer's Society (n.d.a; n.d.b) has created a hub of online resources and information.

Independent mental capacity advocate

The Mental Capacity Act (2005) established the legal right to advocacy for those who lack mental capacity. This means people with dementia can be supported by an independent mental capacity advocate during their capacity assessment and best interest meeting, if they do not have family or friends to support or represent them or when there are concerns regarding safeguarding (Mental Health Capacity Act 2005. s.1(35)(1–6).

How does the Mental Capacity Act relate to personalisation?

Personalisation is concerned with people having rights, choice and independence. People living with dementia have the same human and legal rights as those who do not have dementia; this includes the right to have choice, control and freedom. A diagnosis of dementia does not mean that the person cannot make a particular decision at a particular time. The first statutory principle of the Mental Capacity Act 2005 is the assumption of capacity (Department for Constitutional Affairs, 2007, p 20). This means we must assume that a person living with dementia has the capacity to make decisions, unless it is proven otherwise.

This view is supported by the work of Williamson (2010) who stated: '*People with dementia, including people with severe dementia, are able to express their views about what is important to their quality of life*' (Williamson, 2010, p 10) and '*maintaining a good quality of life is perfectly possible after a diagnosis of dementia*' (Williamson, 2010, p 10).

This section on the Mental Capacity Act has highlighted the absolute right that a person has to be at the centre of any decision-making that is about them. When we work in a manner that is in line with personalisation, we learn that the person, and those close to them, have a good sense of the kind of care and support that will work well for them. This has led to the recognition that those who are in receipt of health and social care support are well positioned to give input and steer regarding the services and support needed within a local area. The idea of co-production puts this thinking into practice.

Co-production

Co-production is an approach to identifying, commissioning and developing local community-based supports and provision. It brings people together to discuss, explore and identify how a person or a group of people can be supported. As a collective of people, the concept of *good support* is explored and discussions are held to identify how this can be achieved. In the context of dementia care and support, the people who would be involved in the co-production process would include:

- people with dementia;
- family members of people with dementia;
- people who organise community initiatives within local areas;
- service providers;
- commissioners;
- funders;
- members of the local community

to collectively identify the solutions to strengthen the community that people reside within.

A co-production group is involved in the delivery of the solutions through commissioning projects and services. They would continue to be involved in overseeing the outcomes achieved via the commissioned projects and services. Working together in this way is a paradigm change to how services have been traditionally commissioned and brings people together to broaden the perspective of the discussions taking place and the representation in the decisions being made.

There are a number of definitions of co-production; here are some of the most commonly known.

> *Coproduction means delivering public services in an equal and reciprocal relationship between professionals, people using services, their families and their neighbours. Where activities are coproduced in this way, both services and neighbourhoods become far more effective agents of change (Boyle and Harris, 2009, p 11).*

As a delivery model for health services, coproduction is based on the sharing of information and on shared decision making between the service users and providers. (Bettencourt et al, 2002 cited in Realpe and Wallace, 2010, p 5)

It [Coproduction] builds on the assumption that both parties [people who work within the local authority and those who do not] have a central role to play in the process as they each contribute different and essential knowledge. (Cahn, 2000) (Cahn, 2000 cited in Realpe and Wallace, 2010, p 5)

Co-production is an approach to the development and design of support services available in communities and for people who access health and social care support. Although the model has been facilitated for a long time in the discipline of sciences, its introduction to public services is still in its early stages. A discussion paper published by Nesta in 2009, 'The challenge of coproduction', stated a key finding: '*The opportunities are huge, but there are plenty of remaining barriers to creating the conditions for coproduction*' (Boyle and Harris, 2009, p 23.).

The barriers relate to the historical decision-making processes that shape the protocols, policies and procedures within local authorities, which are contradictory to the ethos of co-production. During the recent years of austerity, public service reform has had a heavy focus on cost efficiencies and change management has often been led by selecting the lowest cost option. This has resulted in an output-driven delivery model based on what individuals actually receive rather than on the quality of what they receive.

Although there continue to be barriers to achieving a Co-production Model in the delivery of public services, it is recognised that to achieve personalisation, a system-wide transformation will be needed, and this will require a redesign of the existing support and service structures. Co-production is an ideal vehicle to achieve this and continues to be an important development in the approaches available to enable the realisation of personalised practice.

Considering co-production

Co-production makes strengthening the core economy of neighbourhood and family – the central task of all public services. This means:

- *Recognising people as assets because people themselves are the real wealth of society*
- *Valuing work differently, to recognise everything as work that people do to raise families, look after people, maintain healthy communities, social justice and good governance*
- *Promoting reciprocity, giving and receiving because it builds trust between people and fosters mutual respect*
- *Building social networks because people's physical and mental well-being depends on strong, enduring relationships*

(Boyle and Harris, 2009, p 14)

Questions to aid reflection

1) If co-production was fostered as the way to facilitate and distribute public services and funding, what difference would this make?
2) What would be the similarities and differences between the traditional commissioning approach to the distribution of public funds and the approach offered through co-production?

In the context of dementia care and support, co-production could either be focused on a micro approach:

- a support solution that would suit an individual, where the person, family, friends and professionals have worked together to learn what would work best and have collectively found a way to make this possible;

or a macro approach:

- a support solution that would work for groups of people in the community which would include people with dementia, for example, setting up a new social group to attend, resolving a transport issue, or employing a team of people to work as support workers

Within co-production, it is recognised that those actively involved in the discussions regarding the redesign of service structures are to represent the wider population of people with dementia and their family members and carers. Therefore, there can be challenges inherent in co-production in achieving outcomes where all individuals involved feel listened to and heard.

Co-production, the values of inclusion and collective agency

The values of inclusion and collective agency covered in Chapter 1 have a lot of principles in common with co-production.

- It is important to get to know one another.
- A culture of equality needs to be fostered.
- A problem is more likely to find a solution if there is a group of actively interested people involved in the conversation.
- The idea that no one group or person is more important than any other group or person.
- Bringing people together from a variety of backgrounds to support each other to exercise their ability to gain voice, choice and control creates a stronger picture of the strengths and assets of a local area.
- Collectively people can build on the picture of what is currently available in the community to build a stronger place for everyone.

Outputs and outcomes

When making plans for the future or what needs to change to improve the quality of life, it is useful to understand the difference between outputs and outcomes.

Outputs relate to what is delivered. *Outcomes* refer to the difference made.

Outputs

Outputs have a focus on describing and counting activities.

- The number of people who attended an activity.
- How long the activity was delivered for.

For instance a day centre may have 20 people who attend and 12 of those people took part in the cooking workshop which lasted two hours.

Outcomes

Outcomes focus on what has changed in the person's life as a result of the activity or the care and support they have received, the subjective experience of the person and the difference it has made for them.

Developing an understanding of the outcomes of the approach can provide insight into what is needed to improve the experience of accessing care and support.

It is important to remember that it is the person in receipt of care and support who should determine how a *good* outcome is defined.

Quality outcomes for people living with dementia

The Department of Health (2010) developed quality measures in reference to the provision of care and support for people with dementia in England: 'Quality outcomes for people with dementia: building on the work of the National Dementia Strategy'. Within this paper a set of *'I' statements* are presented that have been co-produced between members of the department of health, people with dementia and their family carers who capture what people would like to see in their own lives.

The 'I' statements are put into the following context.

'*By 2014, all people living with dementia in England should be able to say [each 'I' statement]*'.

- *I was diagnosed early*
- *I can enjoy life*
- *I understand, so I make good decisions and provide for future decision-making*
- *I am treated with dignity and respect*
- *I feel part of a community and I'm inspired to give something back*

- *I get the treatment and support which are best for my dementia, and my life*
- *I know what I can do to help myself and who else can help me*
- *I am confident my end of life wishes will be respected. I can expect a good death.*

(Department of Health, 2010, p 12)

National Dementia Declaration

In the same year as the "Quality outcomes for people with dementia: building on the work of the National Dementia Strategy" the National Dementia Declaration for England was published. The declaration was signed by over 100 organisations as a commitment to put the actions set in the declaration fully into practice by 2014. The declaration provided momentum to address the issues surrounding dementia and has ensured that it remains a public policy priority (Dementia Action Alliance, 2010).

In 2014, the All-Party Parliamentary Group on Dementia commended the continued focus on the provision of quality dementia care and support. The report highlighted the areas of dementia care and support which had not reached the aspirations set in the National Dementia Declaration (Alzheimer's Society, 2014). It also noted areas of practice that had improved, which included increased personalised support at the time of diagnosis and the difference this made to people's quality of life, although this continued to vary throughout the country. The report also called for improvements in crisis prevention and funding for services that support '*people with dementia and their carers to live independently in their own homes for as long as they are able and wish to*' (All-Party Parliamentary Group on Dementia, 2014).

The National Dementia Declaration for England put forward seven outcomes to work towards improving the experience for people living with dementia. These were written by those living with dementia and their families and affirm their wish to have choice and control about the services they receive.

The declaration contains a series of 'I' statements, which build on and further those created by the National Dementia Strategy.

The collection of 'I' statements outlined within the National Dementia Declaration can be broadly separated into seven categories.

1) I have personal choice and control or influence over decisions about me.
    - I have control over my life and support to do the things that matter to me, and I can make decisions now about the care I want in my later life.
2) I know that services are designed around me and my needs.
    - There are a range of services that support me with any aspect of daily living and enable me to stay at home and in my community, enjoying the best

quality of life for as long as possible, while my carer can access respite care if and when they want it, along with other services that can help support them.

3) I have the support that helps me live my life.

- I have information and support, and I can have fun with a network of others, including people in a similar position to me.

4) I have the knowledge and know-how to get what I need.

- It's not a problem getting information and advice, including information about the range of benefits I can access to help me afford and cope with living at home and my carer has access to further information relevant to them and understands which benefits they are also entitled to.

5) I live in an enabling and supportive environment where I feel valued and understood.

- I had a diagnosis very early on and, if I work, an understanding employer, which means I can still work and stay connected to people in my life. If I develop behaviour that challenges others, people will take the time to understand why I am acting this way and help me try to avoid it.

6) I have a sense of belonging and being a valued part of family, community and civic life.

- I feel safe and supported in my home and in my community, which includes shops and pubs, sporting and cultural opportunities.

7) I know there is research going on which delivers a better life for me now and hope for the future.

- I am confident that there is an increasing investment in dementia research in the UK and I understand the growing evidence about prevention and risk reduction of dementia.

(Dementia Action Alliance, 2010, pp 4–5)

The outcomes of personalisation

A focus on learning about the outcomes that have been achieved and actively utilising what has been learnt to make any changes needed to reach better outcomes in the future is what will make a difference to the quality of life experienced. A shift to measuring outcomes, rather than outputs, as an indicator of the quality of health and social care provision needs to be established within the various measurement frameworks.

Table 2.1 provides a summary of what has been learnt about personalisation and what it means for people with dementia.

Table 2.1 *Summary: Personalisation*

Personalisation means ...	What personalisation means to people with dementia
Tailoring support to people's individual needs and aspirations.	People with dementia and their informal carers will receive support that they have played an active role in determining and in a manner that works best for them.
Ensuring people have access to information, advice and advocacy to support them to be able to make informed decisions about their care and support.	People with dementia and their informal carers will have the information and support they require to understand what options are available to them and to make effective choices.
Finding new collaborative ways of working (which includes co-production) that support people to actively engage in the design, delivery and evaluation of services.	The person with dementia and everyone else providing care and support will imaginatively and creatively work together to create an effective package of support and care that corresponds to the wishes of the person with dementia.
Developing local partnerships to coproduce a range of services and options for people to choose from which promote opportunities for social inclusion and community development.	Services from the statutory, private, community and voluntary sectors work together, alongside people with dementia and their carers to achieve inclusion and connection in the community.
Developing the right leadership and organisational systems to enable staff to work in creative, person-centred ways.	Investment is made into the culture of the organisations and leadership to realise person-centred approaches. People with lived experience help to shape and inspire leadership.
Embedding early intervention, re-enablement and prevention so that people are supported as soon as it is needed and in a way that's right for them.	People with dementia receive a diagnosis as early as possible, which is clearly explained to them. At the time of diagnosis the person is provided with information and advice which supports them to make choices and plans about the life they want to live.
Recognising and supporting carers in their role, while enabling them to maintain a life beyond their caring responsibilities.	The contribution of informal carers is fully understood and valued, its effect on their physical and emotional health is recognised and, when appropriate, suitable support is offered. Carers are seen as having a life outside of their role as carers, for which they should have every opportunity to enjoy.
Ensuring all citizens have access to universal community services and resources – a total system response.	People with dementia continue to be and are included in all aspects of community life without experiencing any barriers to participation and contribution.

Delivering personalised support to people living with dementia

Those leading on the delivery of services for people with dementia will be aspiring to deliver the best service possible and to implement personalised practices within their organisation. Organisations have access to excellent evaluation tools, for instance the VIPS framework and Dementia Care Mapping™, as well as the frameworks and models introduced in this chapter. These tools provide effective direction on delivering person-centred care, personalisation and self-directed support. The effectiveness of these tools and models is complemented by person-centred planning and approaches, covered further in Chapter 6.

Key lessons learnt

- Personalisation is the accumulation of a number of approaches and developments within health and social care.
- *Normalisation*, one of the roots of personalisation, highlighted the inequalities within society that related to people being placed within large institutional hospital settings due to their mental health or disability.
- The Social Model, developed and led by people who lived with disabilities, recognises that the barriers people face to leading a full and inclusive life are based on society's structures, while the Medical Model captures an approach to the provision of health and social care that is determined by a direct response to conditions and diagnosis.
- Self-directed support and personalisation help people with dementia overcome barriers and achieve a better quality of life.
- The Citizenship Model sees the relationship between the person living with dementia, paid-for carers, the community and the government as equal and balanced, with the person living with dementia having meaningful relationships within the community and an identity that is embedded in these relationships and the contributions they have made to society.
- The Professional Gift Model aligns with the Medical Model and often places people who are accessing the social care system at the receiving end of predetermined professional-led decisions and service provision.
- Personalised practice would be strengthened if there was a strong understanding of the Social Model and the Citizenship Model.
- Co-production brings people together to discuss, explore and identify how communities can become stronger for everyone and the types of investments that would serve the best purpose for local people.

- Personalisation has opened up the opportunity to recognise a bigger picture of what it takes to achieve an outcome of *well-being* and *quality of life*.
- *Outputs* relate to *what we do*, whereas *outcomes* refer to *what difference we can make*. The person in receipt of the care should decide what a good outcome looks like.
- Personalisation is not to be experienced as a one-off planning meeting, response or isolated event but should instead be embedded throughout a person's life.
- Personalisation is at the heart of the vision for the future of the UK's health and social care provision.

Questions to aid reflection

1) What are the main developments over the past 50 years that have evolved into personalisation?
2) What would you say if you were to have a conversation with someone about the areas of your own life that contribute to your well-being and quality of life?
3) Consider all the ideas and models that have been covered in this chapter; out of these which would you find most useful to incorporate into the experience of care and support?

3 The dementia journey

This chapter covers:

- **The different types of dementia**
- **The importance of engaging with the person with dementia**
- **The dementia journey, focusing on the early, mid and late stages in the context of the individual's experience**
- **Personalisation at each stage of dementia**
- **Before a person receives a diagnosis of dementia**
- **The importance of an early and timely diagnosis**
- **Future decision-making using advanced care planning.**

What is dementia?

The word *dementia* has been defined by the Alzheimer's Society (2017a, pp 1–3) as follows: '*a set of symptoms that may include memory loss and difficulties with thinking, problem-solving or language. ... Dementia is caused when the brain is damaged by diseases, such as Alzheimer's disease or a series of strokes. ... Dementia is progressive, which means the symptoms gradually get worse over time*'.

The definition provided by the Alzheimer's Society explains the reality of dementia; it is a chronic and progressive condition with, as of yet, no cure. People who have a diagnosis of dementia will experience the syndrome (a group of related symptoms) in different ways, with progression and the changes in the person's life experience varying from one person to the next.

While dementia is seen as a memory disorder, it is also appropriate to think of the other symptoms of dementia that affect a person's body, behaviour and emotions. The person living with dementia will gradually, over time, experience changes in their ability to manage daily tasks, manage their emotions and maintain their relationships. The decline in ability will vary and fluctuate; it is also important to remember that people can retain their skills and abilities, including making decisions for themselves.

Relating to people on the basis that they are capable is paramount to the person's sense of well-being and health. Ensuring that the person's ability to make decisions about their life and how they wish to be supported or cared for is not underestimated is key to supporting them to maintain and achieve quality of life, as well as keeping with the principles of the Mental Capacity Act 2005.

Retaining control

Controlling practice can come from people and organisations that are well-meaning but are not fully conscious of the negative effects of the approach they have adopted. This approach has the potential to lead to negative consequences for the person living with dementia where they may become passive, dependent, frustrated or disconnected from others.

Ken is a person living with dementia who shares his insight into what good support looks like and his need to retain control over his own life.

> *Decay sets in at the moment of diagnosis – medically nothing can be done – but you can do a lot for yourself. Well-meaning people can destroy your confidence. My wife is technically my carer but you need to continue to do things for yourself. There is a fine line between doing too much for someone and giving them the help they need.*
>
> (Ken Howard, Young Dementia UK, n.d.)

Reflection

- What principles and practices would ensure that the person living with dementia retains control and self-determination?

People diagnosed with dementia will, most likely, experience diminished cognition and an impaired ability to make choices. Despite this, the person must not be treated as though they have lost their ability to fully participate in conversations and to make decisions. Until a time when their capacity is in doubt, a full capacity assessment has been conducted and it has been concluded that the person no longer has the capacity to make that decision at that particular time.

The risk of not engaging

Engaging with others can sometimes feel overwhelming, and often it takes time to build a good relationship with understanding, rapport and trust. It is important to consider the approach to take when getting to know someone to achieve a positive experience.

Living with dementia is a series of stages, from pre-diagnosis and receiving the diagnosis to the middle stages and later stages of dementia, which is referred to as the dementia journey. If a person is not engaged with positively at every stage of their dementia journey, their sense of self-worth is at risk, and this will have a marked impact on their sense of well-being and self-identity, as Seligman (1975) states: '*When this* [not appropriately engaging with people who have dementia] *happens, people with dementia are discouraged and after repeatedly trying to get their voice heard and their wishes granted they will give up and learned helplessness occurs together, perhaps with associated depression*'.

Helplessness and hopelessness

Here are some outcomes that can occur within a person living with dementia if they are not listened to and consequently do not have control and choice over how they experience their own lives. Some of these outcomes will be instilled within a person due to the very nature of dementia, although these feelings and emotions can be compounded or brought on by the way the person is treated and related to by the people around them.

Helplessness is a feeling that any effort made will not change the outcome of a situation. This can be associated with people who have recently received a diagnosis of a chronic disease, such as dementia and, because of this, feel powerless and unable to act independently (Elsevier Mosby, 2005). People could experience helplessness as a result of overly rigid institutional rules or the behaviour of staff members. An individualised approach to care fosters self-esteem and will assist in the prevention of helplessness (Saunders, 2003).

Hopelessness is a loss of confidence that future events or occurrences will be positive. It is '*a subjective state in which an individual sees limited or no alternatives or personal choices available and is unable to mobilise energy on his/her own behalf*' (Peate, 2006, p 476). Hopelessness is associated with poor health outcomes and may be prevented by the maintenance of a positive environment that supports independence and self-confidence (Saunders, 2003).

Reflection

- Consider some of the experiences you have had where a person's actions, a situation or the environment could have created a sense of helplessness or hopelessness.

- If you were able to go back to this time, what would you do differently to achieve a better outcome?
- If a person living with dementia was feeling a sense of helplessness or hopelessness, what could be done to support a better outcome?

How dementia develops

To understand the dementia journey better and to be able to offer personalised support in the most appropriate and positive way, an understanding of what dementia is and how it develops is needed.

Dementia is a progressive disease with patterns and stages. The progression will differ for each individual. This progression can be seen in the context of three stages.

- Early or mild – minor changes in a person's ability, behaviour and memory, for instance:
  - mislaying items around the house;
  - forgetting recent conversations or events;
  - struggling to find the right word in conversation or losing the thread of what is being said.
- Middle or moderate – changes in a person's ability, behaviour and memory become more marked, for example:
  - becoming confused about where they are or walking off and becoming lost;
  - muddling up time and getting up at night because they are mixing up night and day.
- Late or severe – pronounced changes in a person's ability, behaviour and memory and the person becoming increasingly weak, for instance:
  - having difficulty eating and sometimes swallowing;
  - experiencing considerable weight loss, although some people eat too much and put on weight.

Health professionals utilise a variety of scales to measure the stage of dementia a person has reached. These scales address a person's:

- mental ability;
- daily living skills;

- behaviours;
- overall functioning and ability to get on with day-to-day skills.

The Mini-Mental State Examination is the most commonly used *test* for complaints of memory loss and other mental abilities. This test would be conducted with consideration to the person's history, symptoms and a physical examination.

Dementia and personalisation

The way a person experiences the progression of dementia will vary greatly; some stages will overlap, some aspects may come before others, some symptoms from different stages may disappear altogether. Each person living with dementia will experience the condition in their own unique way. To deliver a personalised approach, those providing health care and support should invest time to get to know the person so as to be able to recognise and respond to their individual experience.

The forms of dementia

The different forms of dementia include:

- Alzheimer's disease;
- frontotemporal dementia (including Pick's disease);
- vascular dementia;
- dementia with Lewy bodies (DLB);
- mixed dementia.

Alzheimer's disease

This is the most common form, accounting for between 60% and 80% of cases (Alzheimer's Association, 2020), and it has therefore been studied in the greatest detail.

Various factors may contribute to the onset and development of Alzheimer's disease. The older a person is, the more likely they are to develop it, affecting 1 in 14 people over the age of 65 and 1 in 6 over the age of 80 (Alzheimer's Society, 2016). Genetics also plays a part, and, in a few families, there is an increased chance of developing the condition.

Alzheimer's disease is a physical disease and is caused by the development of *plaques* and *tangles* in the brain. These plaques and tangles lead to the death of brain cells and give rise to various symptoms. In addition, people with Alzheimer's disease experience a reduction in the level of chemicals involved in transmitting messages within the brain essential for body functioning, that is, the messages needed for body movement.

Alzheimer's disease usually develops slowly in people. People in the early stages may experience lapses of memory and have problems finding the right words as well as:

- becoming slower at grasping new ideas and unwilling to try out new things;
- becoming confused or losing track of the day or date;
- showing poor judgement or finding it harder to plan or make decisions;
- having problems judging distance or seeing objects in three dimensions (when navigating stairs or parking the car, for instance);
- losing interest in other people or activities.

(Alzheimer's Society, 2015, p 5)

As highlighted by the Alzheimer's Society, there are a number of indicators for the early stages. Seeking a diagnosis at an early stage can help determine if these behaviours are a result of early-stage Alzheimer's or if they can be explained by other life factors. As the condition progresses, the person may start to get up at night as they confuse night and day, go outside in their night clothes, become very agitated or unknowingly behave in socially inappropriate ways.

The final stage is the late or severe stage. Here, the person living with dementia will become heavily dependent on the people around them to maintain their quality of life and to meet their basic needs. They are likely to be physically weak, their memory will have declined, and may find it difficult to recognise everyday objects, surroundings and those closest to them.

During the final stages, pronounced and fluctuating changes in a person's behaviour are likely, and they may become, even for short periods of time, subdued or frustrated. Any change is due to the heightened confusion and disorientation the person will be experiencing. It can be common for them to lash out aggressively while being supported by close personal care. It is important to remember the person will not be behaving in this way intentionally and to recognise the behaviour as a form of communication and a reflection of the confusion and frustration they are experiencing.

Frontotemporal dementia (including Pick's disease)

This less-common form of dementia is caused by damage to the frontal lobes and/or the temporal lobes. These areas of the brain are responsible for emotions, feelings and language. For example, someone may become less sensitive to other people's emotions, perhaps making them seem cold and unfeeling. They may also lose some of their inhibitions, leading to behaviour that is out of character, such as making tactless or inappropriate comments. There are three types of frontotemporal dementia: one that affects behaviour first and two that affect language first.

When someone is diagnosed with frontotemporal dementia marked changes can be seen in their behaviour, personality or their command of language. These changes would be recognised by those who know the person well but they themselves may not be aware of these changes. The person may develop repetitive habits, gestures and phrases. This can include developing obsessions or hoarding. The person may also appear uncharacteristically:

- selfish and unattached;
- unfeeling;
- rude;
- easily distracted;
- less interested;
- low in motivation.

Other symptoms of this form of dementia include:

- acquiring a sweet tooth;
- uninhibited behaviour;
- compulsions.

As dementia progresses, people whose behaviour and personality changed initially will begin to have trouble with language and, likewise, those who initially had trouble with language will see changes in their behaviour and personality. In the later stages, the symptoms become similar to the later stages of Alzheimer's disease.

People live, on average, seven or eight years after the initial symptoms, depending on when the diagnosis was given. There is no medication specifically designed to treat frontotemporal dementia. Acetylcholinesterase inhibitors, such as donepezil (Aricept), which are normally prescribed for Alzheimer's disease, are not effective. However, there are medications that can help control some of the symptoms, including antidepressants and antipsychotics. There are several support measures and treatments available which can make everyday life easier, including occupational therapy, speech and language therapy, physiotherapy and relaxation therapies, such as music, dance and massage.

Vascular dementia

Vascular dementia is a deficiency in blood flow to the brain due to diseased blood vessels. The brain requires a constant supply of blood to deliver oxygen and nutrients which are delivered through a network of blood vessels. If these vascular systems within the brain become damaged, the blood vessels leak or become blocked, preventing the blood cells from reaching the brain. The symptoms of vascular dementia can sometimes develop suddenly and quickly get worse, although they can also develop gradually over many months or years. People with Vascular dementia may also experience stroke-like symptoms, including muscle weakness or paralysis on one side of their body. If the brain does not receive the right level of oxygen and nutrients, it can affect three elements known as cognition.

- Thinking.
- Memory.
- Reasoning.

Vascular dementia is the loss of ability to manage these three elements, and this begins to affect daily life. There are different types.

- Stroke-related dementia

  A stroke happens when the blood supply to the brain is suddenly cut off. In most strokes, a blood vessel to the brain is blocked or narrowed. The severity depends on whether the blockage is temporary or permanent and where the blockage has occurred.

- Post-stroke dementia

  Twenty percent of people who have had a stroke are at risk of developing post-stroke dementia within the ensuing 6 months (Alzheimer's Society, 2014, p 3). A person who has had a stroke is at higher risk of having further strokes, which then means the person is at greater risk of developing vascular dementia.

- Single-infarct and multi-infarct dementia

  This is caused by one or many smaller strokes as a result of a blood vessel that becomes blocked by a blood clot which quickly releases itself. The stroke is so small that the person does not notice the symptoms and can often believe they have just been a little bit unwell. The blood clot, even triggering a temporary blockage of a few minutes, can cause permanent damage to a small area of brain tissue known as an *infarct*. It is common in these circumstances for many small strokes of this type to occur over a period of weeks or months, which then leads to infarcts spreading around the brain; this then results in multi-infarct dementia.

- Subcortical dementia

  This is the most common form of vascular dementia, and it is caused by a disease of the smaller blood vessels that reside deeper within the brain tissue. The disease causes these smaller blood vessels to have hardened walls and to become twisted, reducing blood flow within this area of the brain. This disease can also affect the nerve fibres that carry signals around the brain, also known as *white matter*. It can cause infarcts at the base of the brain.

Dementia with Lewy bodies

This form of dementia gets its name from microscopic deposits that are in the brain, which can cause damage and eventually the death of the brain's nerve cells. DLB is a progressive condition and usually develops over a period of years. People with DLB will usually have some features of Alzheimer's disease and Parkinson's disease and may experience the following.

- Impaired attention and alertness.
- Spatial disorientation causing difficulty in certain activities, such as planning and coordinating mental activities.
- Memory is often affected, though less so than in people with Alzheimer's disease.
- Slowness, muscle stiffness, trembling of the limbs, a tendency to shuffle when walking, loss of facial expression and changes in the strength and tone of their voice (features of Parkinson's disease).
- Detailed and convincing visual hallucinations (seeing things that are not there), often of people or animals.
- Fluctuating abilities day by day
- Falling asleep very easily by day and having restless nights with confusion, nightmares and hallucinations.
- Fainting, falling or having funny turns.

Mixed dementia (vascular dementia and Alzheimer's disease)

People can have a diagnosis of several forms of dementia, and at least 10% of those diagnosed have a combination of Alzheimer's disease and vascular dementia (Dementia Matters, 2018). In these circumstances, people will experience a mixture of the symptoms inherent to each form of dementia.

Before the diagnosis of dementia

The onset of dementia can be a different experience for each individual. Multi-infarct dementia may start suddenly and then progress in a stepwise manner as a repeated series of mini-strokes occur. The person often has periods of lucidity when they are more engaged with others and can take part in everyday activities. Whereas when someone has Alzheimer's disease, the onset and progression of dementia are usually more gradual, though in many ways it is often indistinguishable from multi-infarct dementia.

The period between the onset of dementia and its diagnosis is a difficult time for people living with dementia and their family. It can take a long time to reach a diagnosis with many factors influencing this, for instance:

- the recognition and acceptance, on behalf of the person and their family, that an appointment with a general practitioner (GP) is required;

- the ability and confidence to communicate the person's experiences to a GP;
- the length of time available to speak to a GP during an appointment period;
- the GP being alert to the signs of early-onset dementia.

The need to promote the early diagnosis of dementia and ensure the availability of information and support is an important priority in the National Dementia Strategy.

Understanding the symptoms

The very early symptoms of dementia may be mild and the changes experienced may only be gradual. Therefore, the early signs of dementia can be difficult to detect. The person may not notice the early indicators of dementia, and they, as well as the people close to them, may not notice these changes, only taking action when the changes have become prominent and noticeable. The symptoms, and the speed at which these affect someone, will depend on the form of dementia, as well as their overall health. Each person will experience the symptoms of dementia differently.

Early and timely diagnosis

Early diagnosis involves methods to determine the nature of a disease or disorder at its early stage of progression. Generally, an early diagnosis improves prognosis and access to treatment. The case for timely, as opposed to early, diagnosis is identified as being of the utmost importance, in order for the benefits to be balanced against the risks (Nuffield Council on Bioethics, 2009, p 43). Receiving a diagnosis of dementia does hold potential risks for the person; therefore, the timing of the diagnosis needs to be carefully managed and delivered with their well-being, rights and circumstances as a primary focus. According to the *Journal of Alzheimer's Disease*, a timely diagnosis '*refers to a diagnosis at the stage when patients come to the attention of clinicians because of concerns about changes in cognition, behavior, or functioning and can be still free of dementia and functionally independent*' (Dubois et al, 2015).

Receiving a diagnosis at any stage of the dementia journey still means that the person can begin to receive good and timely advice, guidance, support and treatment. A personalised approach from this point is crucial in enabling a positive experience of receiving care and support for the person with dementia and their family. The Prime Minister's Challenge on Dementia 2020 (Department of Health, 2015, p 16) states: '*everyone should be offered high quality support after receiving a diagnosis of dementia*'.

A personalised approach at the point of diagnosis is complementary to the Citizenship Model, as covered in Chapter 2. This approach recognises that people are a part of their community, where they have developed and built up meaningful relationships within their lifetime. Alongside those people who are important to them, the person can address some of the challenges or difficulties they are facing. Personalisation and the Citizenship Model advocate for people to play an active role in shaping their care and support, moving away from being a passive recipient of services, as identified in the Professional Gift Model, to taking the lead in shaping how they wish to live their life and the care and support they receive.

The National Dementia Strategy (Department of Health, 2009) has placed greater emphasis on early dementia diagnosis, prevention and risk reduction. Dementia is not currently screened within the whole population. Health and social care in England has introduced case findings in high-risk groups, including:

- people over 75 years of age, as age is the strongest risk factor for dementia;
- those with high vascular risk;
- people with Parkinson's disease;
- people with learning disabilities.

(Bamford et al, 2007)

Providing an early diagnosis offers an opportunity to:

- inform people what it means to have dementia;
- allow for the delivery of therapy and the prescription of medication;
- signpost people to sources of information, local and national support groups;
- provide advice about driving;
- provide advice regarding financial matters and making appropriate plans for the future;
- provide guidance regarding the benefits available, when a person would be eligible to apply and the application process;
- start the process of gathering information and planning to ensure that the person continues to experience a good life and maintains optimum control;
- provide guidance on advanced care planning (ACP);
- provide help with setting up a lasting power of attorney.

Referral to other professional input can also be provided once a diagnosis is confirmed; this could include referrals to community mental health teams, speech and language therapists, dietitians and occupational therapists.

When to seek a diagnosis

Sometimes someone in the very early stages of dementia will not want to admit to themselves that they have been experiencing changes to their ability, emotions and memory and will not want others to notice or find out. The changes in their ability to manage day-to-day life can lead to family, friends and neighbours becoming fearful that the person or others are at risk, especially in situations where the gas tap has been left on and unlit or the front door left unlocked overnight. Situations like this can cause considerable concern, which leads to them contacting the person's GP.

Barriers to diagnosis

One of the difficulties with the provision of appropriate and timely support to people living with dementia is the need to first receive a diagnosis. There continues to be a lack of awareness and understanding regarding dementia, which can lead to stigmatisation and barriers to receiving a diagnosis (World Health Organization (WHO), 2019).

Diagnostic process

Receiving a diagnosis can take time. Depending on the person's presenting stage of dementia, a diagnosis can take between 4 weeks to 12 months, especially if the person is in the early stages (Social Care Institute of Excellence (SCIE), 2015).

A wife's story

Here is a story that has been shared by a woman whose husband was diagnosed with early-onset dementia.

My name is Janet. I am a retired Finance Director and I am a world expert on dementia ... more correctly, my husband's dementia. This complicated disease affects everybody in different ways and everybody's journey is different. This is the story of our journey.

First of all, my husband was, and is, a lovely man and that makes it both easier and also so much harder.

How our journey started

Very slowly at first as Martin instinctively compensated for his failing ability to cope for a while before I noticed

- *Avoidance of handling change*
- *Difficulty telling the time*
- *Forgetting how to use various computer programmes*
- *Blaming the tax man for increasing complexity*
- *Not remembering how to play crib*

- *Becoming less able to manage monetary affairs*
- *Forgetting our anniversary (my emotional low!)*
- *Stopping smoking after 40 years because the taste changed*
- *Becoming quieter and more withdrawn.*

In retrospect I think it was more stressful before we got an official diagnosis and 'came out'! I started helping Martin to mask his increasing confusion and spent a lot of time planning how to remove the risk of failure from his life, without upsetting him further.

But Martin wouldn't accept that there was anything wrong and we avoided the subject, until a couple of crisis points after which Martin agreed to speak to the doctor (but for my sake, not his!).

(Janet, Young Dementia UK, n.d.)

Reflection

- What support could be provided to those who are preparing to have a discussion with their GP about the changes they are experiencing?
- Should family members be able to be part of this discussion? What would be the benefits of this, and what would be the disadvantages?
- What thoughts does this story give you regarding hopelessness and helplessness, as explained on page 75?

An accurate diagnosis during the early stages of dementia can be difficult as a person's *dementia-like* symptoms can be caused by other health conditions. Appropriate assessment and investigations can detect the root cause of the symptoms. The appropriate treatment for the health condition can then be provided to the individual, and the symptoms become fully or partially reversed, depending on the root problem. For instance, the symptoms experienced by the person could be due to the side effects of the medication they have been prescribed, a combination of medications they are taking or an infection or a brain tumour. When seeking a diagnosis, the person and their family may find that they have to be persistent with tests and assessments to eliminate any other factors and to confidently reach a fully informed and accurate diagnosis, followed by appropriate support.

A thorough assessment can also help to accurately diagnose not only dementia but the form of dementia the person has. There are a number of ways that a person may begin to be assessed for and receive their diagnosis of dementia. During a visit to hospital, most people aged over 75, who have been admitted urgently to hospital, will have an initial assessment on levels of confusion and memory loss. The outcome of this initial assessment can lead to a full assessment if there are any concerns and if the person has given their consent for this to take place. This is deemed good practice within hospital settings, and it has been put in place to make sure that an early diagnosis is possible. Caution is needed while undertaking an assessment within a hospital setting, especially if the person has been admitted urgently. They may be experiencing confusion and memory loss as a result of an illness or accident. The confusion may also be due to the sudden change in their environment rather than as a symptom of dementia. During a routine visit, a GP may now ask about memory problems, especially if the person is over 60 or had a stroke, heart condition or diabetes.

Screening and assessment

After the initial screening assessment and discussion at the hospital or GP, further assessments and tests will be carried out.

Stage 1: Visit the general practitioner

Generally the first step for anyone who is concerned about memory loss, confusion or changes in behaviour or mood would be a visit to their GP. This visit could take place in the surgery, or the GP may prefer to make a home visit as it is easier to observe changes and assess someone's behaviour in their own home. The person will be in familiar surroundings, and any problems with managing or navigating these surroundings will become clear. The GP will use the following procedures for the assessment:

- **Mental ability tests –** These are designed to test thinking, memory and orientation. This could be in the form of an interview, a written test or a series of questions that test cognitive ability and often comprises a Mini-Mental State Examination.
- **Physical examinations and tests –** These are likely to happen if another medical condition is suspected, that is, stroke or Parkinson's disease. The GP will also take blood and possibly urine samples for testing. Through these examinations, they may identify other conditions that are the cause of the symptoms.
- **Looking at *history* –** The GP will spend time with the person to talk about when the symptoms began and how they are influencing the person's life now. The GP may also talk with someone who knows them well. They will read the person's medical history and those of close relatives and will do a full review of any medication being taken.

Once the assessment is completed the GP would explain their findings. If they are confident and experienced in the diagnosis of dementia, they would provide the diagnosis at this stage and, although this is not common, '*occasionally a GP or specialist nurse will make the diagnosis, depending on their expertise and training*' (Alzheimer's Society, 2020).

It is more likely that the GP, if they suspect dementia, will make a referral to a specialist service, such as a memory clinic, or a consultant.

The GP is more likely to be able to provide the diagnosis if the person has reached the advanced stages of dementia or if the person is displaying symptoms of a common form of dementia, such as Alzheimer's.

Providing the diagnosis

A briefing paper for the Faculty of Older People and the Dementia Action Alliance produced guidelines regarding the communication of the diagnosis of dementia in 2013:

> *However, even though the statement 'You have dementia' is only one part of the framework of knowledge for an individual, this particular piece of information is the confirmation of what is happening and the gateway to treatment. Therefore the disclosure of this information needs to be given 'in a sensitive, compassionate way that instils realistic hope' (Lee and Weston, 2011, p 852). To do this takes great skill, as it crosses medical and social boundaries.*
>
> (Murphy and Gair, 2013, p 5)

Practical and creative approaches to sensitive diagnosis

To provide sensitive and person-centred support at the stage of diagnosis will require practical and creative approaches. Here is an example of a model of delivery adopted in Dudley.

Integrated Dementia Care in Dudley Council, which, working in partnership with NHS Dudley, has developed an innovative, integrated approach to the diagnosis, care and support offered to people with dementia, their carers and families. They have developed three dementia gateways located across the borough, which provide care and support for those affected by dementia throughout all stages of the condition. If dementia is suspected by a GP in Dudley, they will refer the person to the borough's Dementia Pathway. The pathway will ensure that a formal diagnosis is made by a dementia specialist and care and support is then offered by a dementia nurse or dementia advisor – this will be a lifetime contact developing a plan of support, help and advice – unique to each person. The advisors and nurses are based in the dementia gateways and work closely with people, families and carers on an ongoing basis, developing a plan of support, help and advice – unique to each person. Through attention to the individual needs and wishes of the person, the gateways ensure tailored care, as well as providing extensive support and advice for families and carers. The gateways aim to ensure those affected by dementia enjoy life to the full, and they offer a wide range of sessions and therapies, from crafts and memory exercises to gardening. There are also day sessions available to provide a break for family and carers (Dudley Metropolitan Borough Council, 2020) (Dinsdale, 2013).

Reflection

- What else would be required at the stage of diagnosis?
- What types of communication and interaction would work best for people at this stage of their dementia journey?
- If you or a family member or friend were going through an assessment for dementia, what would you like this experience to be like?

Stage 2: Referral to a specialist

It is usually the GP who would make the referral to the specialist. If the person or their carer feels that this referral is needed, but it is not offered by the GP, they should ask for a referral to be made, to either one of the following.

- The Memory Clinic.
- The Community Mental Health Team.

Specialists have specific training and therefore have the knowledge base and experience to be able to diagnose dementia accurately. Due to the specialism of their role, they will be able to utilise and access specialised investigations based on the person's age, symptoms and availability. There are main consultants, including the following.

- Neurologists who specialise in diseases of the brain and nervous system and some who have specialisms in diagnosing dementia. It is typical for neurologists to see younger people, below 65, who are displaying symptoms of less-common forms of dementia.
- Geriatricians specialise in the care of older people in relation to physical illnesses and disabilities. If the person is in poor general health, the GP may refer them to a geriatrician to eliminate the possibility of the symptoms being connected to another illness or to establish if the person has a physical illness as well as dementia.
- Old-age psychiatrists specialise in the mental health of older people, including dementia. They can also offer support to younger people with dementia if a suitable specialist is not available for the younger age group in the person's area.
- General adult psychiatrists diagnose and treat a range of mental health issues and generally work with younger people who are under the age of 65, and they

would be involved in supporting the diagnosis of young dementia, which is dementia diagnosed in people under the age of 65.

Consultants form part of a specialist team, which would include doctors at various stages of their training. It is possible that the person may not always have appointments with their consultant, but the consultant is responsible for the care of the person and they will talk to the doctor the person has seen.

The consultant and their team will work in a multi-disciplinary team with other health care professionals to ensure the best care for the person who is being assessed. This team would include psychologists, occupational therapists, social workers, speech and language therapists and dementia advisers, and it would involve any health care professional particular to the person's circumstances and symptoms they are presenting.

Stage 3: Assessment

The actual assessment for dementia can be confusing and daunting for the person. It is good for people to have the opportunity to talk the assessment through with a professional, and lots of memory clinics offer this support to people. These are often referred to as pre-diagnostic counselling sessions. The sessions are available to the person and their family and carers, and are a good opportunity to talk about what people already know about dementia and to chat about concerns. These sessions can broaden people's understanding of:

- why the person has been referred for an assessment;
- what the assessment process involves;
- what support is available if a diagnosis of dementia is given.

An assessment can happen in a variety of locations, and it is not always necessary for the person to go to an unknown place for the assessment to be undertaken, such as a hospital, as it is possible for the assessment to take place at the person's home. If an assessment does take place in a hospital, while the person is there as an inpatient, then the assessment will look at the same areas a GP would consider as part of their assessment, that is, history, physical examinations, mental ability tests and scans (please see the following box for more information about scans).

The test of mental ability will be more detailed when this takes place in a hospital setting, looking at aspects of memory orientation, language and visuospatial skills (eg, copying shapes). The results of these tests undertaken during the assessment process can be utilised as a way to measure future changes the person experiences with their memory, which can further aid the diagnosis in the early stages of dementia. These tests are usually conducted with a mental health nurse or occupational therapist. If the experiences of the person are quite complicated, a neuropsychologist would be involved.

Commonly used scans

These scan types are widely used, and they show changes to brain activity.

- CT (computerised tomography).
- CAT (computerised axial tomography).
- MRI (magnetic resonance imaging).

Some conditions have symptoms similar to dementia, such as tumours and brain bleeds, and CT and MRI scans can identify these conditions, which then rule out dementia. These scans can also show changes to the size of the brain, which can indicate dementia and an MRI scan can show changes caused by diseased blood vessels in the brain, indicating stroke or possible vascular dementia.

If a scan shows no unexpected changes in the brain, it does not rule out dementia as the early stages of the disease can be difficult to distinguish from normal ageing.

Less-common scans

- SPECT (single photon emission computerised tomography)
- PET (positron emission tomography)

These are specialised scans, and they can highlight reduction in brain activity, for instance blood flow or metabolism. If the diagnosis of dementia is unclear after a CAT or CT scan, then a specialised scan may be used.

Mild cognitive impairment

A diagnosis of mild cognitive impairment may be given if the symptoms are mild and the symptoms could indicate depression rather than dementia if the person is maybe experiencing trouble thinking and remembering, but these symptoms are not severe enough to be diagnosed as dementia.

Stage 4: Receiving the diagnosis

The final diagnosis will be given by the consultant or other professionals within the team, though occasionally the consultant will write a letter to the GP and the GP will make an appointment with the person to give the diagnosis.

The diagnosis will be based on the information gathered during the assessment, and the diagnosis should be communicated in a manner that is sensitive to the person's situation and needs. It is important that the person understands the diagnosis and is provided the opportunity to talk through this and ask any questions they have.

The person has a right to know the outcome of the assessments for dementia, although they should be asked if they wish to know the outcome before being provided this information. Ideally this conversation should be held during pre-diagnostic counselling.

If the consultant believes the person would find their diagnosis too distressing, or they may not understand the meaning of the diagnosis, these concerns should be discussed with their close family and friends. The purpose of this discussion would be to reach a conclusion, collectively, about what would be in the person's best interests regarding how they should be informed and when. This does not commonly happen but may be the case when:

- the person may also have another serious illness;
- the person has found the assessment particularly distressing;
- they have recently been bereaved.

It is important when the diagnosis is given that everyone can understand the terminology used and is given the opportunity to ask questions.

During the diagnosis process, people often feel considerable uncertainty. On receipt of a confirmed diagnosis, people can wonder what is going to happen to them as dementia progresses. People can also feel unsure about the type and amount of support they will need and receive and who will provide this support.

Any questions asked should be responded to sensitively and at a pace that works for the person, explaining any terminology and providing space in the conversation for the person to ask questions.

Most memory services offer sessions, running for several weeks after diagnosis, at which the person, and those close to them, can talk through the next steps in more detail and receive further written information. These sessions usually cover medication, living well, driving, benefits, local support services, planning ahead, how the person is feeling and their emotions.

An example of good practice in memory clinics

The Royal Society of Psychologists College of Psychiatrists' Centre for Quality Improvement (CCQI) has developed an accreditation programme for services providing memory clinics, and this is called the National Memory Services National Accreditation Programme (MSNAP) (Copland et al, 2018). The accreditation programme provides a clear quality framework for professionals to work within and assurance to those who are accessing the services. It approves the services being delivered with a focus on quality that is associated directly with the experience of the people who access the service. The effectiveness of this accreditation is strengthened by the involvement of those who have accessed the memory clinic in the design of the accreditation; those who utilise memory clinics are also directly involved in the accreditation process.

Stage 5: Ongoing assessment

The GP will remain responsible for the ongoing care of the person with dementia, and in the initial stages of the diagnosis, people will have access to a local memory service. This may be run privately or by the NHS and can include the Community Mental Health Teams for Older People. The memory service is usually short term, and once the person is discharged, their main contact will continue to be their GP. A referral can be made back to the memory service if the person's symptoms change, and for advice and support during difficult times.

After receiving a diagnosis of dementia, it is important that the person continues to receive support from knowledgeable and trained professionals. Continued medical and psychiatric consultation is an important step in the journey and will help them identify the changes that are occurring and recognise them as part of the stages of dementia.

Although professional input is important, it is possible for this to be delivered in a manner that aligns with the Social Model and the Citizenship Model, where the person is listened to and is at the centre of all decisions and actions.

Medication

During the early stages, medication that has proven to slow the development of the condition may be prescribed. Good standards of practice determine that the person living with dementia must be involved in any discussions and decisions regarding accessing and receiving treatment, including the prescription of medication. As part of the decision-making process, accurate, clear and detailed information and advice regarding the treatment, including possible side effects, needs to be shared with the person in a way that they can understand.

Initially, the specialists involved during the assessments will prescribe the medication with the routine prescriptions coming from the GP, who will be the person's main contact after they have been discharged from the memory clinic. Medication with follow-up reviews should then take place every six months.

Support during assessment and diagnosis

It is important that the person who is undergoing examinations and receiving the diagnosis is supported throughout. They may find the examinations difficult, and, if the person is diagnosed with dementia, they may find hearing the news and its implications stressful. '*Different people will have different experiences of receiving a diagnosis and therefore they will have different ways of coping afterwards*' (Ken, Social Care Institute for Excellence, 2020). The person may experience a mix of emotions at the point of diagnosis, and it is important to be aware of these and to support the person appropriately. This support should include always striving towards the person continuing to be and feel respected, capable and an important part of people's lives.

The news may be devastating, '*The first time they said, "You've got Alzheimer's disease", it was a hell of a shock. When they said, "There's no cure", I defy anyone to say that's not a shock*' (David, Social Care Institute for Excellence (SCIE), 2020). The response from the person and the people close to them at this stage is fundamental.

The experiences in the early stages of dementia are not fully determined by the biomedical changes that happen; they are also influenced by what people do and say and the decisions that are made, including how the decisions are made. A person who has recently received a dementia diagnosis may:

- fall into a *sick role* and disengage from all the activities they were capable of before the diagnosis;
- have concerns about how they will be cared for in the future;
- be aware of how the relationships they have in their life may change;
- be concerned about becoming a burden on the people close to them;
- be in denial regarding the diagnosis;
- become anxious and fearful about what the future holds.

It is difficult to accept the diagnosis and to come to terms with what this means for life now and in the future. '*No one has asked me about my feelings ... 'Are you feeling frightened?' We need emotional counsellors, there needs to be tests for emotional wellbeing alongside blood pressure etc.*' (Pete, Social Care Institute for Excellence (SCIE), 2020).

Denial of the diagnosis is not uncommon, including questioning whether the diagnosis is accurate and whether the tests were conducted correctly. The person could be of the opinion that what they are experiencing is simply the natural signs of aging. Equally a diagnosis of dementia can cause feelings of fearfulness about the future, frustration at how life is changing and upset at the loss of skills and abilities.

There can be a sense of shock, anger, isolation, loneliness, helplessness, sadness, despair, bitterness, shame, guilt and grief, as people may realise that the future plans that they had in place will now need to be reconsidered. Emotions may also fluctuate, going from one extreme to another. Not all the emotions are negative, as this example illustrates: '*Well you know for me it was a big relief – knowing that I could give it a name*' (Peter, Social Care Institute for Excellence (SCIE), 2020). For some, being diagnosed is a positive thing as it places a reason and explanation for the changes they have experienced. Research demonstrates that although there are negative reactions and feelings at the stage of receiving the diagnosis, a lot of people go on to respond positively.

Pratt and Wilkinson (2001) found in their study of 24 individuals with dementia that some people could remember few concrete details about receiving their diagnosis but recalled initially feeling shocked, angry and depressed. At the same time, many individuals felt that the diagnosis had validated their experience of cognitive difficulties and had provided positive opportunities for personal growth.

Realising it is not the end

I was diagnosed with Alzheimer's disease about five years ago in my mid-50s. Being diagnosed with dementia is brutal. It is horrendous. Only someone who has been through it can understand. You are given a mental death sentence.

I felt the doctor left me in that frame of mind and left me to pick up the pieces of my life. Someone needs to give you hope, and tell you that you won't be a burden. You have to realise that this is not the end. You walk away and nothing's changed but everything is different.

(Ken Howard, Young Dementia UK, n.d.)

Reflection

- What can be done to support people receiving a diagnosis of dementia to remain positive, in control and well connected to their community?
- What is important within a professional practice to ensure that people feel positive about managing their dementia and their future?

Responding to the diagnosis of dementia

It may be wrongly assumed that the person who has received the diagnosis is no longer able to make decisions for themselves or participate in their usual everyday activities, including attending the clubs and organisations that have been a big part of their life. Those close to the person can start making decisions on their behalf and doing everything for them. This may be due to concerns about their ability to carry on doing things for themselves and their safety. However, this level of caring can result in a negative outcome. The person would lose their involvement in their regular activities and the opportunity to maintain their skills and abilities. This poses the risk of them becoming detached from those around them and losing their confidence to do things for themselves. This situation can lead to dependency on others developing at an early stage in the dementia journey.

It is important for the person with dementia to:

- continue to do all the things that they are capable of;
- participate in the activities they are interested in;
- maintain the relationships that are important to them;

- have the opportunity to express their concerns and talk these through;
- make plans for the future that are positive.

In the early stages of the dementia journey, it is essential to have a focus on what the person can do and what they want to do. Making time to discuss what good care and support would look like during the early stages of the dementia journey is vital to ensure that any support and care planned and provided going into the future is personalised and in keeping with the person's wishes and preferences. These discussions are better held at a time when the person can engage and those involved in the conversation can focus on the discussion to hear the person's voice, ideas and preferences. The person living with dementia should be, wherever possible, the lead in shaping their future and making decisions about the care and support they wish to receive. Others could be involved in the discussions at their discretion.

Advanced care planning

The Prime Minister's Challenge on Dementia 2020 stated that every person living with dementia in England should be able to agree with the following statement: '*I am confident my end life wishes will be respected. I can expect a good death*' (Department of Health, 2015, p 6). This aim for dementia end-of-life care is currently adopted globally, with initiatives in Europe, the USA and Australia.

One of the quality standards set by the National Institute for Health and Care Excellence highlights the importance of personalised care plans, which play a vital role in making the statement set out earlier a reality: '*People with dementia are given the opportunity to discuss advance care planning at diagnosis and at each health and social care review*' (National Institute of Health and Care Excellence (NICE), 2019, p 5).

Advanced care planning (ACP) is an approach to end-of-life care planning that supports the achievement of this aim and standard. An ACP is different from an advanced decision, living will or an advanced directive, all of which state the treatment a person would or would not want to receive no matter how sick they are. For the purposes of this chapter the term *advanced decision* will be used to represent these living wills and advance directive.

Advanced decision

> *An advanced decision (sometimes known as an advanced decision to refuse treatment, an ADRT or living will) is a decision the person makes now to refuse a specific type of treatment at some time in the future.*
>
> *It lets their family, carers and healthcare professionals know their wishes about refusing treatment if they are unable to make or communicate those decisions themselves.*
>
> (NHS, 2020)

An ACP is a record of the person's future preferences and decisions about their care and treatment, including the circumstances in which they want to refuse treatment. The completed plan can then be shared with those who are responsible for the person's care or treatment. It is best to complete the ACP at a time when the person is able to be fully involved and in control of the information added to their ACP and if possible soon after receiving a diagnosis.

In Chapter 6 we look at how the techniques and tools from person-centred planning can complement ACP.

Key lessons learnt

- The dementia journey is covered by three stages: early/mild, middle/moderate and late/severe, with symptoms associated with each stage. The dementia journey is experienced differently by each person living with dementia.
- Receiving a diagnosis can take a long time due to a number of different reasons; access to specialist diagnosis teams, the person recognising the signs of dementia to then seek a diagnosis.
- There are standard assessment tools and approaches for diagnosis.
- Good, practical and emotional support at the time of diagnosis is of high importance.
- ACP is a method to capture a person's wishes for their future care and support.

Questions to aid reflection

1) If you are to be actively involved in the support or care of a person with dementia, what would you want to know, or need to know, about them to make sure that the approach you offered was thoughtful and personalised?
2) If you had invested time in getting to know a person, how they communicated and their preferences for the future, how would you share this with other people to make sure this knowledge and insight was not lost along the dementia journey?
3) When supporting a person to plan for the immediate or distant future, how would you ensure they were fully informed about all the options available to them and aware of the level of choice and control they have?

4 Great support in the later stages of dementia

This chapter covers:

- **The carers' perspective and rights**
- **Carers' eligibility for support**
- **Finding the right support**
- **Advocacy**
- **Beyond service-based respite, what taking a break looks like**
- **The dementia journey, the mid and late stages in the context of the individual's experience**
- **Summary table – the dementia journey and personalisation.**

Continued support at home

A person living with dementia may wish to remain in the family home. With careful planning and consideration for everyone involved, including other family members, the right support can be put in place to make this possible. This could come from immediate family, friends, members of the community, community groups, paid-for support and professionals. While living within a family setting, the person with dementia may already be receiving support from family members. Initially, this may not be obvious, covering a whole range of practical, physical and emotional support, which may include:

- checking that the person has everything they need with them before they leave the house;
- changing the environment so the person can remember where they have put their items;

- making sure the person is not in danger of hurting themselves – for instance spatial awareness may have declined and support may be needed to manage the stairs;
- helping to address physical needs, for example, getting dressed;
- assisting with preparing and eating meals;
- ensuring everything has been left safely, for instance locking the door or switching the gas off;
- encouraging and supporting the person to take part in everyday activities.

It does not have to be the family members living in the same home who provide the support; other members of the family, friends and neighbours may provide worthwhile support too, such as:

- occasional social visits;
- telephone chats;
- help with shopping;
- arranging and attending appointments.

Each person with dementia will be living in their own unique situation; their family arrangements, the number of friends they have, how frequently they see them and how well they are connected to the local area they live in will all differ. Therefore, the access they have to support within their family and social networks will vary greatly. Equally, the circumstances of those providing care and support within the family home will also fluctuate greatly. The factors that create these differences include:

- the relationships that exist among family members;
- the physical environment, the home and the surrounding area;
- existing caring arrangements, for example, children, grandchildren, and other elderly relatives;
- work commitments;
- the caregivers' own health conditions.

It is important that professional involvement is sensitive to potential issues within families when working alongside people with dementia. Invest time and energy into developing a good knowledge of the circumstances, a biography of the family and an appreciation of the varying perspectives of each family member. Each family member is likely to have their own unique perspective on the circumstances and insights regarding what support and care they want to provide and what they are able to do for the person. Gathering the information and developing a detailed understanding is one step to ensuring the support and care provided is *personalised* and suitable for the person with dementia and the whole family.

It is important to appreciate that, although the terminology *personalisation* could lead to the assumption that it requires a focus on the person with dementia and getting it right for the individual, in practice it is important to have a much wider perspective that considers the person and the people around them.

Family and friends

It can be challenging for those close to the person to accept the person's diagnosis. Supporting a family to come to terms with it and the changes they can see happening while also encouraging them to recognise and appreciate all the things that the person can continue to do, as well as their skills, past times, interests, knowledge of subjects and passion.

The person living with dementia, with support from friends and family, can begin to document details about their life. This can help inform future decisions and how future care is provided. Chapter 6 provides guidance on how to record information and what type of information is useful.

When in discussion, remember to keep communication positive. Focus the conversation on what is possible. Think about what arrangements and approaches would make sense for everyone and talk about what people would like to do. Positive communication can be challenging as people can find the change of circumstances difficult to come to terms with, so make time for people to share how they are feeling. It may be difficult for them to express themselves, and their emotions may prevent them from thinking or acting rationally. Recognise this, and, when the conversation takes a turn to focusing on a negative, give the time necessary for people to voice their thoughts and then try to bring the topic of the conversation back onto the positive.

If the people you are speaking to are focusing on a negative or their emotions are preventing them from thinking or acting rationally, you could help them by trying to be sensitive to what the person may be feeling by:

- helping them to pinpoint what feelings they are experiencing and showing empathy, while letting them know what support is available;
- looking out for non-verbal signs of emotion;
- recognising the emotions they are feeling and not rushing off this onto the next subject and making time for expression;
- avoiding telling someone that they don't need to feel upset or concerned; this could lead to the person feeling ignored or misunderstood;
- creating the space and the time for the person to process the conversation and the questions raised and for them to be able to form a response;

Recognising carers

Carers' organisations are recognising the increase in the number of people who are caring for a family member, with 10% of carers caring for a person with dementia (Carers UK, 2019, p 8). It is important to recognise the support carers need too: someone to listen to them and provide advice and time to relax, continue to pursue careers, relationships and interests and meet other responsibilities. There are a number of carers' organisations across the UK already providing invaluable support.

The Care Act 2014 has improved carers' rights and the likelihood of carers receiving support from the local authority. More information about carers' support from the local authority is available later in this chapter.

The stresses of caring

Family members and carers can find looking after a family member with dementia worthwhile and fulfilling yet stressful. There are difficulties that family carers commonly experience in the early stages of dementia, which include their relative with dementia:

- leaving the house and becoming disoriented;
- becoming lost when they are accompanied shopping or visiting public places;
- having restless and sleepless nights;
- having repetitive behaviour, for instance continually asking the same question.

The boundaries of the relationship can also change significantly; for instance providing personal care to a relative can change the relationship dynamics.

These difficulties and increased responsibilities as a result of caring lead family carers to dedicate much more time to their relative. Over time the caring role can become consuming, and it can place restrictions on the caregiver's life, preventing them from:

- having some time for themselves;
- maintaining other relationships;
- being able to take care of other responsibilities;
- maintaining work commitment;
- following interests and hobbies;
- being able to exercise and take care of their own health.

The family member providing the care may reach a stage where they need to assess the demands in their life and prioritise them. This may result in reaching the conclusion that they will need to give up other commitments, such as work, hobbies, friendships or spending time with other family members. If they feel they are no longer able to maintain work commitments, either having to reduce their hours or give up their working role completely, this will impact their income and therefore the finances of the whole family.

It needs to be recognised that providing care to a loved one is often something people find themselves doing, not through choice, but through circumstances. When supporting a relative with dementia to plan for the future, the wants and needs of those providing care need to be taken into consideration too.

It cannot and should not be assumed that a family member is prepared or able to provide the care and support their relative needs on an ongoing basis. It needs to be recognised that providing care over long term can lead to the family member struggling with their own health, identity and sense of wellbeing and this must be prevented.

In the Carers UK, 'Caring & family finances inquiry – UK report (full report)' (UK report 2014a, p 44), it was highlighted that almost one in three (30 percent) of carers had seen a drop of £20,000 or more a year in their household income due to caring. This illustrates that the pressure of providing care to a loved one is not only physical and emotional but also financial.

In an annual report produced by Carers UK titled 'The state of caring 2013' (2013, p 4), it was stated that: '*Two in five (42%) carers felt they had missed out on financial support as a result of not getting the right information and advice early enough*'. This presents a further issue for those providing care within the family home as, without the necessary support and guidance, carers will not access the support that is available to them.

'The state of caring report 2014' (Carers UK, 2014b, p 9) highlighted that 75 percent of carers found it hard to maintain relationships and social networks because other people do not understand the impact that caring has. Therefore, many carers may gradually begin to feel isolated and lonely, which, in turn, has a negative impact on their wellbeing.

Supporting the carer

A husband, wife, son or daughter may be providing the care and support a loved one needs; they will be responding to the changing circumstances of the person with dementia. They are likely to be fulfilling their role to the best of their abilities and as much as the circumstances will allow. Being aware of their rights and the support available to them requires a family to have some background knowledge of health and social care, and quite often people are living in difficult circumstances, unaware that there is help available to them.

The caring responsibilities can grow over time, as the condition of the person being cared for progresses. This means that those providing care do not immediately recognise they have become a *carer* or that support may be available for them. When carers do access support, they enter into a complex system with new terminology to learn and it is only at this stage that they may be referred to, or labelled, as a *carer*. This can understandably cause mixed reactions and feelings.

Reflection

- At what stage does someone become a *carer*?
- What do you think is the most useful form of support for carers?
- How do you think a professional offering health and social care support should approach discussing any areas of sensitivity in the most respectful way?
- If you were providing care to someone but felt no longer able to maintain this caregiving due to the impact it was having on your own health and wellbeing, what steps could you take? What questions would you need professionals to answer?

Capturing memories

Capturing memories, important moments, events and occasions can be valuable for people with dementia. If someone enjoys reminiscing and having the opportunity to do this, it is worth spending time bringing memories together in the form of photographs, stories, keepsakes and videos.

Technology, for instance iPads and tablets, can be a good way to develop a memory/reminiscence aid.

Some people find it useful to put together a memory box, where they can store all the items to look at when they want to. There are tools and resources available on the internet that are useful ways to store photos, stories and videos, and you can search to see what is available. Within the collection of memories, include information about important dates/special occasions to encourage the person to remember and celebrate these.

The middle stages of dementia

As dementia progresses, the person with dementia will become more physically and emotionally dependent. They need more support to ensure good physical care, such as a good diet and adequate fluids, and may need help dressing and maintaining good personal hygiene. Some families will be willing and able to continue to provide this increased level of care, but this cannot be assumed or expected. For the person or people providing care, it can become tiring and stressful and will impact their quality of life and wellbeing to a greater degree.

A balance needs to be made between the level of care the family members want to and can provide and the provision of support from other sources, which could include other family members, people from the community or paid support.

There are many reasons why a family member may not be able to continue to provide the care and support required, some of which include:

- being physically unable to provide the care required;
- a decline in the family member's mental health, which could have been directly linked to the impact of providing the care/support required;
- the family member being at risk of losing their job;
- the family member being unable to maintain relationships, putting them at risk of becoming isolated.

It is during the middle stages of dementia that further support from the Local Authorities Older People Team, Community Mental Health Team or Clinical Commissioning Group may be required. The online resource from NHS Choices titled 'Your guide to care and support' (2015) states: '*most local authorities will have a social care team devoted to older people. These teams can provide support that enables older people to remain living independently in their own home*'. There is therefore a focus on ensuring that people can remain within the family home and that the first form of support a person receives should start from this perspective.

If it does reach a stage after all avenues have been explored, for example, making adaptations within the home or paid support coming into the home, where it is not possible for the person to remain within their own home, the local authority's team for older people will guide people through the options available to them, for instance sheltered accommodation, extra care housing or care and nursing homes.

Carers' rights

The number of carers within the country far supersedes the number of people who are employed in the health and social care systems. The 2011 census figures for the UK showed an 11% rise in the number of carers since the 2001 census – increasing by over 620,000 to 6.5 million in just ten years and this number continues to rise (Carers UK, 2012, p 2).

This could be explained by the increase in the older population and the increased awareness of what it means to be a carer, leading to more people identifying themselves as a carer.

Every year over 2.1 million adults become carers, and almost as many people find that their caring responsibilities come to an end (Hirst, 2014, p 5). This *turnover* means that caring will touch the lives of the majority of the population as we all need or provide care or support to a family member at some stage, as the figures from Carers UK (2019, p 2) indicate: '*3 in 5 people will be carers at some point in their lives*'. The research illustrates why it is important to ensure that there is a good support network in place for those who find themselves providing care to a loved one.

An analysis of the 2011 census showed that 3.7 million people provide 1–19 hours of unpaid care per week, 775,000 people provide 20–49 hours of unpaid care per week and 1.4 million provide 50 hours or more unpaid care per week (Office for National Statistics, 2013). The figures gathered and presented by the 2011 census bring to the forefront how heavily dependent the health and social care systems are on those who provide care on an unpaid basis within people's own homes. If all carers were to state that they could no longer meet their caring responsibilities, there would be a huge issue around capacity and sustainability in the provision of health and social care. Carers deserve the support and recognition for the care they provide to loved ones, and professional interactions should be respectful and considerate.

Carers have rights too, and these are enshrined in law, covering England, Scotland and Wales. In England, the rights of family carers are identified in the 'Care Act 2014', which received Royal Assent on 14 May 2014. In Scotland, carers' rights are identified in the 'Carers (Scotland) Act 2016', which commenced in 2017–2018. In Wales, the 'Social Services and Well-Being (Wales) Act 2014' represents carers and their rights. As a result of these acts, local authorities have a duty to provide:

- support to carers based on the identified needs of the carer;
- relevant and timely information, advice and guidance;
- appropriate access to support for adult carers and young carers;
- access to advocacy.

The Care Act 2014 grants carers the right to request support; on this request the local authority has a duty to complete a carers assessment with the carer. Those who are assessed as eligible have the right to access support that is available or to request a personal budget. The intention of the support being provided to the carer is to meet their own support and care needs and to reduce the stress of providing care. Carers UK (2014c, p 1) stated how the Care Act 2014 strengthens the recognition and rights for carers in the social care system, and this includes the rights for carers to access support and services.

In England, anybody identified as a carer should be offered a Carer's Assessment. These are designed to capture the circumstances of the carer and areas of their life where support is needed, followed by a discussion regarding the support that would work well for them. The approach taken to complete it should follow the principles of personalisation; the carer should be central to the process, the Assessment should capture the carer's perspective and the carer should be fully aware that an Assessment of them is being undertaken with an explanation about what will happen after the Assessment is completed.

The carer can invite other people to be involved in the assessment, such as other family members and friends. Upon completion, the information gathered determines whether the carer is eligible for social care support and they have a right to a copy of their final Assessment.

Eligibility for carers in England

The Care Act 2014 removes the requirement for the carer to be providing substantial care on a regular basis. The only requirement is that the carer has a need for support, either now or in the future. The carer's eligibility threshold is based on identifying:

- whether a carer's needs are a consequence of providing necessary care for an adult;
- to what extent the carer's needs affect their ability to achieve specified outcomes, as covered later;
- to what extent their caring responsibilities are putting their health at risk;
- whether, and to what extent, the caring role they fulfil impacts on their wellbeing.

The eligibility decision is based on the carer's needs and should not reflect the needs of the person they care for, even if the person they care for is not eligible for social care support.

The eligibility of the carer is determined by the local authority, using a set of specific outcomes to establish entitlement. This set of specific outcomes is outlined in the Care Act 2014 Carers' Eligibility Social Care Institute of Excellence (SCIE) factsheet (Social Care Institute for Excellence (SCIE), n.d.), a link to which is provided in Bibliography at the end of the book. If these outcomes, such as the carer being unable to engage in work, training, education or volunteering, apply to the carer due to their caring role, they then become eligible for support.

If the person providing care is deemed as eligible for social care support, they would be able to make decisions about how they would like to be supported, through the services available, via a personal budget or a mixture of the two.

A carer can utilise the personal budget available to them to shape up the support in a manner that would work for them and they could use part of their personal budget alongside service provision. As an example, a carer may wish to engage with a local agency to provide support in the home while utilising a personal budget to cover the cost of attending a weekly activity. Before the support is put into practice, a Care and Support Plan would be completed which should cover the following areas.

- What the carer wishes to change and achieve.
- What support the carer wants to receive.
- How the budget available to the carer will be used.
- How the budget available to the carer will be managed.

Here are some examples of how a budget could be utilised.

- To employ someone to come and spend time with their family member so they can have a rest.
- To pay for someone to do household tasks.
- To pay for an item of equipment to reduce worry or concern, such as a non-intrusive monitor.

- To pay for something that helps them to relax, for example, a pond in the garden or yoga sessions.

Throughout the process of completing a carer's assessment and a care and support plan, a carer has the right to access and be supported by an advocate.

Advocacy

Mind (2018) states that advocacy '*means getting support from another person to help you express your views and wishes, and help you stand up for your rights*'. Advocacy Focus (2020) add to this by furthering the definition: advocacy is a process that supports people to:

- *Have their voice heard on issues that are important to them*
- *Protect and promote their rights*
- *Have their views and wishes genuinely considered when decisions are being made about their lives*
- *Express their views, thoughts and concerns*
- *Access information, advice and guidance*
- *Explore choices and options for services and care*

Meanwhile, Wells (2006) notes that there are many definitions and approaches towards advocacy. The National Development Team for Inclusion (Advonet, 2018) sees advocacy as:

taking action to support people to say what they want, secure their rights, pursue their interests and obtain services they need. Advocacy providers and Advocates work in partnership with the people they support and take their side, promoting social inclusion, equality and social justice.

Killeen (1996) alternatively highlights advocacy as a process of empowerment in which it

means making the case for someone or a group of people or helping them to represent their own views, usually to defend their rights or to promote their interests. The concept has a special relevance to people who are disadvantaged and as a consequence are less able to speak for themselves.

The definitions presented demonstrate that advocacy is underpinned by human rights, social justice and equality. Advocacy is a vehicle to achieve outcomes that align with the values of inclusion, self-determination and personalisation.

An advocate can provide valuable support for those who are feeling overwhelmed about their circumstances. Accessing health and social care support is a daunting and complex experience. It helps to be supported by a knowledgeable advocate who has a focus on reaching the best outcome for the person who can act as a guide through the health and social care processes. The input from an advocate can be reassuring, especially for people who feel that they have not been heard.

Involving an advocate can be valuable for people with dementia, whether they are living at home, in residential care, in a hospital or in a nursing home. The involvement of an advocate to support people with dementia and their carers can make a considerable difference and provide the much-needed support at certain crucial times of the person's life, for instance:

- when someone requires health care intervention;
- during Assessments and Care and Support Planning;
- during a Capacity Assessment or Best Interest meeting;
- when a person is moving, for example, from home to a supported living scheme or care home.

Advocacy is available in most local areas, and information about accessing advocacy should be shared with people with dementia and their carers as soon as the person has received a diagnosis.

Older People's Advocacy Alliance is the only UK-based national organisation supporting independent advocacy services for older people. Their website provides up-to-date information regarding advocacy and rights. International organisations also exist for advocacy, including Dementia Alliance International.

Where can support be found

Many people with dementia remain living in their own home, and they are likely to want to do so for as long as possible – to be in a familiar environment and surrounded by people who love them and who know them well. A number of factors will determine someone's ability to continue to live in their own home, including:

- if they live on their own or with other people;
- the ability, capacity and willingness of the people they live with to offer practical and emotional care and support;
- if the right level of paid or unpaid support can be offered from outside the family home to make it possible to remain living there;
- if the environment is suitable or can be adapted to be made more appropriate;
- if there are any significant risks identified regarding the person continuing to live at home and no practical way can be found to manage these risks.

To remain living at home the person will require care and support to varying degrees. The introduction of personalisation and personalised budgets means that they now have the freedom to create a support arrangement that would work best for them. This could include utilising the budget available to employ a support worker directly or to cover the cost of equipment to aid independence in the home (when this equipment is not available through the local occupational therapy team) or to purchase aids for communication which are not available through the local speech and language therapy team.

Respite

Respite, as a term, is not always used, and over recent years this has been replaced by terms such as short breaks. What respite and short breaks refer to is a source of funding or service that provides the opportunity for the person providing care to have a rest or a break from caring. Respite applies when people continue to live at home supported by a family member(s). In these circumstances the family member may need a break to take care of their own wellbeing, to rest and recuperate. Respite is designed to meet this need, where the person with dementia can continue to receive support and care while their carer has a break. It can be achieved in a manner that works well for the person and the carer. The length of respite support time should be determined by the carer, and a period for a break could range from a few hours to a fortnight away. Traditionally, respite has meant that the person with dementia has left the home for a period to stay somewhere, which is usually a local residential care home offering respite accommodation.

Families of people with dementia have often reported that respite, following this model, may provide rest and self-care for themselves but at the cost of safety and comfort for the person they care for. They may '*feel torn between the necessity to have a break and their anxiety about the impact of institutional respite care on the person with dementia*' (World Health Organization, WHO, 2012, p 8). This has often created further problems and stress for the carer rather than alleviating it.

The change of environment when receiving respite, getting accustomed to the layout of the respite provision, finding where things are and receiving care from strangers can be a frustrating and confusing experience for the person with dementia. In large and institutional respite settings, there is usually a high turnover of carers and different carers working each day. This level of constant change can be frightening and frustrating for a person with dementia. They may then find it challenging to adapt back into their familiar routine when they return home, especially if things have changed in the home environment while they have been away. This situation poses insurmountable difficulties for their family member(s) who are caring for them.

Carers and people with dementia often report that the anticipation of going into respite can lead to feelings of anxiety, confusion, guilt, disorientation, concern and frustration (Leocadie et al, 2018). Respite, when provided in this way, can be more exhausting for the carer than having no break at all. When a carer has reached a stage where they need a break, it may seem that the only option is for the person they care for to attend a respite service, even if this is not what the person or their family wants. A report by Bamford et al (2009, p 176) found: '*Data from the focus groups and interviews with people with dementia and carers suggested that a limited range of services was available locally, with people being "fitted" into available services*'.

A report conducted by the National Co-ordinating Centre for NHS Service Delivery and Organisation (NCCSDO) (Arksey et al, 2004) explored the different models of respite service delivery commonly found in the UK, North America and Europe. These included:

- day care services;
- home care services;
- host-family respite;
- institutional/overnight respite;
- respite programmes, offering multiple forms of respite care;
- multi-dimensional carer-support packages, where respite care is one option;
- video respite.

The report also provides a detailed insight into the benefits to carers and care recipients of each model.

When supporting a family in this situation it is important to recognise that traditional respite provision is not their only option. In line with the ethos of choice, control and flexibility embedded within personalisation, respite can happen in a way that makes more sense for the person and their family. As Bamford et al (2009, p 176) stated: '*Little information is available about the distribution of different types of respite care and short breaks nationally*', and there continues to be a focus on traditional forms of respite care and short breaks.

Approaches to respite

Day care

Day Care centres usually open each day of the working week, depending on the area, and tend to be open during the day time. They offer care, support and activities, and people find them a good option for a number of reasons.

- Offering a link between the person with dementia, their family and health and social care employees.
- Specialist support.
- A varied range of recreational activities, some of which will be in keeping with the person's interests and hobbies.

- A chance to meet new people and form new relationships for the person with dementia and their carer.

Day care is a planned provision that has become the main source of community-based support for people with dementia. *Day care* is a term that embraces a range of activities delivered outside the home in a number of different settings, including day centres, community centres, residential care and hospitals.

The measurement of value and benefits has usually been from the carer's perspective. Many carers place a high value on such services, perceiving benefits for both themselves and the person with dementia. There is also evidence to suggest that day care attendance might have a preventative effect on entry to long-term care (Arksey et al, 2004, p 4). So it could effectively support people to continue to live within the family home and prevent the need for residential care provision. This can support the person with dementia to continue to be around people they know well, reducing the level of confusion and frustration that can be experienced when in unfamiliar surroundings. It is worth noting that Arksey et al's report does state that the evidence is limited and at times contradictory.

Home care services

A care or support worker will come to the family home and spend time with the person with dementia while their carer has a break. The person with dementia does not have to leave the home and spend an extended period of time in a care setting, therefore reducing their potential level of anxiety and distress. Home care can be provided flexibly, whether this is for a few hours or a few days. This option also works well for people who are uncertain of service provision and feel more confident if they can be supported in their own home. In this situation the carer or support worker is most likely to be employed by a voluntary organisation, through a local home care agency or directly by the family (Levin et al, 1994).

Reports and evaluations have demonstrated that those in receipt of care, funded by the local older people's team, within the home often receive very few hours of care; '*Carers reported that they would have liked the service more often, and liked visits to last longer as the relatively short periods of respite constrained the type of activities they could undertake*' (Arksey et al, 2004, p 4).

Evidence collated from national and international published and grey literature about the effectiveness and cost-effectiveness of respite services for carers of people with dementia suggested that home care respite could assist in maintaining family routines and roles and the person with dementia's sense of self (Arksey et al, 2004, p 5).

Sitting service

An alternative to paid-for respite is a service usually called a *sitting service*. This is provided through a network of local volunteers who will come to the family home and spend a few hours with the person, while their main carer has the chance to have a break.

Shared lives schemes or host family respite

This respite option offers a greater level of personalised approach compared to traditional respite provision. In a shared lives or host family scheme, the person with dementia would stay with a specially trained carer in the carer's home. The person with dementia and the short break carer have the opportunity to build a positive relationship, and the environment remains consistent with the aim of providing a greater sense of stability. This provides peace of mind as the person with dementia is receiving the care and support they need as well as one-to-one interaction. '*Care recipients preferred a break in a homely environment to a stay in a residential home*' (Arksey et al, 2004, p 5).

Video respite

This approach was developed in the 1980s as a method to provide a short break. Introducing the idea of the video tape as a form of engagement for the person with dementia provided a break for the carer. This approach would now be via DVD or an online download. '*The tape was well received by carers and care recipients, and was used regularly to create respite time*' (Arksey et al, 2004, p 6).

The idea of utilising technology as a resource for people with dementia has progressed a great deal. Technology is used to support, entertain and inform. This proves especially useful when the person with dementia lives a greater distance away from their main carer. '*Used sensitively and thoughtfully, technology enhances rather than replaces human relationships and interactions* (Social Care Institute for Excellence, 2017).

Multi-dimensional carer

The term *multi-dimensional care* refers to interventions that consist of a set of support services. In addition to respite care, other services may be incorporated, for example, education about dementia-related issues, training in lifting and handling techniques, a support group for carers or accessing individual counselling. This is designed to address the multi-dimensional problems and needs that carers are likely to experience and provide practical community-based services. This approach gives carers a choice regarding what is included and whether this would be service or community-based. Carers believed they had benefited from this approach, and results of a research report conducted in 2004 suggested no gains in terms of psychological health of the person with dementia but positive effects on the person's behaviour (Arksey et al, 2004, p 6).

A personal budget to purchase respite

People who access a personal budget can make their own decisions about the care and support that they receive. This applies to respite too, although, with a personal budget; it may look very different from the traditional provision or any of the models presented earlier.

People can choose to use their personal budget to cover the cost of having a break in a way that would work best for them, while achieving the outcome of improved wellbeing and having a change from the usual routine of caring duties. The budget could be used to go to the coast for the day or for going out for the evening with a neighbour or a friend. Direct payments as a method to receive a personal budget and voucher schemes were welcomed as a way of increasing the flexibility of respite provision, and there was support for greater use of these options (Arksey et al, 2004, p 7).

The schemes were considered perfectly appropriate for people with dementia, as they themselves could articulate what they wanted in the early stages of the dementia journey and for as long as they could. At the stage in the person's dementia journey where their capacity has been reduced, the decisions about accessing respite provision should be based on the best interest basis informed by knowledge of them, which has been gathered through good records of previous choices and their likes and preferences. This information can be recorded in their person-centred plan, advanced care plan or, if power of attorney had been established, by the attorneys.

Carers may be offered vouchers rather than a service or a personal budget. Vouchers can then be utilised to choose from a range of options available. The principle with the vouchers is to offer more choice to the carer, although what is available could be more restrictive than via a personal budget managed as a direct payment (Think Local Act Personal, n.d.).

Vouchers can be exchanged for services, such as those offered by care agencies or residential homes. Often the services and support that can be accessed are those listed on the voucher, which may not be suitable, leading to the vouchers remaining not being used. A recipient might be able to use vouchers to pay for extra costs associated with their holiday, including live-in care workers or short-stay residential care (Able Magazine, n.d.). Vouchers are not offered everywhere.

Having a break does not always mean the carer and the person with dementia having to spend time apart. The opportunity to spend time together, away from the house, or visiting a place of interest or importance can be equally as beneficial and re-energising as having a break from one another. Personal budgets can be a positive way to pursue an interest or spend time together in this way. By having a personal budget to cover the cost of having a break, it is possible for the carer and the person with dementia to be free to spend their time together how they please.

Coping mechanisms for carers

It is important to recognise approaches to coping with the caring role and what helps to reduce the level of stress experienced. Research has shown that a reduction in expectation appears to help carers manage their situation, while having time to watch TV and read helped the proportion of carers involved in the study to relax and manage any distress (Saad et al, 1995, p 496).

Carers will employ different coping styles; for example, some may adopt a problem-solving approach to address difficult situations that arise associated with caring, while others might rely on emotion-focused styles that enable them to feel less stressed by situations.

However, many carers may not have developed effective coping skills. The provision of guidance to develop these mechanisms needs to be considered as part of the support carers are offered. Groups that may be able to offer some assistance in these areas include carers support groups and dementia support groups.

Later stages of dementia – moving on from home

In the later stages of dementia, the person is likely to experience:

- memory loss;
- loss of communication skills;
- loss of movement;
- eating and weight loss;
- problems with continence.

Memory loss

Memory loss is often very severe in the later stages of dementia. The person may still appreciate and respond to stimuli such as music, scent and touch, and this stimulus may trigger related memories. The person with dementia may:

- find it difficult to remember the people who are closest to them;
- struggle to navigate around environments that were previously familiar to them;
- have flashes of clarity for short periods of time;
- be reliving previous life experiences and be looking for people or things that have not been a part of their life for a long time.

When the person is reliving moments from their past, it is important to make use of these times to support the person to reminisce and step back into that time with them to provide reassurance.

Loss of communication skills

The person with dementia is likely to find it difficult to communicate with others. It is important that they continue to experience a warm, respectful and reassuring connection with those around them. The communication will move from responding to words and clear signs of communication to conveying thoughts in different ways, such as visible cues, body language, expressions and gestures.

Movement

The ability to walk will gradually decline, and performing everyday tasks unaided will become challenging. The person may begin to shuffle, walk unsteadily and seem slow. These are the first indications that their mobility is declining. Bumping into things, dropping objects or falling are common and may be more severe in people who have had a stroke or arthritis. Input from a physiotherapist and occupational therapist is important at this stage.

Eating and weight loss

Towards the later stages of dementia, people are likely to lose weight. This can lead to a reduced ability for the immune system to function effectively, as well as an increased likelihood of falls. It is important to support the person's nutrition and diet and seek advice on choosing and preparing nutritious food, maintaining hydration and how to offer physical assistance with eating. The person may find it difficult to swallow due to the deterioration of muscles and reflexes. This can lead to choking, which, in turn, can lead to chest infections. At this stage the GP can make a referral for a speech and language therapist or nutritional specialist who can assess the person's diet and identify what is going to work well for them, signposting them to specialist diets or equipment.

Problems with continence

During the later stages many people lose control over their continence. This is not inevitable, but there are many reasons why it may be experienced.

- Severe constipation.
- Not remembering to go to the toilet.
- Side effects of medication.
- Urinary tract infections.
- Not recognising the physical indicators that they need to go to the toilet.

The GP can make a referral to a community nurse or a continence specialist, who can provide advice on personal care and the equipment and products available.

It is in the later stages of dementia that it becomes important to draw on what has been learnt in the earlier stages of the dementia journey about the person's wishes and preferences.

End of life

Problems with capacity and communication, at the later stages of dementia, mean that it would be difficult for the person to make their wishes and preferences known.

It is at this stage where the information gathered in any future planning documents, completed in the earlier stages of the dementia journey, would help guide those involved in the person's life. This includes information gathered on person-centred plans, advanced decisions and advanced care plans.

These plans can capture the following information.

- Where would the person want to be?
- Who would they want to have with them?
- What treatment would they receive?
- What kind of environment would they want to be in?

Understanding and respecting the individual's wishes and preferences is as important for them as it is for those around them. Loved ones and carers can experience a sense of ease during an emotionally challenging time if they know what to provide and how to provide their care and support.

This is a difficult time, emotionally and physically, for everyone involved. To be able to approach and experience the end of life in a manner that upholds respect for one another and the dignity of the person, while creating an environment that brings people together and provides comfort, is of the greatest importance.

The dementia and personalisation journey

The different stages of the dementia journey are summarised in this table:

Dementia journey	Personalisation journey
Before diagnosis – 1–3 years	Beginning to recognise changes in the person; these will either be recognised by the person themselves or by those around them.
Getting diagnosed – 1–2 years	Making the appointment to see the GP. Visiting professionals for advice and guidance. Going through the assessment process. Seeking further guidance and information from organisations that support people with dementia.

(Continued)

(*Continued*)

Dementia journey	Personalisation journey
After diagnosis – early days	Accepting and being supportive of the emotional reactions that everyone involved can experience. Emphasising the need for a positive approach and to think about the future and utilising the approaches from person-centred planning and practice. Beginning to have the conversations that are needed to ensure good future care and support. Capturing the information in a way that can be shared with others and referred to at a later date.
Middle stages	The person will experience some changes in what they are able to do for themselves, and the people around them will be able to see these changes. Ensuring that the person's environment is still a positive one that supports the person's wellbeing. Continuing to capture the information about how the person wants to be cared for and supported. Considering the development of an Advanced Care Plan. Thinking about setting up a power of attorney. Beginning to recognise when the person has become eligible for health and social care support and pursuing this if it is wanted.
Later stages	The person will need a significant amount of care and support. Implementing everything that has been learnt in the prior conversations and planning. Ensuring that the care and support a person receives is respectful and responsive, taking into consideration everything that can be understood about the person's preferences, choices and communication.
End of life	Being there for the person and ensuring that their end of life was one that they wished for. Recognising the signs of the end of life and being able to respond in a way that eases any anxiety and confusion. Being able to go through this time with a person who results in a feeling that everything was done in the right way for them.

Key lessons learnt

- Carers have rights and may also be eligible for support. The importance of recognising the contribution made by carers has been addressed, as has the need to provide appropriate and timely support, including emotional support and access to information and advice. It cannot be assumed that carers are prepared or able to continue to provide the care required.

- Respite is a provision that provides support to carers, enabling them to have a rest and a break from caring. Respite has evolved, and there are now a range of options to access respite including creative and personalised approaches.
- The Care Act 2014 defines the eligibility for carers support and access to a personal budget with the option for people who are carers to lead on their own assessment.
- People have a right to access independent advocacy, and this should be available in all local areas.

Questions to aid reflection

1) People with dementia are equal citizens with rights. Advocacy can support people to have a voice and to have their rights protected. In which laws are these rights enshrined, and how do these apply to people with dementia?
2) How can it be recognised when a person who is a family member or a friend of a person with dementia has become their carer? How can this person be supported in a way that makes sense to them, and where they have choice and control over how they receive this support?
3) What do carers have the right to be aware of, and what do they have the right to access?

5 The shape of care and support

This chapter covers:

- **The settings available for the provision of care at the later stages of dementia**
- **Legislation and eligibility for health and social care support**
- **Personal budgets and personal health budgets**
- **Personalisation in care settings and services for people with dementia.**

Settings for care at the later stages of dementia and end of life care

There could be a range of settings where the person is living during the later stages of dementia, such as:

- in their own home, with or without family;
- on their own in a house/flat or bungalow that is part of a residential complex;
- in a specially designed village for people with dementia;
- in a room, as part of a supported living scheme;
- in a room within a residential care home;
- in a room in a nursing home;
- temporarily on hospital wards, offering acute provision of care, which is neither intended for nor appropriate for people with dementia.

Care and support in a hospital setting

During emergency or crisis situations, people living with dementia can find themselves admitted to units on hospital wards when they are not able to gain appropriate alternative accommodation. A report by Public Health England published in March 2015 (p 1) shared the key message that there has been a '*48% increase in emergency admissions involving people identified as having dementia since 2008/09*'. There were a total of 292,200 emergency admissions in 2012–13 where a reference to dementia was recorded and 83 per cent of these were through accident and emergency departments (Public Health England, 2015, p 2). In February 2020, the proportion of patients aged 75 and over who were initially identified or given the case finding of potentially having dementia and who were admitted as an emergency for more than 72 hours was still worryingly high at 81.7 per cent, rising from 81.5 per cent in the previous month (NHS England, 2020, p 2).

Being in a hospital for a person with dementia, or preparing for a hospital visit, can be frightening and disorientating. The hospital environment can be difficult to navigate; it can be loud and very busy. To make the stay at hospital as stress free as possible for the person with dementia, their carer, family and friends, it is important that the hospital staff get to know the person and their needs. Sharing information with the hospital staff can help them get to know the person, for instance, providing information about:

- approaches to communication that work well, which can be recorded on a communication chart;
- details about the decisions the person will make, which can be recorded on a decision-making table;
- information about the important people in a person's life, which can be recorded on a circle of support;
- detail about the person and what people like and admire about them, which can be recorded on an 'All about Me' profile;
- understanding about the person's important day-to-day routines, which can be recording using good day and bad day.

The above charts, tools and profiles will be explained further in Chapter 6.

The Alzheimer's Society (2017b) produced a leaflet called 'This Is Me' which can be used to record useful information about the person with dementia which in turn helps the hospital staff to understand them as an individual. This includes:

- the name by which they wish to be known;
- brief details of their normal routines, including whether they need reminders or support with washing, dressing, going to the toilet, eating and drinking or taking medication;
- details about food they particularly like or dislike, or any difficulties they have eating;

- facts about illness or pain that may bother them;
- details about any cultural or religious needs;
- knowledge about sleeping patterns;
- whether they like to be active or inactive, for example, if they walk about, and what can calm them when they are agitated;
- whether they have an advance decision or a personal welfare lasting power of attorney.

Residential care and support

Personalisation promotes the idea that people with dementia should have control and choice and that they should be supported to make those choices a reality.

This includes the choice of where to live, or whether to remain within familiar surroundings in the family home and within their local community. There are times when other factors play a part in influencing this, for instance, the onset of other health issues, changes in family dynamics, a reduction in the support and care available from family and friends or the physical environment posing difficulties. In these circumstances, the person with dementia may have to reconsider their choices to find the next best option.

The options available may include sheltered accommodation, supported living or residential care. The decision should not be rushed and all options need to be considered, with the necessary support from family, friends, advocates and attorneys, as appropriate and following the best interest principles if the person is assessed as not having the capacity to make this decision. Those involved in such conversations should refer to any past discussions and information that has been recorded while the person had capacity.

Being prepared for the eventuality of moving to a residential home earlier on in the

dementia journey and having discussions, as early as possible, about a person's preferences can help to inform any decisions that need to be made at a later stage.

The discussions need to have a focus on the future and what the person's preferences and wishes would be when they reach the later stages of the dementia journey. These discussions can be strengthened, and will feel more purposeful, if the person is aware of the range of options available to them and that their decisions are recorded for future reference.

The public perception of residential care

High-profile media coverage of abuse within care home settings, such as the Panorama programmes on the 'Undercover Care: The Abused Exposed' (BBC, 2011) and 'Nursing Homes Undercover' (BBC, 2016) scandals, drew attention to the neglect and abuse of disabled people and older people, respectively. This is likely to have contributed to a change in public perception of care homes; a poll of 2050 people by think tank Demos (2014, p 26) revealed that:

- more people associated a care home with a place of abuse rather than a place of safety;
- only one in four people said they would consider moving into a care home if they became frail in older age.

In addition to the Demos think tank findings above, a YouGov survey (2013) commissioned by the Alzheimer's Society demonstrated that 70 per cent of people fear going into a care home. The serious and devastating insights into abuse within residential settings have prompted closer inspection of the quality of provision and the following areas of weakness have been identified.

- Hospitals and care homes are organised through regimes and routines that often take precedence over the wishes of individual residents.
- There is a lack of understanding regarding dementia among the team working within residential settings.
- The arrangements regarding sharing information are not adequate.
- In the worst cases, the practice of the provision of care is not adequate or person centred. People with dementia experience being treated like objects and find themselves moved about without any discussion or agreement.
- The safeguarding and whistleblowing measures lack influence in practice. In extreme cases, people find themselves emotionally and physically abused.
- There is very little time, if any, for the staff working within the care home to have quality time with the people living there.
- Basic needs are the main consideration and, even if these are met, there is very little consideration for how the people want these needs to be met or for any other need a person may have.

A report conducted by the Care Quality Commission (CQC) in 2014, titled 'Cracks in the Pathway', stated:

> *In 29% of care homes and 56% of hospitals we visited, we found aspects of variable or poor practice where assessments were not comprehensive in identifying all of a person's care needs.*
>
> (p 16)

and

> *In 34% of care homes and 42% of hospitals we found aspects of variable or poor care regarding how the care met people's physical and mental health and emotional and social needs.*
>
> (p 6)

These findings will add to people's concerns about admittance to a residential care home or hospital. The CQC has made a commitment to improve the experience of receiving care in these settings. As a result of this report, the CQC is aiming to:

- appoint a new national specialist adviser for dementia care;
- train inspectors across all inspecting teams to understand what good dementia care looks like so that their judgements of the performance of care providers are consistent and robust;
- include a separate section in hospital inspection reports that shows how well the hospital cares for people with dementia.

In addition to this, the questionnaire results for a survey report 'Home from Home' carried out for the Alzheimer's Society in 2007 found that:

> *of twelve nursing homes using Dementia Care Mapping to understand the quality of care over the six-hour daytime period of observation, people spent more than 69 minutes (19.2%) asleep, but less than 29 minutes (7.7%) talking (or communicating in other ways) with staff or other residents, outside care tasks. In addition, this latter figure is skewed by a small proportion of residents with higher levels of social interaction.*
>
> (Alzheimer's Society, 2007, pp 16–7)

The average resident spent less than two minutes engaged in social interaction. In the same survey, 54% of people said their relatives living within the care home setting did not have enough to do during the day. Comments included: '*I found my Father's files full of trite observations, minute detail of his bad language etc, but never found staff sitting with him or holding his hand*' (Alzheimer's Society, 2007, p 16). Previous studies produced similar findings (Hancock et al, 2006).

Interestingly though, within the same study, carers did provide positive responses regarding the level of interaction provided:

> *We have recent experience of an event tailored to engage us and my brother-in-law and another resident. We all walked to the local pub in the company of the Activities Organiser. Three hours invested in two residents! Excellent.*
>
> (Alzheimer's Society, 2007, p 17)

Clearly the above findings demonstrate that residential care settings vary in their quality of provision. The national drive for improvements within care home settings should have now made a difference within these settings. If the care home is managed well, the opportunity for the residents to get involved in activities they enjoy and to have meaningful time with others is more likely to occur. If the home has a person-centred approach, the skills, interests and passions of the residents will be taken into consideration.

So, what are the positives of care homes that are worthy of recognition? The CQC report also found some good examples of quality person-centred care; for example, Professor Gillian Leng stated:

> *As the report makes clear, there are some examples of excellent care across hospitals and care homes in England. These are services that recognise that a Personalised approach is the key to high-quality care for people with dementia. They know that care must be delivered by knowledgeable and skilled staff who have time for the individual needs of the person with dementia. They make sure that comprehensive assessments are carried out, updated and then shared when someone moves between services. Where we find services like this we find an open and transparent culture, focused on the needs of individuals, willing to look for innovative and creative solutions, seeking out good practice to adopt and constantly keeping its own performance under review. We want all services to be like this, but sadly we know that is not always the case.*
>
> (CQC, 2014, pp 3–4)

The following statements given by professionals and people with dementia and their families demonstrate examples of good person-centred practice within a care home setting:

> *We saw that the trust had made efforts to increase the profile of people with dementia and improve their care by encouraging involvement of non-medical staff, relatives and volunteers from the local community. They visited patients on wards during mealtimes to help people to eat their meals and have a 'chat'. Open visiting times had also been introduced and this enabled more flexible and enhanced contact for people with dementia.*
>
> (CQC, 2014, p 25)

> *Mum now has an appointed carer who liaises with all the carers who were on duty, her care plan is clearly updated [and] we have a 'go to' person. There are lots of activities and the home is run as a 'family', the carers are her family and mum's wellbeing and dignity is maintained. She is nurtured.*
>
> *(CQC, 2014, p 33)*

These examples of person-centred practice demonstrate that good-quality care and support can be achieved within a care home setting. To achieve this high standard, good leadership is required, which creates a culture based on well communicated and clearly understood values. The examples given show how important good communication is along with an environment that is welcoming to families, friends and members of the community. These approaches help the care home setting to become an active and integrated part of the community rather than an isolated building with isolated activities.

Here are some further considerations regarding residential care settings:

- The provision within a care home setting is externally inspected and regulated by the CQC and this should have been strengthened further since the intention is to train all inspectors in dementia.
- According to regulation 18 of the Health and Social Care Act 2008 (Regulated Activities) Regulations 2014, the staff within a residential setting must receive the

support, training, professional development, supervision and appraisals that are necessary for them to carry out their role and responsibilities CQC (2015, p 74).

- Medication is prescribed by a GP and dispensed by a pharmacist who is involved in the residential care practice and should be administered and managed by trained and competent staff.
- Specialist clinical input can be provided from physiotherapists, speech and language therapists, occupational therapists and dental hygienists.
- Since the publication of the CQC 'Cracks in the Pathway' report (2014), it is recognised that residential care settings should provide a choice of nutritious, appetising meals that meet the needs and choices of individuals and support with eating where needed (CQC, 2017); the Nursing Times (2017) produced a resource that also has a focus on eating and nutritional care in practice and this resource also highlights the importance of routine regarding mealtimes and the opportunities regarding social connections at meal times.
- The person should be able to make their room into an environment that they are happy with.
- There are no concerns regarding utility bills and upkeep as this is all managed by the residential setting; these costs are incorporated into the overall residential fee, which can range significantly – some care homes do charge the residents for additional services and a report published by the Citizens Advice Bureau titled 'Hidden Charges in Care Homes' found that 40% of homes charge for the installation of a telephone and the phone calls made (Greenhalgh and Whitham, 2016, p 19).
- The person living in the care setting will have access to 24-hour care and support.

There are positives to receiving care within a residential setting and it is important to recognise that each care setting has its own strengths and style of care delivery.

It is important for the person with dementia and their family to have the opportunity to visit different places and to decide which home best suits them. The level of choice available to a person depends on the availability of rooms within the care home as in some areas demand is very high.

It must be taken into consideration that the negative press surrounding residential care homes, nursing homes and hospitals does not mean that these are the only areas of health and social care where issues occur and where it can go wrong; it can be equally as problematic within a day care setting, shared lives schemes and when someone employs their own people as a support and care team.

There is the potential for a positive or negative outcome from all the options available to a person with dementia and their family.

The following points are recommended to achieve a positive outcome:

- The person is actively involved and taking the lead in deciding where and how they want to be cared for and supported.
- Everything about the person is understood; how to communicate with them meaningfully, their interests, their background and biography, their culture and practices, important relationships in their life, how they follow day-to-day routines and their preferences on lifestyle choices. Understanding this detail is built into the way the person is supported and cared for.
- Everyone involved – those within the dementia care triad – continues to talk about how things are and address any areas of concern or areas that can be improved.
- The person with dementia and their carers/family know that if the care and support they receive is not working for them it can be discussed and changed.
- The person with dementia is treated with dignity and respect always, no matter where they are and who is providing the care and support.
- The people providing the care and support experience a good environment to work in with a culture that is supportive and encouraging; they are also given the opportunity to be trained in the areas that would make a difference to the people they provide care and support to and that they are given the support needed to fulfil their role well and confidently via team meetings and supervisions.

Personal budgets

In the previous chapter, the concept of personal budgets for carers was explored. In this chapter, they will be explored further in the context of the person with dementia.

Developments in the delivery of health and social care have seen a move towards providing more choice and control to those accessing the system, with a move away from a purely service-based provision to one that recognises the strengths and opportunities available through community-based options. In 2004, Duffy (2004, pp 7–13) noted that families would like to have more power in the planning and delivery of services. As a way of providing the resources to achieve the care and support a person wants in their life, personal budgets and personal health budgets have been successful in helping people achieve greater control and choice.

Providing the opportunity for people to find their own solutions regarding the care and support they want and need, while also broadening the focus from services to options and solutions that reside in a person's community: This approach means that people can maintain the connections they have to people and places that are important to them within their local area.

People with dementia who are eligible for support from their local authority or clinical commissioning group (CCG) have had the opportunity to access a personal budget or a personal health budget for a number of years. In this time people have shared stories about how they have utilised their budget and the difference this approach has made to their quality of life.

> *We didn't want to consider Mum going into a home and agreed as a family that she had the right to stay in her own home. We visited Residential Care Homes and Nursing Homes on the advice of the Social Worker but found none we felt would be good enough. Equally I had past experience of managing homes and knew Mum would not get the 1:1 attention she needed in those environments. Use of local respite and homecare services also reconfirmed to us that 1:1 support would give Mum the quality of life she deserved.*
>
> (Leslie, 2016)

People have shared how accessing a personal budget or a personal health budget has enabled them to:

- maintain the relationships that are important to them;
- make choices about how they are supported;
- have a break in a way that works for them;
- live in their own home;
- continue to fulfil meaningful roles in the community;
- plan for a future that matches their aspirations and goals;
- pursue their interests.

Eligibility for health and social care

Understanding the eligibility criteria for health and social care is essential in assisting someone to access the support available to them.

Once eligibility has been determined, the exploration around the person's preferences regarding how they utilise the support available can begin; including the option to access a personal budget or personal health budget to set up their care and support in their own unique way.

Eligibility for social care

At the time of writing, the Care Act 2014 states the eligibility threshold for people living in England. Under this Act local authorities in England now have a duty to make sure that people living in their areas receive: preventative services, the information and advice they need and the option of a range of provision of high-quality, appropriate services (Department of Health and Social Care, 2016a).

The aim of these duties is to ensure that people receive the support they require at the time they require it, moving away from lengthy processes that cause people to wait too long to receive the support they need. Prevention is the key message, working in a manner that avoids the need for people to access care home settings or hospitals by offering responsive and person-centred support.

In Scotland the national eligibility criteria for social care were agreed upon by the Scottish government and the Convention of Scottish Local Authorities (COSLA) in 2009, which were designed to be applied across the whole of adult social care in Scotland. Each local authority has their own eligibility criteria for managers and practitioners to refer to. As part of the development of the Scottish Self-Directed Support Strategy, concerns were raised regarding the fairness of the national distribution of resources when the emphasis was placed on localised processes and decision-making. The Scottish government's National Eligibility Framework employs a four-criterion approach, categorising risk as being critical, substantial, moderate or low:

- **Critical risk** – Indicates that there are major risks to a person's health, well-being and independent living, which calls for immediate or imminent provision of social care services.
- **Substantial risk** – Indicates that there are significant risks to a person's health, well-being and independence, which calls for immediate or imminent provision of social care services.
- **Moderate risk** – Indicates some risks to a person's health, well-being and independence, which calls for some provision of social care services.
- **Low risk** – Suggests that there may be issues surrounding quality of life, but these are low risk to the person's health, well-being and independence, which may require limited provision from social care services, possibly alongside alternative support or advice.

The approach to measure eligibility in Scotland mirrors the approach that was in place in England prior to the introduction of the Care Act 2014, also called Fair Access to Care. A threshold approach sets a definition between one threshold to the next, which would, in turn, determine the level of support the person being assessed would receive. In practice, it can prove challenging to 'fit' people into these thresholds as people's lives are so uniquely different from one another and are not often consistent from week to week or month to month.

In Wales, the eligibility to access social care is determined by the statutory document 'The Care and Support (Eligibility) (Wales) Regulations 2015'. This document states that an adult would meet the eligibility criteria if the need arises from the adult's physical or mental ill health, age, disability, dependence on alcohol or drugs or if the need relates to one or more of the following:

- ability to carry out self-care or domestic routines;
- ability to communicate;

- protection from abuse or neglect;
- involvement in work, education, learning or in leisure activities;
- maintenance or development of family or other significant personal relationships;
- development and maintenance of social relationships and involvement in the community;
- fulfilment of caring responsibilities for a child.

The eligibility for social care support is determined in the instance where the need is such that the adult is not able to meet that requirement, either alone, with the care and support of others who are willing to provide that care and support or with the assistance of services in the community to which the adult has access.

There are similarities between the eligibility criteria stated in the Care Act 2014, which applies in England, and those of the Welsh eligibility criteria. This approach is not dependent on a threshold, as is the case in Scotland, but instead relies on gathering information and making a decision about a person's overall situation, which takes into account wider considerations other than the person's health.

In Northern Ireland, the eligibility for social care is defined by the Department of Health, Social Services and Public Safety. The system in Northern Ireland is similar to that in Scotland, where the eligibility criteria are determined in each local area for managers and practitioners from that area to refer to. This is based on a national eligibility model based on the four thresholds of low, moderate, substantial and critical.

Well-being principle

The Care Act 2014 establishes the 'well-being principle' – an overarching approach that local authorities should take when exercising their responsibilities under the Act.

Well-being covers a range of outcomes such as:

- physical well-being;
- mental well-being;
- emotional well-being;
- participation in work, education and training;
- social and economic well-being.

(Care Act 2014. s.1(2) (b)(e)(f))

Local authorities must ensure that all aspects of well-being are taken into account when supporting a person through assessment and care and support planning. To establish whether a person is eligible for social care support, firstly a referral would need to be made to the social work team under the appropriate local authority, which could be the:

- older people's team;
- mental health team;
- generic/neighbourhood team.

Most local authority areas now have a single point of access to request an assessment and the team would refer this to the appropriate internal team to complete an assessment. The referral could be received directly from the person with dementia, somebody on their behalf or from another professional such as a general practitioner.

The Care Act 2014 gives local authorities a duty to carry out a Care Act Assessment for all people presenting a need for care and support. The assessment process would determine whether an adult is eligible for care and support. The assessment should be carried out regardless of the person's financial position and any initial opinion the local authority has regarding the person's level of need (Department of Health and Social Care, 2016b). The assessment process must address the outcome areas, as identified below, and the completion of the assessment must fully involve the person, while utilising appropriate communication skills.

The Care Act calls for strengths- and assets-based approaches to assessment, which aims to capture the skills and capabilities of the person, as well as the people and places that are important to them.

Assets – In this context, assets are the relationships the person has and their connections within the local community, which could lead to finding ways the person wishes to be supported.

Strengths – Here, strengths refer to the skills and knowledge the person has and how the person would like to make use of these within their life and ongoing support.

This approach recognises the individual as a person with a history, talents, skills and important relationships, rather than purely defining a person by their diagnosis of dementia. The approach also acknowledges the outcomes that would work for the person as well as the areas in their life that currently pose a challenge to them.

The Care Act 2014 stipulates that people can complete their assessment, either on their own or with their family and friends, with support as they require from a local authority-based, appropriately trained assessor:

> *If the person agrees and has capacity, they may also carry out a self-assessment, where the person takes the lead in identifying their needs and outcomes. The local authority will still be involved to help support the process, and to be satisfied that the person has identified all of their needs, but the person can take more control.*
>
> (Department of Health and Social Care, 2016b)

This provides the opportunity for the person to decide what needs to be recorded on their assessment and the flexibility to complete this at a time and pace that works best for them, involving the people of their choice to complete the information as accurately as possible providing the level of detail necessary to capture their circumstances.

People are not always aware that they have the option available to them to fill in their own assessment, consequently, the assessment process can still be experienced as a professional-led exercise. Those working within local authority settings can often be pushed to capacity and therefore the time needed to complete an assessment thoroughly and at a pace that works best for the person is not available, resulting in the information collected being gathered at a time that may not be best for the person and the resulting information being sparse and inaccurate. On the other hand, those accessing social care for the first time can find it reassuring to have support and guidance from a professional through the assessment process.

Assessments can be challenging to complete as a person's abilities can change and fluctuate each day. One day a person with dementia may be completely confident in their home and feel able to make lunch and go about day-to-day activities and the very next day they may feel disoriented and confused. It is important that an assessment captures this, the person's recent history and how their day-to-day experiences fluctuate. Where the level of an adult's need fluctuates, the local authority must take into account the adult's circumstances over a period of time to accurately establish the adult's level of need.

After completion of the assessment, the local authority will determine whether the individual has *eligible needs*. Under the Care Act 2014, a person is eligible for social care support if the following are true for them.

- They have needs due to a physical or mental impairment or illness.
- Those needs mean that they are unable to achieve two or more specified outcomes (which are detailed below).
- As a consequence, there is, or is likely to be, a significant impact on their well-being.

The Care and Support (Eligibility Criteria) Regulations 2015. s.2(1)(a-c).

The *specified outcomes* are:

- managing and maintaining nutrition

  (The assessment should consider whether the adult has access to food and drink to maintain nutrition, and that the adult is able to purchase, store, prepare and consume the food and drink safely.)

- maintaining personal hygiene

(The assessment should take into account the adult's ability to manage their own hygiene themselves, maintain hygienic standards and routines and launder their clothes.)

- managing toilet needs

  (The assessment should consider the adult's ability to access and use a toilet and manage their toilet needs consistently, hygienically and safely.)

- being appropriately clothed

  (The assessment should review the adult's ability to dress themselves and to be appropriately dressed, for instance, in relation to the weather and to maintain their dignity.)

- being able to make use of the home safely

  (The assessment should examine the adult's ability to move around the home safely, which could, for example, include using the stairs, kitchen facilities or accessing the bathroom. This also includes the immediate environment around the home such as access to the property, for instance, steps leading up to the home.)

- maintaining a habitable home environment

  (The assessment should consider whether the adult is able to maintain a clean and safe home. A habitable home is safe, clean and has the essential amenities, such as water, electricity and gas.)

- developing and maintaining family or other personal relationships

  (The assessment should observe whether the adult is lonely or isolated, either because their needs prevent them from maintaining the personal relationships they have or because their circumstances prevent them from developing new relationships.)

- accessing and engaging in work, training, education or volunteering

  (The assessment should consider whether the adult has an opportunity to involve themselves and contribute to society through work, training, education or volunteering on a basis of their interests and the opportunity being meaningful to the person. This includes considering the physical access to any facility and support the person needs in order to participate in the work training, education or volunteering of their choice.)

- making use of necessary facilities or services in the local community, including public transport and recreational facilities or services

  (The assessment should take into account the adult's ability to get around in the community safely and consider their ability to use such facilities as public transport, shops or recreational facilities.)

- carrying out any caring responsibilities the adult has for a child

  (The assessment should consider any parenting or other caring responsibilities the person has. The adult may, for example, be a step-parent with caring responsibilities for their spouse's children.)

An adult is to be regarded as being *unable to achieve* an outcome if the adult:

- is *unable* to achieve it without assistance or

  (This includes situations where an adult would be unable to do so even when assistance is provided. It also includes where the adult may need prompting, for example, the person may be physically able to wash but they need reminding to do so.)

- can achieve it without assistance *but doing so*:

  – causes them significant pain, distress or anxiety

  (For example, an older person with dementia may be able to prepare a meal, but may become confused with where items are kept in the kitchen which leads to anxiety and distress.)

  – endangers or is likely to endanger health or safety or

  (If the health or safety of the adult or another member of the family, including any child, could be endangered when an adult attempts to complete a task or an activity without relevant support. For instance, if the person is likely to leave the gas on after making some food.)

  – takes significantly longer than would normally be expected

  (For example, an adult with a physical disability is able to dress themselves in the morning, but it takes them a long time to do this, leaves them exhausted and prevents them from achieving other outcomes.)

If the management of the above outcomes are a concern for the individual and they cannot achieve two or more of these, then they would be deemed as being eligible for social care support.

The Care Act also provides local authority discretion to meet needs that are not covered under the eligibility definition stated above. This would be in circumstances where the person is at risk or support would be preventative to a person's circumstances or condition worsening. The decision to provide support in these circumstances is at the discretion of the local authority if sufficient evidence and details are provided to support the decision.

Once a person's eligibility for social care support is established, a social worker is assigned to work with them and their family. The social worker's involvement will have a focus on ensuring the person is supported and cared for in a manner that meets the outcomes required, as set out in the person's assessment. The care and support plan is written at this stage. During the development of this plan, the person with dementia, with support from any other person they would like to have involved, will be actively deciding how they would like to be cared for and supported. Information published by the Department of Health and Social Care in 2016(c) stated that the local authority must do everything it reasonably can to reach an agreement with the person as to how their needs should be met.

As part of the care and support planning process, the local authority will inform the person with dementia how much budget is available to them to meet their social care needs. This will be calculated based on the information provided in the person's assessment and set at an amount that the local authority believes will meet the identified needs of the person. This should be equivalent to the cost of any service-based option, that is, day centre or home care support, that would have been offered through a traditional approach to social care provision. At this stage, the level of budget communicated to the person is known as the indicative budget, an indication of the budget the person will receive. The indicative budget provides a guide for the person and their family when developing the care and support plan; this supports the development of the plan in these ways:

- exploration of the options available to the person;
- the opportunity to make the best use of the resources available to them;
- consideration about what is possible rather than just what is available.

The plan can then be written demonstrating how the budget will be utilised. The person may also wish to consider all the resources available to them such as friendships, relationships, clubs they are involved in, funding and grants available to them and eligibility for welfare assistance, as part of their care and support plan.

It is important to have a focus on meeting the outcomes the person is wishing to achieve as it may be possible that some of these outcomes can be met in ways that do not require the use of the budget; for instance, a friend may be happy to help the person go shopping, or a neighbour may be happy to support the person with their garden.

The person is entitled to a copy of their assessment and their care and support plan. Having access to a copy of the completed assessment will prove useful when completing the care and support plan as reference can be made to how the person's outcomes and needs, as identified in the assessment, are going to be met.

Recognising the frustrations people may experience

When people access their local authority for support and care, their experience can feel frustrating and out of their control.

- They may have to wait for a social worker to be available to complete an assessment with them, without being informed of their option to work on an assessment themselves.

- When the assessment process starts with a social worker's involvement, there may be limited time available to complete the assessment.
- The person with dementia and their family may not be aware of the options available or have the opportunity to explore which option would work best for them due to the lack of time the social worker has available for them.
- If there hasn't been the opportunity to explore the options available, the care and support plan may not be based on the best option to meet the outcomes the person needs or wants.

If this is the experience for the person, all parties of the dementia care triad (introduced in Chapter 1) should communicate to remind everyone involved that the focus should be on the person and the outcomes that would work best, making sure the process from referral to a completed care and support plan, and the implementation of care and support, is managed in a timely manner and fully engages the person with dementia.

Crisis

People may only access services when they have reached a point of crisis. At this stage, the local authority may need to respond rapidly to meet the immediate need and to avoid any risk, or further risk, of harm to the person or those around them.

This results in accessing the services with immediate capacity. The social worker involved would have completed an assessment, although it may not have been possible to fully involve the person, or their family, in this process due to their circumstances.

Once the support and care is put in place, and the immediate risk has been mitigated, it would then be possible to start to plan in a meaningful way with the person. This plan should lead to a review of how the person is being cared for and supported. The immediate arrangement put in place at the point of crisis may not be the best long-term solution.

Financial assessment

Access to social care support is means tested; once a person's eligibility has been determined this would be followed up with a financial assessment. This would be carried out by the financial team within the local authority and they would determine the person's position to make financial contributions towards the cost of their care and support.

The financial assessment should take into consideration all aspects of the person's finances. A person's assets, which include income, savings, property and pension, would be calculated as part of this process. The person's expenses would also be calculated and this would include any disability-related expenditure (an expense the person has as a direct result of their disability).

What is the difference between a personal budget and a personal health budget

A personal budget comes from social care and is available to meet assessed social care needs and outcomes.

A personal health budget comes from the clinical commissioning group and is available to meet identified health care needs.

Health funding and personal health budgets

The 2010 whitepaper 'Equity and Excellence – Liberating the NHS' outlined new initiatives to improve outcomes and to transform NHS culture by increasing choice and control through the offer of personal health budgets to those eligible for Continuing Healthcare and to encourage the integration of health and social care services (Department of Health, 2010). The guidance on the legal rights to have a personal health budget highlighted that, from October 2014, people have had the right to ask for a personal health budget as an alternative to receiving service provision (NHS England and NHS Improvement, 2019, p 4).

Due to successful outcomes achieved via personal health budgets, the NHS is now rolling out this approach and offering personal health budgets to people with long-term health conditions, learning disabilities or people with mental health conditions. This is relevant for people with dementia as people with long-term health conditions that require a consistent level of health intervention and care may be eligible for Continuing Healthcare funding. To access this, a referral to the local clinical team is required for an assessment of eligibility. The referral needs to be sent to the clinical team by the person's GP or social worker.

Checklist tool

For most people, the first step to establishing whether a person would be eligible is to have an assessment with a health or social care professional using a screening tool called the checklist tool. This helps health and social care professionals figure out whether the person's care needs may be of a level or type that indicates that they may be eligible for NHS Continuing Healthcare. If this screening suggests that they may be eligible for NHS Continuing Healthcare, the person's local CCG will write to them to confirm that they will be referred for a full assessment for NHS Continuing Healthcare, which is called a decision support tool (DST).

Decisions support tool

In this assessment, information will be gathered regarding the person's circumstances and diagnosed conditions. The person should be fully involved in the assessment and decision-making process. Their views about their needs for care and support should be taken into account. If they feel that they need help to explain their views, they may want to involve an advocate or ask a friend or relative for support.

The full assessment will be carried out by a multidisciplinary team made up of a minimum of two different health or care professionals who are already involved in the person's care. The involvement from professionals helps build an overall picture of their needs. In some cases, more detailed specialist assessments may be required from these professionals.

The DST is used to assess whether the person's main or primary care needs relate to their health, by looking at the following areas of care need, referred to as the 12 domains:

- behaviour;
- cognition (understanding);
- communication;
- psychological/emotional needs;
- mobility (ability to move around);
- nutrition (food and drink);
- continence;
- skin (including wounds and ulcers);
- breathing;
- symptom control through drug therapies and medication;
- altered states of consciousness;
- other significant needs.

Once the assessment is completed, the multidisciplinary team will make a recommendation to the CCG about the person's eligibility for NHS Continuing Healthcare. For individuals who need an urgent package of care because their condition is deteriorating rapidly, the fast track tool may be used instead. This enables the CCG to arrange for care to be provided as quickly as possible.

Care and support planning

When a person has been identified as being eligible for either health or social care support through the assessment process, they would then go on to develop a care and support plan. This is aspirational and focused on what the person would like to happen now and in the future.

Before starting to write it, the person would know the level of budget available to them, that is, the indicative budget.

The person taking the lead

The Care Act and the Right to Ask scheme state that the person must be at least involved in developing their plan, and they must take the lead where appropriate and possible for them to do so. local authorities must also provide an independent advocate to help the person take part in the planning process, if that person would otherwise have substantial difficulty in doing so. Where it has been determined that the person lacks the capacity, through the appropriate capacity assessment process as highlighted in Chapter 5, any person who is interested in the adult's welfare should be involved in the development of the care and support plan, while involving the person directly in the most appropriate way.

A care and support plan should provide information about the following:

- Who the person is and what is important to them – It should be clear within the wording of the plan that it has been developed with the person as the main focus. The plan should be written in a way that represents the individual, their personality and character. The reader of the plan should be able to get a real sense of who the person is.
- What the person would like to change and achieve – This provides an exploration of the aspirations the person has in regard to that they would like to achieve, this could include maintaining aspects of their life as it is now, or achieving a goal or making changes in their life where the current arrangement is not working well for them.
- How the person wants to be supported and cared for – All the ideas about what good care and support would look like should be presented in the plan. This is where the ideas of what is possible should be represented. Ideas should be written down about what would work well for the person and where this support would come from. When developing the plan, the range of options regarding good care and support can be explored. With the details of the exploration and the conclusion of the best option presented in the plan. Care and support could be found from a range of options including technology, equipment, care and support agencies, employing a personal assistant (PA), activities and community association, within the person's informal community and the support from their family and friends.
- How the budget will be utilised – This section should clearly outline how the person is going to utilise the budget available to them. This can include all the resources available to the person. The costs should be represented as yearly amounts and weekly amounts for ongoing costs, such as support or activity fees. Any costs that are one off, such as purchasing equipment or the cost of training, should also be recognised under a section titled one off costs. If the person has identified a way of being supported that has no cost attached to it, this should also be represented here with a nil amount attached to it.
- How their support and care will be managed – If the person has chosen an agency to provide all the support they require then one would expect the agency to provide some of the ongoing management of the team they employ. If the

person is going to utilise the budget they have available to them to commission the service, then how is the person, or the family, going to have some involvement in managing this? Would it be possible to have regular meetings with the agency to discuss progress, and to be involved in the selection of the team members? If the person has decided to employ their own PAs, what needs to be put in place to manage this arrangement, for instance, training, supervisions and meetings?

- How their budget will be managed – There are a range of options available which are described in Chapter 2. If the management option is stated on the care and support plan it means that steps needed to transfer the budget from the local authority can begin as soon as the care and support plan is agreed, reducing any potential delay in setting up the support.
- Contingency plans to cover when things could go wrong – A contingency plan is important for a number of reasons, assuring the local authority or CCG that the person's assessed outcomes will continue to be met under these circumstances and that the person and their family have had a chance to think through how to manage this situation if it happens. For instance, if PAs are going to be employed would it be an idea to employ a few people so that back up support is available when needed or would a family member be happy to be available at these times?
- An action plan for how the care and support plan is going to be put into practice – this can help to reassure those signing off the plan that it can be put into practice. It is also helpful for everyone involved to have a sense of what they need to do once the plan is agreed on. This may include:
  - recruiting PAs or support workers;
  - liaising with the chosen agency;
  - organising the activities;
  - setting up the community-based arrangements.

The people involved in supporting the person to implement their plan could be varied and it does not have to be dependent on one person to oversee everything. For instance, the person may take the lead on certain parts of their plan, while the social worker, friends and family may help with other aspects. This would be agreed with the people involved at the time of writing the plan.

When developing the action plan, it is useful to consider people's strengths, skills and knowledge to help to decide who would be best to take on each task.

Care and support plan templates

CCGs and local authorities have a template document that is used as the care and support plan and this would be the final version that is submitted. However, it is important to remember that this is the person's plan and they should have the opportunity to develop it in whatever format suits them; this could be on big sheets of paper using colourful pens or it could be typed up on a computer. The important factor is to find a way of developing the plan so the person is able to be fully involved and has a sense of ownership over their own plan. The information that has been put together using this approach can be transferred onto the template document at a later date, once the person and their family feel that they have captured everything they have wanted to within that plan.

In 2014, National Voices, a coalition of health and social care charities, worked with a wide range of people who use services to develop a common understanding of what is meant by care and support planning. The guide they produced highlights a four-step approach:

Care and support planning guide

Prepare – getting ready for the care and support planning discussion.

This stage is about:

- thinking about what matters most to the person to whom the care and support plan belongs;
- getting any useful and important information before the discussion;
- taking time to think and talk to other people about the different choices the person has.

Discuss – talking with the care and support partner.

This stage is about:

- the person and their care and support partner working together;
- talking about staying well and living well;
- talking about what they are going to do;
- talking about what care and support the person might need from other people.

Document – writing down the main points from the discussion.

This stage is about:

- writing down all the main points that the person talked about with their care and support partner;
- making sure that the plan belongs to the person and is easy for them to understand and use.

Review – checking on how things are going.

This stage is about:

- seeing how the person is getting on;
- reviewing the plan with the care and support partner and making any changes.

Reflection

- How can the plan be developed and recorded in a way that makes sense to and is accessible to the person?
- What would 'good' look like for the person?
- Consider who would be the best people to involve?

Reviewing and monitoring

In the early stages of a support package, the CCG and local authority would want to ensure that everything is working well for the person, their outcomes are being met and the budget is being utilised well. Therefore, the first review would take place within the first three months and would consider

1. if the person's assessed needs and outcomes are met, whether they are receiving a good quality of support and if the arrangement is working well for the person;
2. if the budget is being utilised well and records are being kept.

At the first review, everyone involved will get the chance to share how they feel things are progressing. The focus will be on the person, their family and any other people involved in providing the care and support. If this review demonstrates that things are going well, the ongoing reviews will then take place on a regular basis, usually half-yearly or yearly depending on the circumstances.

The person and their family may also find it useful to find their own way of checking how things are going, arranging to get together with the specific focus on discussing what is working well for the person and if any areas need to be addressed. Sometimes these gatherings are given a name, such as a circle of support or a circle of friends. More information about circles of support can be found in Chapter 6.

How a budget can be used

A personal budget or personal health budget can bring a great deal of flexibility regarding how someone is supported and the person can use the budget as creatively as they wish. For instance, they may choose to use it on the following:

- the services of a care agency chosen by the individual;
- a PA (instead of a carer arranged by the local authority);
- visit to a community or social activity, such as going to a club, concert or sport event;
- an educational activity;
- an item of equipment to meet an outcome shown in the care and support plan;
- complementary therapies, such as aromatherapy or music therapy, to improve well-being;
- transport to visit family and friends or attend a leisure or educational activity;
- support to get to a café to meet friends, or to go to a place of worship;
- taking a break with a carer.

A budget cannot be used for expenses that would be deemed as everyday living costs, for example:

- food;
- rent;
- utility bills;
- toiletries.

A personal budget or personal health budget cannot be used:

- for any illegal or unlawful purpose;
- to buy services from a CCG which are delivered on the founding principles of the NHS, free at the point of delivery;
- to pay for anything that is not directly related to meeting an eligible social care need as set out in the assessment.

Key lessons learnt

- There are eligibility criteria for Adult Social Care and Continuing Healthcare, which outlines when a person would become eligible.
- When people become eligible for health and social care support, they do have the option of receiving a personal budget or a personal health budget.
- Residential care is one of the options for people with dementia and the strengths and weaknesses of this option have been explored in this chapter.

- To achieve a personalised approach to care and support, it is also important to have insight about the following:
  - the services and support available;
  - the rights of the person and what they are entitled to;
  - the range of people and professionals who will be involved and how to involve them;
  - the options available to a person and how to make decisions that can be honoured.

Questions to aid reflection

1. People with dementia are equal citizens with rights. Advocacy can support people to have a voice and to have their rights protected. In which laws are these rights enshrined and how do these apply to people with dementia?
2. If you are to be actively involved in the support or care of a person with dementia, what would you want to know, or need to know, about them to make sure that the approach you offered was thoughtful and personalised?
3. If you had invested time in getting to know a person, how they communicated and their preferences for the future, how would you share this with other people to make sure this knowledge and insight was not lost along the dementia journey?
4. When supporting a person to plan for the immediate or distant future, how would you ensure they were fully informed about all the options available to them and aware of the level of choice and control they have?

6 Skills for personalised support

This chapter covers:

- **A toolkit to develop skills and approaches to achieve personalised support in dementia care**
- **Enhancing positive interaction**
- **The promotion of respect and dignity**
- **Hearing the voices of people with dementia**
- **Person-centred approaches to gathering information**
- **Promoting creative thinking, self-determination and community connecting through person-centred planning.**

The skills presented in this chapter aim to encourage readers to advocate for and adopt an approach where the person with dementia is in the driving seat with regard to planning their life now and for the future. This chapter discusses the aspirations and dreams that people with dementia have for their future and the future of their loved ones (Green and Lakey, 2013).

People first

So far, this book has recognised people with dementia as *people first*. People who have their own unique expectations and wishes should be recognised and understood as a fundamental human right and a part of achieving personhood.

Although not used previously, the term *people first* shifts the focus of service or care interventions to recognise the individual, the person. This position requires an understanding of how dehumanising the experience of being diagnosed and then receiving health care intervention and prescribed services can be. Whether the dehumanisation is real, subconscious or perceived, the term *people first* encourages everyone to continue to relate to the person as an individual first with their own identity and preferences, and this should shape the defining characteristics over their disability or diagnosis.

Planning

The approach to planning introduced in this chapter achieves the goal of seeing people as *people first*.

Good planning has the person at the centre and at the heart of the conversation, and it includes the people who care most about that person. It is captured and recorded in a way that is meaningful to the person.

Good planning recognises and builds on the person's community, where a tapestry of meaningful connections can begin to emerge. This is sometimes referred to as the circle of support or circle of friends (which is explained later in this chapter).

Good planning goes beyond the framework of making decisions about the predetermined services and support available to the person to a much wider conversation about achieving a good life. A plan that is developed on these principles is a useful source of information for those who will provide care and support in the future, whether in a paid or unpaid capacity. It helps those providing care and support to do so in a person-centred, respectful and dignified way. Having the opportunity to plan ahead means that the person's voice is central to the delivery of care and support going into the future, helping to prevent errors, misunderstandings and even avert crisis.

The thoughtful, sensitive and sometimes intuitive use of the skills needed for planning leads to a well-connected and informed dementia care triad + 1 (as discussed in Chapter 1), consisting of the person, their family and friends, paid professionals and the community.

These planning approaches have been separated into three *skills boxes* below.

Skills box 1: skills that promote respect and dignity

Skills box 1 contains a range of basic skills initially outlined by Tom Kitwood (1997) in '12 Positive Interactions'. The aim is to prevent the objectification of people with dementia and to stop treatment and interactions that lead to the person feeling like an object. The intended outcome of adopting the 12 positive interactions is for people to feel valued and respected.

Celebration

Taking time to celebrate and recognise the things that are happening in a person's life that bring happiness, comfort and a sense of purpose. This requires mindfulness when spending time with the person and embracing a cheerful and conversational approach, which helps them recognise what is happening in their life and the good things that are taking place. It is about being observant of what creates a state of happiness, comfort and a sense of purpose within the person and about mindfully creating opportunities for these events.

Collaboration

A recognition that the purpose of the collaboration is to work together to achieve the best outcomes and life experience for the person with dementia and their family. The person with dementia is treated as an equal with a right to be heard, and their opinions are understood by those around them. Such an approach creates a balance in which family, paid-for carers and the person with dementia (the dementia care triad) are equal.

Creativity

Opportunities to get creative and to be engaged in activities that feed the creative spirit – finding creative opportunities that suit the person: singing, dancing, making something, painting, baking and many more. Involvement in something enjoyable is supportive of the person's well-being and their expression, and it can unlock creative thinking for other areas of their life.

Facilitation

To really know a person is to understand their subtle gestures and simple body language and to have the level of insight and knowledge to respond positively. Good facilitation to lead a good life day to day is to provide just enough support for the person to interact with others to complete conversations or to complete actions.

Giving/Accepting

Being ready and willing to give and accept gifts of good will or help from the person. The size of the gift or the level of goodwill given and received is of little importance.

It is the sharing of these moments that hold significance and create meaning and memories within relationships.

Creating closeness

Spending dedicated time with the person and, while with them, creating a safe space which is soothing and comforting for them. This could include considering the immediate environment: the music, the ambience, the temperature and what else is happening in that environment at the time.

Negotiation

The person will have a number of options available to them. Good support will work with a focus on the best outcome for the person and will fully involve the person in reaching the decision of what most suits them. This requires meaningful interaction and conversation based on listening and acting on the person's responses.

Playfulness

Based on the principle that everyone likes to have fun. People with dementia can play games, tell stories and interact in ways that they find enjoyable. This may be planned or spontaneous and is a great opportunity for self-expression.

Recognition

This means having an open and unprejudiced attitude and recognising people in an open and positive way. It is important to make sure we work with them from their point of view and the perspective of their life and the world around them. Any practice that places assumptions on what the person would want or any judgement on what they do actually want would go against this positive interaction.

Relaxation

A chance to stop or slow down for a period of time. This may refer to an activity or conversation. People may want to relax by themselves or alongside other people. The relaxation time is determined by the person and may involve listening to music together, watching birds or animals or just listening to the conversation of other people.

A physical sensation that a person feels when they have become so relaxed that they *float away*. This may be achieved by doing something soothing like having a warm soapy bath, having hands massaged or being in a multi-sensory room that stimulates the senses.

Timalation

This interaction emphasises finding what is pleasurable for the person. It could include engaging the person on their different sensory levels, such as providing different taste sensations during meals, smell sensations via aromatherapy or, where appropriate, kinaesthetic sensations via massage therapy. These types of interactions provide contact, reassurance and pleasure without placing any demands on the person. Engaging in sensory stimulation in this way can support the person to be or feel more present.

Validation

Involves being sensitive to when the person is experiencing heightened emotional states and demonstrating empathy at these times. This is observed by making each experience for the person with dementia a robust one, accepting and acknowledging their reality and the power of that experience to them on an emotional level.

> *It also involves developing a high degree of empathy for them and trying to understand the person's frame of reference, no matter how chaotic, paranoid or hallucinatory. For example, if the person with dementia is distressed about a person who is absent, acknowledge their distress and ask them about the person or what about this person is upsetting them.*
>
> (De Bellis et al, 2009, p 28)

Achieving the outcomes aimed for through the positive interactions set out by Kitwood (1997) would require those interacting with people with dementia to develop skills of interaction, planning, organising, communicating and sensitivity.

To support someone to celebrate would require an insight into what has been happening in that person's life, an understanding of how the person would like to celebrate and an ability to share this information with others to ensure that they can also join in the celebrations.

Collaboration would require people to have developed skills in communication and the art of connecting with others through the dementia care triad + 1 in a way that supports the importance of equal relationships between the person with dementia, the family and paid carers.

The achievement of facilitation could be supported if those involved utilised the communication map and decision-making table as given in Chapter 3.

Through his work on person-centred care, Kitwood encouraged those supporting and caring for people with dementia to develop an understanding of the effects of negative and positive interaction on the person. Studies have demonstrated that the person's quality of life and well-being increase significantly when person-centred support and care are provided (Matthews, Farrell and Blackmore, 1996; Burgener and Dickerson-Putman, 1999).

Skills box 2: skills that help people with dementia make choices

Skills box 2 contains skills that develop the understanding of a person's preferences, support them to make choices and help them to maintain control. They are underpinned by the values of inclusion, covered in Chapter 1, and have been developed through person-centred practices and approaches.

All About Me profile

An All About Me profile captures essential information about the person that anyone providing care and support would need to know. It is really useful to anyone who is new to providing care and support to the person, as it provides detailed and succinct information about the most important things to know and do. The All About Me profile helps people to provide a good level and good approach to their care or support, a foundation to build a positive relationship with the person and, over time, build a more detailed understanding.

An All About Me profile can be developed from a preformatted form with defined areas of information. A template can be found in Appendix 2.

Although this approach can prove useful as a guide to the type of information that should be gathered and shared, it can become a box-filling exercise, which loses the essence and purpose of developing a profile. It is important to maintain focus on creating a profile that records and shares the information that the person with dementia would like to share about themselves and what they see as the essential information that somebody new to caring and/or supporting them would need to know.

The profile should be short and concise, not more than two pages long, providing a real insight into the person that is easy to digest, understand and put into action. It could contain all or some of the following information.

- How the person likes to be addressed.
- The important parts of their daily routine.
- The non-negotiable aspect of their day-to-day life.
- What needs to happen for the person to be and feel safe.
- What creates a state of happiness within the person.
- What can cause upset for the person.
- What others like and admire about them.
- Their skills, interests and passions.
- The important people in their life.

When supporting someone to create a profile, remain mindful of the purpose, which is a short and concise introduction to the person. Support the person to choose carefully between what should appear in the profile and what information belongs elsewhere, perhaps in their support plan or ACP.

Focusing on the positives can significantly change the way the person experiences the care and support they receive. If their All About Me profile includes information about what to avoid or what upsets them this information can be used in a positive way to avoid these circumstances.

Doughnut Sort

The Doughnut Sort was designed by Charles Handy (2002) to support organisations to become good at achieving outcomes and organising their main resource, which, in the majority of cases, is the people that work within the organisation. Following it creates a clear sense of each person's role, responsibility and purpose within the organisation or the community of people who are working together to achieve a common goal.

The Doughnut Sort has been utilised within the context of community, health and social care as a way to identify and define the roles and core responsibilities of all the people involved in the care and support a person receives. This would include people from within the dementia care triad + 1.

As the Doughnut Sort creates clarity regarding the role and responsibilities, it can in turn help to improve the achievement of the desired outcomes and improve the effectiveness of the contributions people make to these outcomes. This approach can increase the sense of satisfaction and purposefulness people feel within the role they play for the person with dementia.

The doughnut provides a method to achieve a balance between what a person has to do within their role, the areas where they have scope to indulge in thinking and acting creatively and where their involvement would be valuable and, finally, the jobs and tasks where they need not have any involvement.

How to complete a Doughnut Sort:

Imagine, if you can, an American-style doughnut with jam in the middle:

1. The jam in the centre represents the tasks and responsibilities a person has to do within their job or role to fulfil it successfully. The tasks mentioned in the 'jam' of the doughnut would be a person's core responsibilities and what they are expected to do well. These are the areas where people may need to follow guidance and instruction to achieve a good outcome. The guidance and instruction may be provided by the person with dementia, their immediate family or professionals involved in the care of the person.
2. The jam is not the whole of the doughnut, and the surrounding doughy areas represent the opportunities people have to make a difference, be creative and go beyond the bounds of duty to live up to their full potential. This would include opportunities for people to use judgement and creativity and to try out new things to see what could work. These are areas where people can use their imagination

when working alongside the person with dementia to help find new ways of doing things that work well for the person.

3. Areas that are not people's responsibility are signified by the area outside the doughnut. This determines the responsibilities or tasks people should not be involved in as it is not their area of knowledge, skill or passion. Someone else who is better placed would have already agreed to take on these responsibilities.

Using the Doughnut Sort helps to build a better understanding of the roles people have to play and when they will be involved. It helps to build a stronger and connected network of people who are making sure, together, that all aspects of the support and care the person with dementia requires will be provided for. It can also provide clarity when there are a number of individuals and/or organisations involved.

Please see Appendix 2 for the 'Doughnut Sort' resource.

Relationship mapping

At the root of person-centred practices, there is an appreciation of the importance of relationships and connection. Spending time together to map out the relationships in a person's life helps everyone to recognise the important connection they have, the people with whom they have had long-standing and meaningful relationships. Finding ways to support those relationships can lead to a greater sense of well-being, now and into the future. Keeping relationships alive and maintaining and enriching these connections lead to a support network that is enduring and purposeful.

The people who form this relationship network also offer a wealth of knowledge and information about the person's life, which can be found through holding meaningful conversations, with questions that aid exploration, discovery and learning.

Conversations of this kind also lead to identifying potential solutions to meeting the outcomes the person, and the people around them, would like to achieve, including ways to set up and organise care and support in a way that makes sense to the person.

On the reverse side, not investing the time to understand the important and meaningful relationships in the person's life could lead to a greater sense of loneliness and isolation for the person, leading to negative effects on their health and well-being.

Please see Appendix 2 for the 'relationship map' resource.

Conversations help to identify the important people and the key relationships in a person's life. When conversations are focused on the person's life rather than the person's 'needs', a lot can be learnt about what really matters to them and what a good life looks like. Talking about interests, past achievements, celebrations and recent events and who shared these moments with the person can all provide insight.

The relationships we learn about will be current as well as people from their past. The relationship map may include:

- those who have an intimate relationship with the person, whom they have known over a long period of time or with whom they feel the most comfortable and the most understood;
- good friends; this includes those the person sees or contacts on a regular basis or has known for a long time – perhaps from their school days. These friends will be people they have built memories with or have a shared mutual interest;
- those they see and spend time with through association, for example, through sharing an interest, hobby, sport or faith group;
- those paid to be in the person's life, for instance their GP, nurse, optician, carer, support worker, personal assistant or cleaner, all of whom serve a vital role in maintaining the quality of life.

A completed relationship map can help to identify:

- the number of meaningful relationships the person has and the close network of support they have around them;
- who the person wants to have involved in planning, support, care and future decision-making;
- who would be good to have been involved in the context of representing a person's best interests, especially if the person has been assessed as not having the capacity for a particular decision (see more detail regarding capacity in Chapter 7);
- any issues that exist within the relationships a person has and what support is needed or wanted to resolve these;
- the friendships and relationships the person wishes to maintain, for which they may need support to maintain in the future;
- the people who have been identified on the relationship map whom the person would like to develop a closer relationship with; this may be someone who they see, or used to see, within a community setting whom they would like to build a friendship with based on their mutual interest;
- the people who would like to invite onto their circle of support (a circle of support is explained in greater detail later in this chapter);
- those who would be good to talk to and involve in gathering information and planning for the future.

Developing a relationship map can be a really empowering experience for the person with dementia as they see the number of people they have in their life. It is however important to be considerate as, for some people, this process can emphasise the lack of connections they have. This is especially true for someone who has already been isolated or segregated from their community and relationships as a result of the way care and support have been provided to them. In these circumstances a person may find themselves in a position where they have no close family, friends or connections with people in the community. For instance, if a person has moved away from their community to a care home setting, they may not have been able to maintain the connections that were important to them, especially if they have not been supported to do so.

A person who has led quite a solitary existence or has had no family of their own may have a limited number of connections within their relationship map. If developing a relationship map would highlight a person's lack of connections or connections that used to be much closer, these questions may be worth exploring.

- If the person wishes to, how can they regain the relationships they have lost and how can they be supported to do so?
- How can meaningful relationships be built from the people who are in the person's life right now?
- What opportunities are available to a person to develop friendships and connections?

It is important not to forget in the haste to support someone to achieve a better quality of life that it may be the person's preference to have limited connections and friendships; they may choose and prefer a solitary life. This can only be discovered through getting to know the person well.

Circles of support

Circles of support, sometimes called circles of friends, consist of a group of people who form a connection between themselves as an intention support network around the person who is the focus of the circle. Together the circle of support holds the purpose of supporting the person to achieve a good quality of life, reach their full potential and overcome the challenges they face along the way.

Mary A. Falvey, Marsha Forest, Jack Pearpoint and Richard L. Rosenberg co-wrote a book titled: *All My Life's a Circle Using the Tools: Circles, MAPS and PATHS* (2003), which explains how intentional circles of support function in a meaningful way.

In an article for Indiana University, Kim Davies (2005) stated that, from birth, people create an intricate network of relationships in their lives consisting of people who are there in times of trouble, sorrow and celebration. Davies goes on to suggest that these friendships are born from shared common threads that bind people to one another. It is these people who become part of a circle of support or a circle of friends as these are the people who are valued in a person's life and who offer support to achieve dreams or to provide help when needed. The relationships that develop into this level of meaning can be formed in many ways and from meeting people in different places and environments, which often occurs naturally and throughout life. In her article Davies wrote about:

- the **circle of intimacy** – the name of the person whom the circle belongs to would be written, along with a photograph of them, if wanted. Within this area of the inner circle, the names of the people who are most important to them are written down;
- the **circle of friendship** – would be where all the friends the person has would be recorded;
- the **circle of participation** – record all the people the individual knows through a shared interest, hobby or place where they spend time in this third circle. For instance, if the person goes to the gym, it may be the people they see there. These are the people where a close friendship has not been forged, but perhaps the potential is there for this to happen;
- the **circle of exchange** – all the people who are involved in the person's life in a paid capacity would be recorded in this fourth circle. This could include paid support workers, opticians and gym instructors.

Please see Appendix 2 for the 'circles of support' resource.

Negotiables and non-negotiables

Utilising this approach helps capture the 'negotiables and non-negotiables' within a person's life to identify what must be there for life to make sense to the person: what is essential and non-negotiable. The approach also captures what would be good to have in place if possible; although not absolutely essential, these areas are negotiable.

Developing an insight into what is negotiable or non-negotiable for the person provides the details required to inform those around the person, including those providing support or care, about what works well for the person and how to strive towards achieving a good quality of life.

This approach recognises that the small things really matter and make a difference in achieving a quality of life and happiness. Paying attention to the finer details of a person's daily experience and respecting the preferences they have can make the difference between a good day and great support and a bad day and support that does not fully recognise or respect the person.

To gather this information requires engagement in a conversation that enables the person with dementia to share what really matters to them – to hold conversations with the people who know and understand the person well. Listening intently and actively to what the person and people around them are sharing establishes an understanding of what has been learnt from the conversation. When the information has been gathered, it can be sorted under the headings of 'non-negotiable' and 'negotiable'.

If the person with dementia is not able to fully engage with a conversation, it is possible to achieve this insight through gaining information from the people who know the person well; this would include the people who would sit within the person's circle of intimacy and circle of friendship. It is still important to involve the person with dementia in the conversation wherever possible and to engage them in a meaningful way and recognise their contribution to the conversation through listening to and observing the person's reactions.

The information gathered as a result of the conversations should provide the details needed by those caring or supporting a person to be able to fulfil their roles well. For instance, if this approach was utilised as a way to understand the person's preferred morning routine, it could include asking and exploring the following questions.

- What makes a good start to the day?
- What is the person's preference around how they get ready for their day?
- What is missing at the moment that is important to the person?
- How could the person's experience be better than it is now?
- Is there anything about now that needs to be maintained into the future?

The attention to the smaller details can often be overlooked. Honouring simple everyday preferences makes a difference to how a person feels: their well-being, self-esteem and sense of security. The following story illustrates this point.

> *While on clinical placement on a general medical ward in my first year of training, I helped to care for an older patient, whom I will call William.*
>
> *The nursing staff had described William as confused and 'wondersome'. He seemed anxious and was touching his face constantly. Frequently, he could be found walking towards the bathroom in his dressing gown, so the nursing staff would help him back to his bed.*
>
> *My dementia training at university, along with my role as a 'dementia friends champion', led me to believe that William was not wandering without cause, and that there was something of interest to him in the bathroom.*
>
> *After talking to him, it became apparent that all he wanted was a shave. William was accustomed to shaving every Sunday but had not shaved in weeks. He had been wearing his dressing gown to go to the bathroom, which had a shaving brush and a safety razor in the pocket but had not yet managed to have a shave.*
>
> *William was not aware that he was able to shave, or that the staff could help him, so I found some shaving foam and walked with him to the bathroom. I helped him to foam his face, and then left him to have a shave, checking in on him regularly to make sure he was okay.*

> *Although William was with dementia, he was not at risk of falling or a danger to himself with the razor. He was clear on what his needs were, and I helped him to meet them. For the rest of the day William was calm and chatty, and there was no wandering or anxiety.*
>
> *This experience reaffirmed the importance of treating patients as individuals and supporting their choices so that they can be cared for with compassion, dignity and respect. I also have a better understanding of how my actions affect others and am committed to developing my nursing practice with the patient at the centre of all care decisions.*
>
> (Perez-Merino, 2014)

From this story it is clear that a 'non-negotiable' for William is to be able to have a shave on a Sunday morning. It would also be a 'non-negotiable' that William receives support in the bathroom to get set up and ready to have a shave. The 'negotiable' would be discovered through having further conversations with William or observing his responses to situations or options given to him. The 'negotiables' may include the brand of shaving foam he uses or the time when he has a shave on a Sunday morning.

Investing time and energy in conversations to learn about the person's preferences results in a greater level of understanding. The information gathered through these conversations can assist in the person being cared for and supported in a way that makes sense to them. Gaining this level of insight among the people supporting the person with dementia can help avoid misunderstanding, frustration and potential relationship breakdowns.

Please see Appendix 2 for the 'negotiables and non-negotiables' resource.

Working/not working

The working/not working conversation captures the aspects of a person's life that are:

- 'working' for them – where they are happy and satisfied. The areas that need to be maintained;
- 'not working' for them – the areas where they are frustrated and dissatisfied. The areas of the person's life that need to improve and a commitment is needed to address these areas.

When holding the conversations to gather the information to learn about what is working or not working, it may start with focusing on an area of the person's life, for instance: where the person is living or how they are being supported. The conversation can also have a wider holistic view of the person's life to achieve a big picture understanding.

Such conversations can also capture the perspective of those on the dementia care triad + 1. The unique perspective of each contribution to the conversation is valuable in creating a deeper understanding of what is happening in the person's life.

This information can be gathered as part of a planning meeting or through a series of separate conversations coordinated by one person who then does an initial sort of the information under the categories 'working' and 'not working' to be shared among those who have been involved. It is then for those who have contributed to share ideas and thoughts about how to:

- make sure the information has been sorted accurately;
- maintain the aspects of a person's life that is 'working' for them;
- move the elements of a person's life that is currently 'not working';
- resolve differing opinions; for example, the person may really enjoy the morning walk they have, the fresh air and the chance to see people, so this is working for them, but, likewise, the person's carer becomes anxious when the person is away from home for a long time so for them it is not working. This would then open a discussion to find a solution to the question 'how can the person be supported to continue their morning walks whilst reducing the anxiety of the person who is providing care?'

Addressing the areas that are not working in a person's life provides an opportunity to generate unique ideas and solutions. Often it is the creative and individualised ideas that suit the person and the people around them. Exploring all the options available, including those that are based within communities or are yet to be created, and identifying which ones would provide the best solution can be a good experience for those striving for a solution.

Here is an example: A person who is living at home and being supported by a support worker can no longer get out of bed independently, and they are offered additional home or domiciliary care so there are two people with them each morning. This provision is often the standard solution offered in these circumstances, yet there are other options that could be considered. Exploring this issue further and discussing the details of what the person is struggling with could lead to a different solution; for instance changing the height of the bed, investing in a rise and fall bed, setting the warmth of the room for when the person rises, having a chair positioned closer to the bed, the person making changes to their night time routine or their sleeping environment could be the key to maintaining their independence each morning.

Once some good solutions and ideas have been found that are worth investing time to make them happen, an action plan can be developed to identify how to put the ideas and solutions into practice. If these actions are successful and the ideas implemented improve the situation, the outcome is likely to improve the quality of life for the person with dementia and the other people who make up their dementia care triad + 1.

Please see Appendix 2 for the 'working' 'not working' resource.

Good days and bad days

Everyone experiences good days where they have enjoyed the company of others and what they have done. A good day is one in which a person looks forward to what it has to offer and feel like the flow and the activities have suited them and their pace of life. Equally, people can have bad days, where everything feels wrong, people do not understand one another, there is communication breakdown and frustration and sadness set in.

Developing an understanding of what a good day looks like and what a bad day looks like from the person's perspective can be achieved through purposeful conversation, observing their interactions and responses to what is happening around them and for them. Exploring and discovering the answers to the following questions helps to build a picture of a good day.

- What was enjoyable about the day?
- What were the person's interactions like with other people?
- Who was present?
- Where did the person find fun and laughter?
- When was the person engaged in a way that meant something to them?

Time spent together, watching, learning and holding conversations where the person is central and others are involved who know, understand and genuinely want the best of them. In this time recognising the details of what makes a 'good day' can help everyone to learn more about the person, what has purpose and meaning for them and what they enjoy. When this understanding has been developed, everyone can work together to take steps to incorporate the enjoyable aspects into more days.

Likewise, these conversations and time spent together can also recognise and observe the elements that make a 'bad day'.

- What causes frustration, and how does the person express this?
- Who was around at the time?
- How were people interacting with each other?
- What was happening, and how was the person involved?
- Which routines were followed?

Utilising what has been learnt together, which would include those in the dementia care triad + 1, enables everyone to recognise what changes need to be made to achieve better experiences for the person and for everyone around them, again creating an action plan to help identify how these changes are going to be made and by whom, with the intention to prevent bad days and move towards more good days. This understanding can help those providing care and support to know what needs to be present and what needs to be avoided in someone's life, while offering ideas that ensure a good or a better experience for the person with dementia on a daily basis.

Please see Appendix 2 for the 'good day bad day' resource.

Life stories

Personal history makes a person who they are today, and an awareness of a person's life before dementia and an understanding of them in their own biographical context is important to maintain individuality in the provision of person-centred care (Stokes, 2000). Kitwood and Bredin (1992, pp 269–87) also highlighted the importance of the role a person's life story plays in developing an understanding about them and as a means to promote personhood and well-being. People build a personal history as they go through their life, and these histories are a unique mixture of *'joys, pleasures, sadness and pain'* (Kitwood and Bredin, 1992, pp 269–87). If they lose their connection with their history, they also lose something of themselves. This is especially the case for people who are living with dementia as they may lose portions of their memory as their dementia journey progresses. People may find themselves trying to make sense of who they are, and it is within this context that a documented life story can prove to be valuable and a guide for those in the dementia care triad.

Life stories document a person's history and provide valuable insight into the person's identity: their experiences, relationships, how they have contributed to the community and society, their joys, sorrows and the person's current reality. This depth and detail of information can provide clear direction and clues when providing person-centred care and support. A person's life story provides other people with ideas and valuable information and can spark meaningful and worthwhile conversations. This includes talking about the person's achievements, their experiences and relationships. Life stories can also be a source of inspiration when exploring the activities available to the person with dementia, helping them to find things that they would enjoy and, in turn, enhance their quality of life and well-being.

Elements of the concept are demonstrated well in the documentary 'Alive inside', which explores how people with dementia respond to music, while capturing astounding reactions in people who have otherwise found it difficult to recollect past events, remember current events, interact with other people, move or speak or recognise loved ones. Learning about the music that has relevance to the person with dementia, through listening to their life story – which would include music from their childhood or from their own special occasions – then creating opportunities to listen to this music can ignite positive and enlivened reactions.

People involved in the documentary, especially those who worked within the nursing home setting, noticed that people with dementia responded better to the music they heard and that had meaning for them than to any other therapy or intervention, including pharmaceuticals. The documentary is inspirational and has brought hope, joy and meaning to many people. This demonstrates that people's life stories can be shared in many lively and engaging ways, such as music, videos and photographs.

Working with a person with dementia to capture their life history opens a window of appreciation and respect. It provides insight about those who have meant a great deal to them, those who are still part of their life and those who are no longer around. It can also reveal fond memories of the good times they have had and important occasions as well as any sadness they attach to memories of difficult and challenging times.

When supporting a person to capture their story, it is worth asking for different perspectives. Naturally, the person themselves is best placed to share their own story as they remember it, including the parts of the story that are most important to them. Other people with an insight into the person's history can also make valuable contributions and add detail.

This work can help those providing care and support to:

- maintain the relationships that mean a great deal to them;
- make it possible to take part in activities that have meaning for the person and are a source of enjoyment;
- make sure that what means a great deal to the person is available to them. This could include music, sounds, photos, gifts, smells, jewellery or anything that holds a memory;
- spend time together to reminisce and talk about the past;
- informs the people providing the support and care.

Appreciations

Developing appreciations identifies the qualities and characteristics that other people value and admire about the person. Appreciations help recognise the person's uniqueness and to acknowledge and appreciate their:

- gifts – the aspects of a person's personality and character that draw others to them, the things they remember about a person and what inspires people to spend more time with them;
- qualities – what others admire about a person, their achievements and uniqueness;
- talents – the things that the person shows an ability in, perhaps they have a natural talent?
- skills – that have been learnt, trained or educated in.

Appreciations enable people, and those around them, to recognise, and have recognised, their positive qualities. Creating a focus on these can shift the dynamic of any conversation and interaction to a space of positivity. It can be enlightening for the person, and those around them, to hear how they are regarded by significant others. They can be gathered individually from people in the person's life and then collated and shared. Alternatively, the start of a meeting can be dedicated to gathering appreciations from those attending.

A round of appreciations at the start of a meeting can form a positive opening, for any form of meeting, which is being held with a focus on the person with dementia. This is a facilitated process where each person present at the meeting is asked to share something positive about the person whom the meeting is for, something they like and admire about them. To record people's contributions, a piece of paper is placed on a wall or on a flip chart stand, with the person's name at the centre and the headings: 'gifts', 'qualities', 'talents' and 'skills' written around the person's name. The facilitator would then ask each person present to contribute something to be added to the poster.

This exercise does not take long to facilitate and helps to set the tone for the rest of the meeting or planning session, bringing a positive perspective for everyone involved, which encourages people to consider the rest of the content of the meeting from a positive perspective. This proves useful when encouraging aiming to find ideas and solutions. Appreciation can challenge people who have previously focused on the negative perspective of the person or their situation. It encourages people to develop a positive outlook, regarding what the person can do and what they do have to offer others.

Please see Appendix 2 for the 'appreciations' resource.

Matching staff profile

It is important that people are well supported and that those providing support in any capacity are a good match for the person being supported. Producing a matching staff profile identifies the skills, characteristics, shared interests and practicalities that would be good for any supporter or carer, paid or unpaid, to have in their offer to create a good match and relationship between them and the person with dementia.

Completing a matching staff profile encourages the person with dementia, and those around them, to think about what qualities they would like people who provide care and support to have. It is a good idea to complete one prior to recruiting care and support, whether this is via an agency, employing directly or via natural support in the community. The information gathered can help to find the right people and the creation of the advert, job description and the interview process.

Investing this time in creating such a profile can help to ensure that:

- the person has a good quality of life;
- the person enjoys spending time with those who are providing care or support;
- creating a long-lasting and enduring relationship between the person and those providing support or care as there is a good match in the relationship they have that goes beyond the action of care and support and into a realm of shared interests, passions and more meaningful connectedness;
- the care or support worker and the person with dementia enjoy spending time together.

The details needed to complete one can be gathered from conversations about what good care or support would look like. This would include a conversation about:

- what skills do the people providing care or support need to have? Do they need to be good at cooking particular meals and involving the person in the preparation; do they need to be confident in using health-related equipment in a way that maintains respect and dignity; do they need to have skills in communication and a creative approach to communication to support the development of a relationship with the person with dementia?
- what interests does the person with dementia have, and which of these interests would be good to have in common with the person who is providing care or support? Having a shared interest can help build relationships, and this is the same for the person with dementia and the people who are supporting or caring for them. Interests can be pursued together helping to develop the relationship further;
- what type of character and personality traits are needed when finding the right people to care and support. What is needed to increase the chances of the person with dementia getting on with them? Discussing and thinking about the people the person has around them now and their past relationships helps to identify what makes the difference between someone they enjoy spending time with and someone they do not. Are there certain characteristics that work well for the person; for example, does the person tend to get on better with someone who is softly spoken and calm, or do they get on better with someone who is bubbly and loud, or does this change depend on how the person feels?
- what practical requirements does the person have of their carers and supporters? It is important to consider if there are certain needs that must be met. This would include times of the day or days of the week that the person needs care or support; does the person need someone who can drive and who has access to a vehicle; do they need someone who can use computers or someone trained in specific areas such as communication?

Please see Appendix 2 for an example of 'matching staff profile'.

My Care and Support Profile

When people want or need care and support, it is good to be clear what areas of their life they want care and support with and how they would like this to be provided. Developing an understanding of this can help the carer or support worker to be informed and confident in their approach. The information that is gathered can be shared in the My Care and Support Profile, which captures the details of how a person wishes to be supported or cared for and the areas of a person's life that they wish to maintain themselves.

Please see Appendix 2 for the 'My Care and Support' resource.

Treasure chest

Developed by New Possibilities, a treasure chest brings people together to discover what opportunities and resources exist for the person within their network of friends and family. This approach opens up the idea that a person's quality of life can be improved through developing closer connections with people around them and the wider community. It captures information about skills, interests, passions and what people would love to learn and is usually gathered at a meeting with all the people present contributing to its development.

The treasure chest can be developed at any time; it is particularly useful when completed alongside a person-centred plan, when people feel ready to start addressing the question 'what needs to happen to make this plan a reality?' The commitment to the person and their person-centred plan is likely to have increased as their plan has developed and everyone involved may have found a new enthusiasm to help the person move towards achieving the aspirations set out in the plan. Following a person-centred plan with the treasure chest builds on this enthusiasm and commitment.

When developing a treasure chest, it helps to have a big sheet of paper divided into four sections with the following headings for each section.

- Useful people to know.
- Passions, interests and hobbies.
- Skills and knowledge.
- Something you have always wanted to learn.

Someone can then take the lead in asking people in the group questions to help complete each section of the paper. It is good for the person leading the meeting to have some useful examples to share to get the process started and to encourage others to contribute, for instance:

- useful people to know – 'I know a man who delivers free papers', 'I know someone who is great at woodwork' or 'I know a solicitor';
- passions, interests and hobbies – 'I am passionate about baking/dancing/live theatre/shopping';
- skills and knowledge – 'I am a good driver', 'I can knit' or 'I'm a good cook';
- something you have always wanted to learn – 'I would like to learn a new language/to play a guitar/to dance the Tango';

The person leading will capture all the contributions or ask people to come and write their contributions onto the sheet of paper, which makes it possible to recognise and appreciate the depth and range of resources available within a person's network. The connections between people will begin to emerge, which enables the development of stronger relationships and developing a sense of community among those involved.

The section of the treasure chest that recognises good people to know helps build the potential to extend a person's network. When people begin to identify the people in their own networks who are 'good people to know' and begin to consider how to link people together, it broadens the possible connections available to the person.

When people share something they have always wanted to learn, there may be connections with other people in the room who wish to learn something similar. This creates an opening for these people to come together to self-organise and pursue this together; for example, 'I love dancing and if Mary would like to have the opportunity to dance on a regular basis, we could go together'.

Whether this is completed as a standalone exercise or as part of a person-centred plan, as people contribute to each section of the treasure chest, it helps them recognise what they have to offer and strengthens the connections that already exist.

A treasure chest is ever-evolving as new connections emerge and can be explored, providing the opportunity to gather and record rich information and to find ideas and opportunities to create stronger connections. Once completed, it supports people to recognise how they can play a meaningful role in supporting the person to lead a life they are happy with, which, in turn, strengthens their relationship.

Please see Appendix 2 for the 'treasure chest' resource.

Solution circles

A solution circle is a facilitated process that helps the people involved to identify new solutions to issues and challenges they are facing. This is intended to be short and focused, lasting usually less than half an hour. It can prove effective in addressing long-standing problems, especially areas that are preventing a person from achieving a good quality of life.

The focus person of the solution circle is the person who presents the problem or issue that they are experiencing. At the end of the process, the focus person can select the idea or ideas that have been generated through the process which they would like to take forward. The underpinning principle is that those who take part have the potential to help regardless of their background, experience or the role they play in the person's life.

Solution circles are supported further when aligned with the values of inclusion, covered in Chapter 1, and the outcome of a successful solution circle exercise demonstrates the value that, together, people are better.

When planning to facilitate a solution circle, it is best to involve five to nine people who can be present and actively engaged. Once you have the people, find a space where it would be possible to hold the gathering. Choose somewhere with enough space to be comfortable, with no distractions and that has somewhere to record the conversation in a clear visual way, either on a flip chart, whiteboard or a room with blank wall space where big sheets of paper can be stuck to the wall (from experience use an adhesive that does not leave marks – masking tape is a good option).

There are four main roles that need to be fulfilled during the development of the solution circle; these are:

- problem presenter – also known as the focus person;
- process facilitator who will manage the people involved and be a timekeeper;
- note taker or graphic recorder who will clearly record all the information shared for everyone involved to see;
- and everyone else – the people who will be supporting the focus person, actively engaging, listening and contributing thoughts and ideas.

Here are the steps, with a recommended six minutes being given to each one.

Step One: The problem presenter outlines the problem they are experiencing. At this stage, the process facilitator makes sure the problem presenter does not run over time and is not interrupted. The note taker takes notes, and everyone else listens. If the problem presenter finishes early, the group stays silent until the six minutes elapses. It is really important to honour this uninterrupted time.

Step Two: The process facilitator opens up the session to the rest of the group and asks them to share their ideas and thoughts. It is important that everything is recorded and the focus remains on sharing the ideas; this is not the time to ask questions, give advice or analyse any of the ideas, and the process facilitator should keep everyone focused and make sure that everyone gets a chance to contribute, ensuring that no one dominates the conversation. The note taker records all the ideas, making sure they use the actual words given and not placing their interpretation onto them. The role of the problem presenter is to listen to the contributions and not to interrupt.

Step Three: The group enters into a dialogue led by the problem presenter, which gives them time to explore the ideas and further clarify the problem. The process facilitator needs to listen to make sure that the content is covering the positive points only and to guide the group away from negativity and anything that relates to what cannot be done.

Step Four: The problem presenter identifies the ideas that stand out as having potential and the ones they would like to put into action. The problem presenter and the group decide what actions are doable within the next three days and at least one action that can be initiated within 24 hours. It is critical to set actions that can be achieved within a short timeframe, such as researching information on the internet or making a phone call. Unless something is achieved soon after a planning meeting of this kind, people lose momentum and get 'stuck'. Someone from the group volunteers to contact the problem presenter within three days to check if they have completed their first action. To bring the solution circle to a close, the group does a round of words to describe the experience and the recorder hands the finished record to the problem presenter.

A solution circle does not guarantee the perfect solution, but it usually gets people 'unstuck' from the problem and helps the problem presenter think about how to address it, with the momentum to keep going until the solution is found (Forest and Pearpoint, 1996).

Please see Appendix 2 for the solution circle resource

Consideration when utilising these tools

It is important to make sure that the information that is gathered and recorded using the approaches described above comes from the focus person, the person with dementia, as a first consideration and then from the people who know the person well and have their best interest as their main concern.

At the heart of personalisation, there is a clear aim to promote a good quality of life. Therefore, if during a planning meeting, or a conversation, someone is talking on the focus person's behalf or interrupting them, the facilitator should bring the attention back to the focus person and remind everyone present about the purpose of the meeting.

Creating the space and opportunity for the person with dementia to take the lead in conversations and planning meetings can be challenging for other people involved for the following reasons.

- During a planning session or a conversation the focus person may need the time to consider how they want to respond to questions or what they want to contribute to the conversation. This time to think and consider may lead to a silence or pause in the flow of the conversation. During these quiet moments of conversations, people can feel a sense of discomfort and awkwardness and their way of addressing this feeling is to break the silence, filling the space with their thoughts and ideas. The process facilitator should aim to encourage everyone involved to recognise that silence is good and that it provides the much-needed time and space for the focus person to think about their responses and to find the right words. Supporting everyone to appreciate the need to go at the pace of the focus person and to recognise that the periods of silence in the conversation may be where best answers and insights can be found.
- When a person has taken the lead within a conversation, they have taken the lead off the focus person. This may be with the well-intended if they may believe that the focus person is finding the conversation too difficult. However the opportunity to learn directly from the person would be missed.
- The long-standing dynamics of a relationship between people who are in the session together may influence the direction and content of the conversation. The dynamics

may also affect the way people engage in the conversation, for instance how comfortable someone feels about speaking up and, likewise, how another member of the group may feel about not taking the lead. When facilitating a conversation, it is important to make sure that there is an equal share of opportunity to contribute among those present and the contributions from each individual are valued and recognised, while recognising that the final decision, wherever possible, should always be made by the focus person or in their best interest.

The importance of hearing the voice of the focus person can be set at the beginning of the planning meeting, or the conversation and people present can be reminded of this as the conversation develops.

The focus person is in the driving seat

In this context, the 'driving seat' refers to a person taking the lead, steering the course of direction of their own life and determining the destination.

Self-directed support supports the idea of the person directing and making decisions about the care and support they receive and how they receive it.

Self-directed support places emphasis on those receiving care and support firmly taking the position of the 'driver' while personalisation focuses on how services and health and social personnel can respond in a person-centred and bespoke way to those in the 'driving seat'.

Before the person with dementia can take the 'driving seat', it may need to be recognised that other people from the dementia care triad + 1 may have assumed a lead role in that person's life. An open discussion with all the significant people from the dementia care triad + 1 is needed to emphasise the importance of the person being able to express themselves, share what is important to them and make decisions for themselves, discussing how the person with dementia could take a lead role in any conversations and planning meetings about their life and the care and support they receive.

Here are some ideas to help maintain the focus on the person during conversations and planning meetings and to shift the focus, so the person is taking the lead role.

Use a talking stick **–** This provides a simple approach to creating focus in a conversation, preventing people from talking over one another. With the understood principle – to contribute to a meeting you need to be holding the talking stick while everyone else present listens. It will also be explained that the talking stick is held by the focus person, and they will pass this onto the person who wants to contribute; once that person has finished sharing the talking stick is then passed back to the focus person who then hands this to the next person who wishes to speak.

The facilitator needs to make sure that the talking stick remains in the focus person's control, and attendees need to be reminded to keep their contributions focused on the purpose of the meeting and positive.

A talking stick can be something from the immediate environment that is easy to hold and pass on to other people, a spoon, a pen. It is best to choose something that stands out visually so that people taking part in the conversation can easily identify and be reminded of who is holding it at any one time.

A talking stick can be prepared in advance of the meeting if it is expected that there may be a problem in maintaining the focus on the person with dementia and with them taking a lead in the conversation. This advanced preparation provides an opportunity to personalise the talking stick to make it significant to the individual; for example, for someone who loves art the talking stick could be a paint brush, or for someone who loves to sing it could be a microphone. It can be designed and made by the focus person to help to build the connection with the talking stick and the purpose of it. It serves to remind everyone that the conversation is first and foremost about the focus person and their life, their aspirations and wants.

When a talking stick is used, it is done so with some rules attached.

- The talking stick starts with the focus person.
- People who wish to contribute to the meeting must signal that they wish to do so and wait until they are given the talking stick before they make their contribution.
- The person holding the talking stick is the only person who can talk.
- Once the person who first held the talking stick has finished speaking, the talking stick should be handed back to the focus person to make sure that they maintain some control over the proceedings at the meeting.
- It is up to the focus person who takes the talking stick next, and the person facilitating the conversation will support in making sure that everyone present is involved and has an opportunity to be heard.

The use of a talking stick brings some order to a conversation; it avoids people talking over others and makes it clear as to whose turn it is to talk. This approach encourages people to listen to one another, and it can create a greater level of understanding between those present and encourages a respectful approach to the proceedings (Seeds for Change, 2020).

Have a facilitator – It is important to have someone who will facilitate the conversation and make sure that everyone present has had the opportunity to contribute when they have requested to do so. The facilitator would make sure that no one person is taking too much of the time available for the meeting to make their contribution. The person taking on the role of the facilitator should be someone who understands the principles of facilitation and should not have an active interest in the conversation taking place, making sure that the focus person remains involved in and leading the conversation. As the conversation progresses, the facilitator should acknowledge everyone's contributions and redirect ideas and thoughts shared by the group back to the focus person for them to consider and make the final decision. The facilitator would aim for the conversation to be smooth, energetic and positive.

Here are some principles regarding facilitation that originate from person-centred planning facilitator.

- Support the group to maintain positivity in their conversation, while recognising that circumstances may lead to addressing negative aspects of a situation. In this instance support those present to reframe the negative into a positive wherever possible.
- Arrange the environment in such a way that people can equally contribute and take part, where people can feel on the same level as everyone else. Plan the seating so everyone can see each other, remove any barriers that mean people cannot see or hear each other and remove the formality of meeting/conference tables by arranging the seating in a circle.
- If the meeting is being recorded using visuals on a flipchart or a big sheet of paper, make sure everyone is able to see the recording.
- Do not try to make a visual recording of the meeting, sometimes called graphic facilitation, and facilitate the conversation at the same time. It is not possible to see the subtle elements of communication when facing away from the group whilst capturing the information on the graphic record.
- A facilitator should place themselves to be able to see everyone to check if people are engaged or if they want to contribute.
- Make sure that all contributions are heard and that no one remains excluded from the conversation.
- Before commencing the conversation, set the scene; remind people about the purpose of the gathering that the meeting is a commitment to listening and developing a greater understanding of the focus person.
- Encourage people to create a positive experience and explain that the meeting is not the place for using jargon or fixing, judging, digging or obsessing.

Preparing for a meeting

The success of a meeting, or a conversation, is largely dependent on having the time to plan ahead with the person with dementia. Preparation can help to build understanding regarding the purpose of the meeting and then for them to exercise control over who they would like to have involved, where they would like the meeting to be held, when would be a good time to bring people together and the finer details of creating a good and positive environment. Here are some areas the focus person might like to consider.

- The purpose of the meeting, what they would like to achieve and what they would like to discuss.
- What approaches to communication they would like to use.
- Who should talk on their behalf if they struggle at any stage – this could be in reference to a decision-making agreement, as explored in Chapter 7.

- Specific points they want to make clear to the group; for instance the person may wish to talk about aspects of their care that aren't working well for them and how they would like this to change.

Time given for preparation can help the focus person be confident about having their views and ideas heard. The focus person is likely to gain greater value from this preparation time if they are supported by someone they trust.

Good questions

The type of questions asked and how they are phrased make a huge impact on the quality of the conversations held and the outcomes achieved. Being conscious of using questions that assist a person to take the lead is key. Making time to reflect can contribute to making the next conversation richer and more meaningful. Were the questions open, positive and supportive or closed, directive and leading?

Assessing the quality of questions being asked

When considering the impact some questions, such as the ones in the Reflection task later, can have on the focus person also consider how the person would feel about themselves as a result of being asked these questions. It comes as no surprise that the outcome of a meeting can be negative for the focus person as a result of the way they were engaged during the meeting. The questions the person is asked and how they are asked can be the very reason why they may have disengaged from the conversation.

Reflection

When talking with someone about what a good start to the day is for them we may incorporate a number of questions.

An open question would be:

'*What does a good start to the day look like for you?*'

A positive question would be:

'*To start the day well, what needs to happen for you?*'

A supportive question would be:

'*To help you to have a good start to the day, what support would you like to have in place?*'

A closed question would be:

'Do you need support to get out of bed in the morning?'

A directive question would be:

'It seems you have reached a stage where you need someone to come and support you in the mornings, is that right?'

A leading question would be:

'Would you like me to arrange for someone to come and support you in the mornings?'

- Consider the following questions: are they open, positive and supportive, or are they closed, directive and leading?
  - If you could do anything, what would it be?
  - Would you like to join the day care group?
  - The respite provision available in the local town has a great reputation; would you like to visit?
  - Often people find it difficult to control their behaviours; is this something you are also experiencing?
  - If you were to go away for a break, what would you like to do?
  - Have you considered taking a place at a care home?
  - Do you think you would find it easier to get around if you could use a taxi?
  - If you could live anywhere, where would you like to live?
- How could some of the closed, directing and leading questions be rephrased to engage with the focus person in an open, positive and supportive way?
- In the approach taken with the above questions, is respect demonstrated to the focus person and recognition of the contributions they have made to society and their achievements?

Skills Box 3: person-centred planning

Person-centred planning provides a range of approaches and processes that help a person to capture detailed and meaningful information about themselves and place them firmly at the centre. The range of approaches covers a breadth of detail, which provides the opportunity for a focus person to consider their past, present and future and share their dreams, nightmares and preferences with people who hold meaning in their life (Inclusive Solutions, 2015).

Receiving an invite to be involved in a person-centred plan provides a chance to be part of an experience alongside other people, including people that form the dementia care triad + 1, to listen to the focus person and hear their story. In doing so, people begin to recognise and learn about what makes sense to the person – to appreciate the person's perspective on their own life and hear the contributions of the focus person and others in moving towards a better experience of life.

During a person-centred planning meeting those present make a commitment to act upon what they have learnt and to support the focus person in addressing what they want to change or achieve in their life. Person-centred planning is built on the values of inclusion, which were covered in Chapter 1, taking them from statements and putting them into action so that they begin to have meaning and purpose in a focus person's life.

The facilitation of a person-centred plan

Careful, thoughtful and skilled facilitation of a person-centred plan is crucial in achieving a positive experience where the focus person is in control of the proceedings and honoured and respected as an individual. Within person-centred planning, there are two distinct facilitation roles.

1. Process facilitator – has a focus on the people, making sure that everyone is present and involved, while also constantly checking that the focus person is taking the lead role in the development of their plan. The process facilitator guides everyone through the planning process, maintaining momentum and enthusiasm. They aim to acknowledge the finer elements of communication within the group, for instance the nonverbal communication such as nods of approval or signs that someone is uncertain or unsure and addresses these as they arise. Everyone is guided through the planning process by the process facilitator to reach an inspiring image and direction for a future designed by and with the focus person. This is accompanied by clear commitments and action to move towards this future. The process facilitator also makes sure that the pace is right for the focus person and the atmosphere is positive and buoyant.

2. Graphic facilitator focuses on capturing the content of the meeting using big sheets of paper and colourful, bold pens and pastels, just like the role of the Graphic Recorder in a solution circle exercise. This is not about creating the best piece of artwork; it is more important to capture the words used by those in the room, images that represent the words but also capture the emotion and the natural connections with other parts of the conversation taking place. The graphic facilitator utilises the opportunity presented by the natural pauses of the conversation to recap on what has been recorded to ensure accuracy. They also involve the people present, and most importantly the focus person, in adding to

the visual record. The graphic facilitator takes a photograph of the completed person-centred plan at the end of the meeting, so this can be shared with those present. The original recording of the plan is carefully taken down, rolled up and symbolically handed to the focus person in a gesture that clarifies the ownership of the plan.

Facilitators of person-centred planning require skills in the following areas to make sure the planning process is positive.

- Listening – This skill can be demonstrated by reaffirming what people have said and creating opportunities to recap what has been recorded on the person-centred planning graphic record, making changes where the original meaning has been lost.
- Recording – Making sure the information is recorded in such a way that people can clearly see that their contributions have been recognised. Capturing exactly what has been shared verbatim, using either the focus person's or the contributor's own words. If the contribution has been lengthy and therefore needs summarising, make sure the focus person or the contributor is involved in deciding on a suitable summary.
- Creating a full picture – The plan is about the focus person, their history, how life is now and their aspirations. The completed plan should capture their individuality and be a true reflection of them with all their quirks and uniqueness reflected within it.
- A commitment to finding a solution – Process facilitators should make sure that time is given to consider solutions to some of the issues faced by the focus person and those close to them, especially long-standing problems, and issues the focus person may face in the future. The aim of planning is to make a positive difference and, as a result, reach real outcomes. The focus person and the people involved in the plan are encouraged to think openly about a range of solutions and not only focus on the services available to them, considering:
  - voluntary groups within the focus person's local area;
  - people who are within the focus person's neighbourhood who may have specific and useful skills and knowledge;
  - the skills and knowledge available in the focus person's immediate network of relationships;
  - funding available via the wide range of funding streams; this could include local authority, clinical commissioning groups, grants and the Department of Welfare and pensions;
  - technology as a form of support and assistance for the focus person;
  - adaptations to the family home to enable the focus person to continue to live there;

- investing time in setting something up that would work specifically for the focus person; this could include recruiting their own support workers or setting up an interest group in the person's local area.

For those involved in facilitating and developing person-centred plans, the following guidelines need to be followed.

- No jargon – Use language that everyone can understand. Avoid service-based language, which needs a translation book to fully understand. Use everyday language that everyone will understand even if this requires the use of more words to fully explain rather than acronyms or initials;
- No fixing – Work from the assumption that people are not broken; they have the capacity to know how to best resolve the issues they are facing they just need some support, space and time to think it through; even if a person is in a position in their life where they are no longer able to express what is important to them, someone close to them will know what is best.
- No obsessing – Give each topic the time and space it deserves but also know when it is time to move on, making sure that the focus person feels in control of their own plan and that they are setting the pace on what needs to be discussed, as well as how much time to spend discussing it.
- No digging – A person-centred planning facilitator will need to create an environment where the focus person and the people close to them feel able to talk about their circumstances openly and honestly, therefore it is important for a facilitator to recognise when someone is being pushed out of their comfort zone by the questions they are being asked or when people have started digging for more detail than the focus person feels comfortable to share, and to then know how to skilfully and gracefully redirect the group onto another topic.
- No judging – Everyone has preferences and makes lifestyle choices; person-centred planning encourages everyone to respect each other's decisions irrespective of personal preference and asks people to see life from the focus person's perspective and to respect whatever the person decides is right for them.

Person-centred planning is a creative and open process that can be adapted to work specifically for the focus person; this can be achieved through:

- altering the layout of the planning tool; for example, for a focus person who loves steam engines the planning sections can be related to a steam engine, such as the fuel depicting what the person needs to stay strong and keep going, the wheels representing the direction the person is going in, and the passengers signifying the people they would like to include on their journey;
- holding the meetings in a different way to create an atmosphere where everyone feels welcome and clear on their purpose within the planning meeting. This can

be achieved through making the meeting relaxed and fun, holding the meeting in a place that has meaning to the focus person, somewhere they enjoy spending time and, where people will be comfortable, making sure everyone coming to the meeting is clear on the purpose of the meeting and their role within it before the meeting takes place. Planning a meeting that is person centred takes consideration to ensure the experience is positive for everyone, for instance considering refreshments, music, accessibility, seating and how the meeting will be recorded.

Who to invite to the planning meeting

The main priority is for the focus person to feel comfortable and at ease to talk openly. Achieving this will largely be determined by how strengthened the focus person is by the people present; therefore, it is important to get this stage of the planning process right. Person-centred planning breaks the assumption that meetings about achieving a good life and finding great care and support involve only the focus person, close family and professionals. Those involved could include anyone whom the focus person wishes to have there, for example, friends, neighbours, work colleagues and members of the community. The focus person may write an invite list or make reference to photographs of the people they would like to invite.

In instances where they may not be able to make this decision, those involved in helping to organise the meeting can consider who the 'right' people to invite would be and who the focus person would want to have there. Here are a few things to consider.

- Does the person get along with the focus person; do they enjoy each other's company?
- Do they have the focus person's best interests at heart?
- Will they listen to the focus person or the ideas contributed without being judgemental?
- Will they concentrate on the focus person and the intention to achieve the best outcome for them?
- Do they have enough understanding about what matters to the focus person?

If, on thinking through these questions, the general feeling is that it would be positive to invite a person, consider:

- what skills or knowledge do they have that they could contribute to the focus person's plan?
- do they have the time and energy to contribute to putting the plan into action?
- are they well connected within their local community?

- have they got a positive outlook, and would they be keen to make a difference?
- do they recognise the skills, positive characteristics and interests of the focus person and what they have to offer other people and the community?

People with dementia who are still living within and have an active part in their community may consider inviting family members, friends, colleagues, former colleagues and neighbours. The range of people to possibly invite could be very different for people who have already moved into a service setting which may have created a distance in some of the important relationships they had while they remained within their community. In these circumstances, developing a circle of support can identify the relationships that have been lost and generate the discussions needed to find ways to re-establish these.

Traditionally, meetings that focused on addressing a focus person's assessed care or support needs would include a range of professional people.

- Social workers.
- Nurses.
- Physiotherapists.
- Occupational therapists.
- Speech and language therapists.

It can be difficult and daunting for anyone to feel comfortable talking openly about themselves during a meeting when the attendees are people they do not know well. In these circumstances people can become so overwhelmed that they do not feel able to talk confidently about themselves, especially when the people present may make decisions about their future care and support.

In recognising this it is then possible to understand that information gathered at meetings that are led heavily from a professional perspective may not lead to developing a good level of insight and understanding of the person and their circumstances. If these meetings form the foundation for the services and support to be put in place for the individual it is fair to suggest that there is a real potential for support and care packages to not work well for the person.

The methods introduced in this chapter regarding person-centred planning could be the answer to ensuring that future care and support work well for the focus person.

More information about graphic facilitation

It is important that the information shared in a planning meeting is captured and recorded in a way that is detailed, meaningful and easy to share. An alternative to a 'note taker', someone making notes which will later be typed and shared with the people attending the meeting, is having someone facilitate graphic while the meeting is taking place. Graphic facilitation entails recording information on large sheets of paper, using colourful pens and pastels to add meaning and depth to the conversation. This approach is a positive one as:

- people can feel more involved and engaged during the meeting;
- people present can see what is being recorded;
- the graphic is creative and colourful, encouraging people to open up their creative thinking, which is valuable when looking for alternative ideas and solutions;
- engages people who think in different ways, such as visual thinkers and auditory thinkers;
- develops clarity in what has been discussed and agreed;
- has a proven track record in making meetings fun, productive and meaningful;
- utilises pauses in the conversation to recap on what has been recorded, making sure that everyone has the opportunity to seek clarity on certain points and to alter inaccurate information;
- gives the focus person confidence as they are reassured that they are being heard. A graphic facilitator would make sure that they only record the decisions and solutions that have been agreed by the focus person or are in their best interest;
- creates a visual record of the topics of conversation and key issues so people can see the links between topics and potential connections/solutions;
- encourages a focus on the topic at hand and avoids wasting time on distractions and tangent conversations;
- addresses the different perspectives of a given situation with the opportunity to work through these to arrive at a mutual understanding and agree on an outcome and solution;
- makes sharing the information recorded easy – the graphic facilitator can simply take a photograph of the visual and distribute this after the meeting while the original is carefully rolled up and handed to the focus person.

Person-centred planning approaches

Every approach to person-centred planning encourages people to be:

- positive;
- creative in generating ideas and finding solutions;
- rooted in the values of inclusion, as described in Chapter 1;

- confident about what they have to bring to the planning conversations and the potential opportunities that could be found through their involvement in the conversation;
- clear on what they have to offer in the way of skills, knowledge and connections.

There are a number of different methods and processes that sit within the family of person-centred plans; these were originally introduced in Chapter 1, and they are described in greater detail here.

PATH – planning alternative tomorrows with hope

Please see Appendix 2 to see an example of a PATH.

This planning approach was developed by Pearpoint et al (2001). A PATH is a future-focused planning process that has the intention of recognising and honouring a person's desired future and collectively finding a way to move towards achieving this. It must be facilitated by a process facilitator and a graphic facilitator. The graphic facilitator focuses on capturing the content of the meeting, while the process facilitator guides the focus person and the people present through the planning process. People are invited by the focus person to gather together to support them to develop their PATH. As part of being present, people take an active role in the conversations and discussions within the PATH meeting.

The meeting begins by welcoming everyone and inviting people to contribute to an appreciation (please see Appreciations earlier in this chapter). This helps everyone present to adopt a positive mindset. Once the group is settled the process facilitator encourages the focus person to explore what a good future would look like for them. This is facilitated in a manner that reduces limited beliefs, assumptions and attitudes about what is possible. Instead, the focus person is encouraged to share what their thoughts and ideas are in the context 'if nothing was going to get in your way' 'If nothing could hold you back'

Once a clear picture of someone's dream is established, the PATH process supports them to bring their dream into a time frame of what can be achieved, '*it is now a year on from today – what have you managed to achieve that has taken you towards your dream?*' This enables people's aspirations to be placed in a time frame that feels positive and possible – realistic, manageable and achievable. The process facilitator encourages the focus person and the rest of the group to talk as though they had already achieved these goals and as though it had already happened, using phrases along the lines of '*imagine that this is now a year on from today, tell me what have you achieved towards reaching your dream*'. The importance of this stage is that the person begins to recognise what their achievement would feel like; this can, in turn, build momentum, motivation and commitment. Once a clear picture has emerged, the questions would then be repeated in the context of a six-month time frame. At this stage it is good to start to create some links between what has been achieved in six months and what has been achieved in a year so that people can start to see the connections and the progression. Producing a graphic record, using arrows or colour to group topics can help emphasise connections.

Once the dream is captured and people have developed an appreciation of what this means for the individual, the focus person is asked what the dream feels like for them and this is recorded on the PATH. The focus person and those around them can begin to feel a sense of enthusiasm and energy.

At this stage a small amount of time is spent on the 'now' section of the PATH. This is intended to capture what life looks and feels like for the person now. It helps to give some measure between the 'dream' and 'now' and begins to highlight any disparity, tension and difference between the two. Only a short length of time is dedicated to this section, five or ten minutes at the most, as the present can be difficult to discuss if there is a big difference between the 'now' and the 'dream'. Listening to the person's current situation can build a sense of urgency towards making the person's dream a reality. Dwelling on this stage of the PATH beyond what the focus person wishes to share can begin to negatively affect the positive energy that was created at the beginning of the PATH planning process. Investing too much time in the 'now' is not going to create the change that may be desperately needed so it is best to move on.

The fifth step is 'enrolling'; this recognises the people with the commitment, skills, knowledge, understanding and connections to help realise the dream. These are the people who are vital to ensure the success of the plan.

First, and most importantly, the focus person signs up to their own plan, whenever possible. It is important that the focus person makes a commitment to work towards achieving their own dreams and aspirations in whichever way they can. They then invite other people to 'enrol' in their PATH to support them in the journey towards achieving their dreams and their desired future. When looking at who to 'enrol' in a plan, it is also possible to think about the people who are not present at the planning meeting who would be valuable in helping to achieve the plan. The planning group could then discuss how to invite people to get involved.

The sixth step is 'building strengths'. This stage recognises that it can take a lot of strength and energy to achieve the goals and aspirations within the plan. Recognising what lifts the feelings and mood of the focus person and the people involved in their PATH, and what gives them the energy to move forward is going to be an important feature of keeping people's energies high. This could include:

- having lunch once a week with a close friend;
- going to church every week;
- making time to read a favourite book one evening a week;
- going for a walk in the countryside on a Sunday.

When working towards a goal, it is possible to overlook making time for the areas that give the focus person and the other people involved in their PATH the enthusiasm and energy to continue and it is important to make sure that these areas of people's lives are recognised and not forgotten as part of the journey.

The final stage recognises the 'first steps' that need to be taken straight after the planning meeting with the emphasis on identifying something that can be done that day or within the next 48 hours. The intention is to make the most of the momentum generated during the planning meeting and to make sure that this is harnessed and maintained to enable the focus person and the planning group to work towards making a difference and achieving the steps towards the focus person's 'dream'.

At the end of the PATH planning process, there is usually a lot of energy and commitment to moving towards the vision of a good future that has been created. People who attended the planning session leave with a clearer insight into what would make a good future for the focus person and the steps they have committed to take to enable them to work towards this.

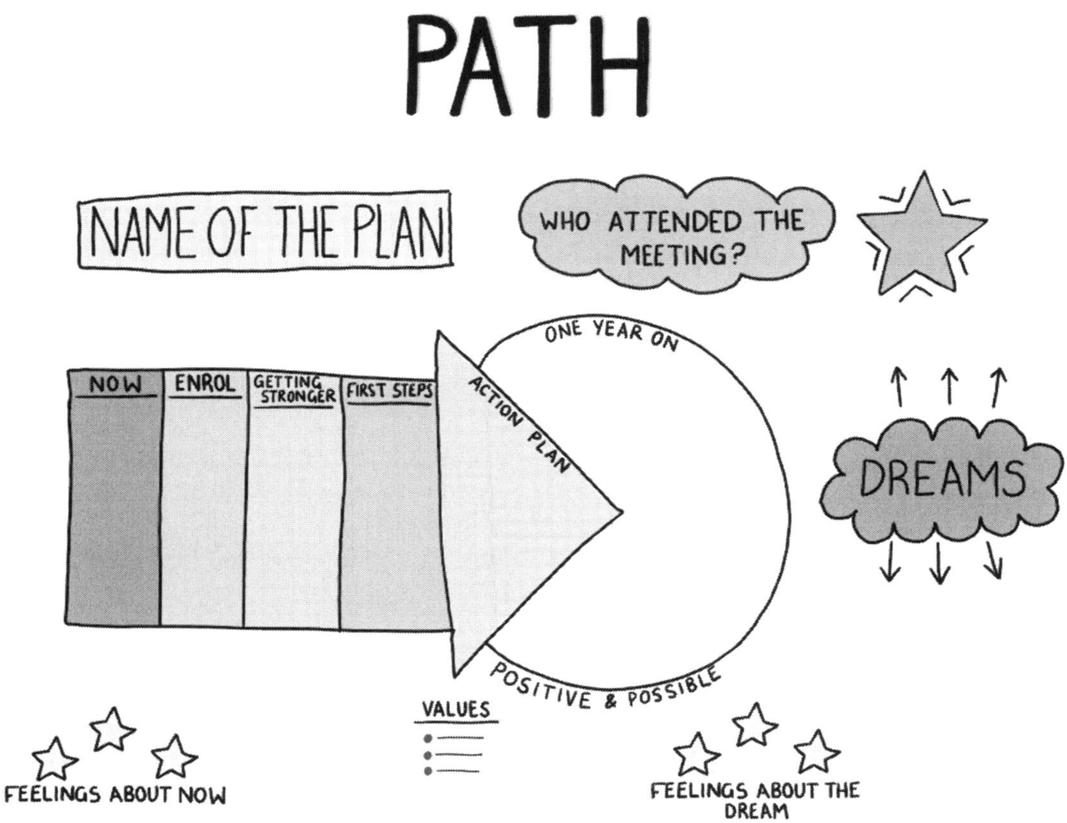

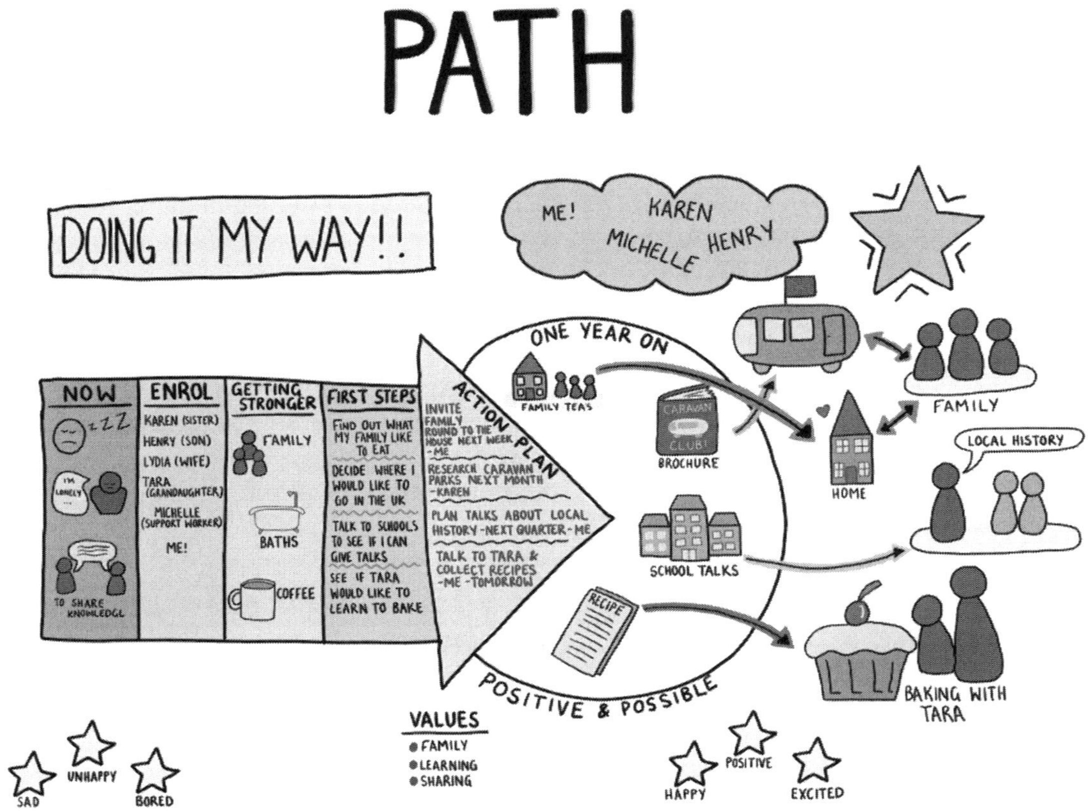

MAP – making action plans

Please see Appendix 2 for a visual representation of a MAP.

This planning process was developed by O'Brien et al (2010) The MAP process works well when a group of people are invited to be involved and come together with a commitment: to listen to the focus person, learn about what the person wishes to change and achieve and be actively involved in creating a better future. Similar to a PATH, a MAP needs to be facilitated by both a process facilitator and a graphic facilitator.

At the start of a MAP planning process, everyone attending is welcomed and invited to contribute to an appreciation about the focus person (please see Appreciations earlier in this chapter). To achieve this, the process facilitator asks each person to share something they like and admire about the focus person.

This first step usually takes about five to ten minutes, depending on the size of the group, and sets the positive tone for the rest of the planning meeting. Opening a meeting this way can fundamentally change how the focus person views themselves, supporting them to be confident and engaged in their own plan.

The second step of a MAP is where the focus person shares their story.

- Proud moments and achievements.
- Important and sentimental memories.
- Places where the person has lived and spent time.
- Influential and significant people and loved ones.
- The roles they have fulfilled.
- Difficult times, loss and grief.

Through listening, those present can learn a great deal about what was, and still is, important to the focus person. The story builds a bigger picture about the focus person and can open a discussion regarding their past and whether they wish to re-establish connections with friendships, family, interests, places or a vocation.

For people who have been supported within the service setting for a number of years their personal story and history can be hijacked by a chronology of the services and medical input they have received, including diagnosis and specialist treatment. When a MAP is developed this aspect of a person's life may be recognised but it does not dominate or over shadow their own personal story. Instead their journey that has got them to where they are today stands out more than any service-based chronology.

The third and fourth steps of the MAP planning process consider the focus person's 'dreams' and 'nightmares'.

'Dreams' – Understanding a focus person's 'dreams' gives everyone an insight of what is important to the focus person; this includes the things they would like to strive to achieve and the things they would like to have in place, on a day-to-day basis. Listening to a person's 'dreams' builds an awareness of their interests, passions and what has meaning for them.

'Nightmares' – Understanding a person's 'nightmares' provides an insight into what the focus person would not want to happen; situations that would cause them fear, anxiety, stress or upset. A focus person's 'nightmares' may refer to negative experiences they have had in the past that they would not want to re-live. Capturing the nightmares as part of the MAP planning process helps to inform people about what needs to be avoided and to plan accordingly.

Step five focuses on the question: 'what does the focus person need to and want to happen on the basis of what we have learnt today?' The intention is to identify what needs to happen to make a positive difference in the focus person's life. Once areas of need and preferences have been identified, an action plan, involving the focus person and the other people present at the planning meeting, is created to move the plan forward. One of the actions would be establishing a time that the planning group can get back together with the focus person to check in on progress towards their plan.

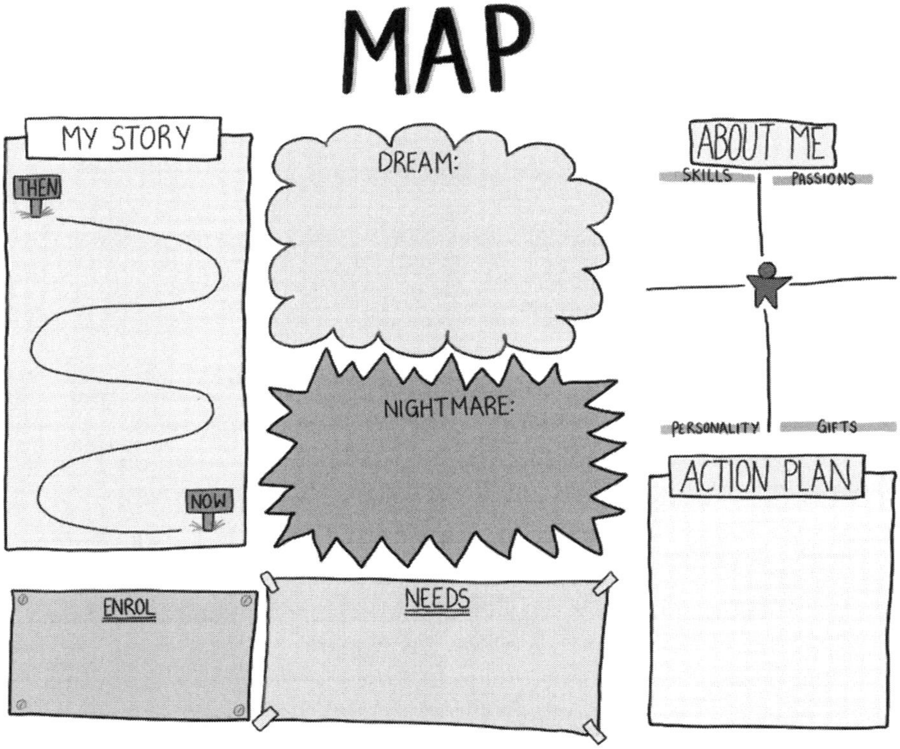
MAP
MY STORY
THEN
NOW
DREAM:
NIGHTMARE:
ABOUT ME
SKILLS
PASSIONS
PERSONALITY
GIFTS
ACTION PLAN
ENROL
NEEDS

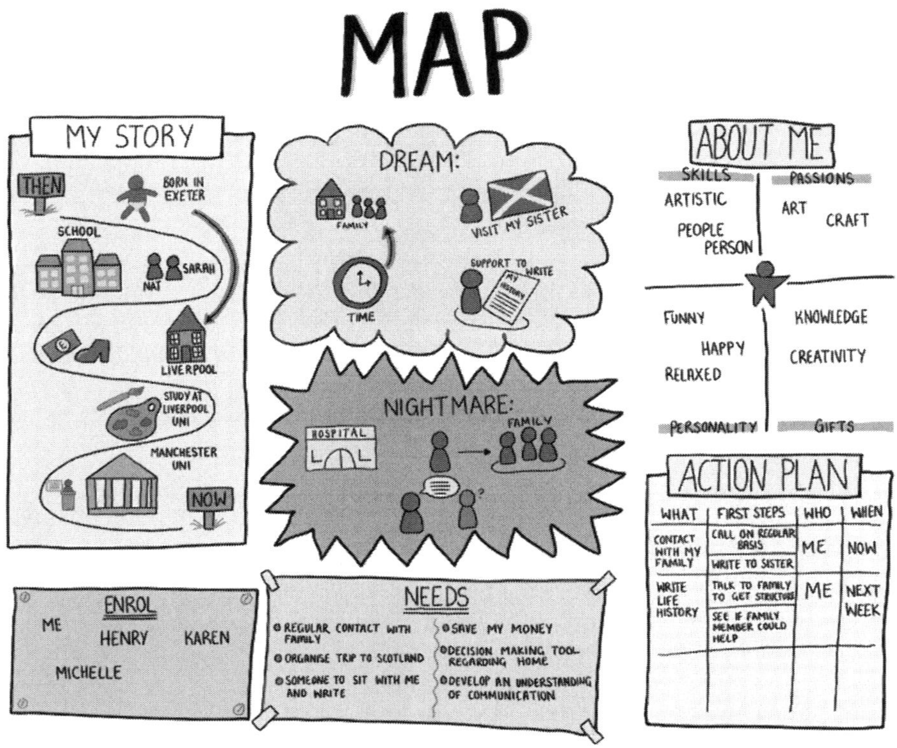
MAP
MY STORY
THEN
BORN IN EXETER
SCHOOL
NAT
SARAH
LIVERPOOL
STUDY AT LIVERPOOL UNI
MANCHESTER UNI
NOW
DREAM:
FAMILY
VISIT MY SISTER
TIME
SUPPORT TO WRITE
MY HISTORY
NIGHTMARE:
HOSPITAL
FAMILY
ABOUT ME
SKILLS
PASSIONS
ARTISTIC
PEOPLE PERSON
ART
CRAFT
FUNNY
HAPPY
RELAXED
KNOWLEDGE
CREATIVITY
PERSONALITY
GIFTS
ACTION PLAN
WHAT
FIRST STEPS
WHO
WHEN
CONTACT WITH MY FAMILY
CALL ON REGULAR BASIS
WRITE TO SISTER
ME
NOW
WRITE LIFE HISTORY
TALK TO FAMILY TO GET STRUCTURE
SEE IF FAMILY MEMBER COULD HELP
ME
NEXT WEEK
ENROL
ME
HENRY
KAREN
MICHELLE
NEEDS
REGULAR CONTACT WITH FAMILY
ORGANISE TRIP TO SCOTLAND
SOMEONE TO SIT WITH ME AND WRITE
SAVE MY MONEY
DECISION MAKING TOOL REGARDING HOME
DEVELOP AN UNDERSTANDING OF COMMUNICATION

Essential lifestyles planning

Please see Appendix 2 for a visual representation of an essential lifestyle plan.

Essential lifestyle planning was developed by Michael Smull and Susan Burke Harrison (n.d.). This approach gathers valuable information about how the focus person wishes to be supported on a day-to-day basis and the finer details of what matters to them in everyday life.

An essential lifestyle plan gathers details about the focus person's important daily routines and rituals. Once gathered, this detail can then be shared to inform those who are providing support or care in the focus person's day-to-day life, enabling them to provide care and support that honours the focus person's preferences for a good life.

The first step of an essential lifestyle plan is to identify the important people who hold the knowledge about what works well for the person and to hold intentional conversations with them to gather the details of what is important to the focus person.

This really is about breaking down all aspects of the focus person's life and especially areas that define a good quality of life for them. The information is gathered through having a series of open conversations with the focus person and the people close to them, this could include people from the dementia care triad + 1.

The second step is to do an initial sort of the information gathered under these headings.

- 'Essential and non-negotiable'.
- 'Negotiable and not essential'.
- 'Would be good if it did happen but the person could live without it'.

Once the initial sort has been completed, a planning meeting would take place. This would be with the focus person and the people they have chosen to invite and who are important to them. At the meeting, the information would be checked to determine if it has been put into the right order of importance. Information may need to be moved around until the focus person and those close to them are happy with how their preferences have been presented.

The second stage addresses the question: 'what would need to be done to make sure the focus person's preferences, both negotiable and non-negotiable, feature in their day-to-day life?' The responses to this question are recorded in such a way that everyone at the meeting would be able to see them using graphic facilitation. The person making the written record needs to first check with the focus person that they agree with the responses before writing them down.

The final stage of the planning meeting is the creation of an action plan that clearly states what is going to be done to make sure that the elements that are 'essential and non-negotiable' to the focus person feature in their day-to-day life. The outcome of an essential lifestyle plan is to gain a greater understanding of the small details regarding how the focus person likes to live their day-to-day life. The details gathered will inform everyone involved to make sure the focus person is supported well and positively in the future.

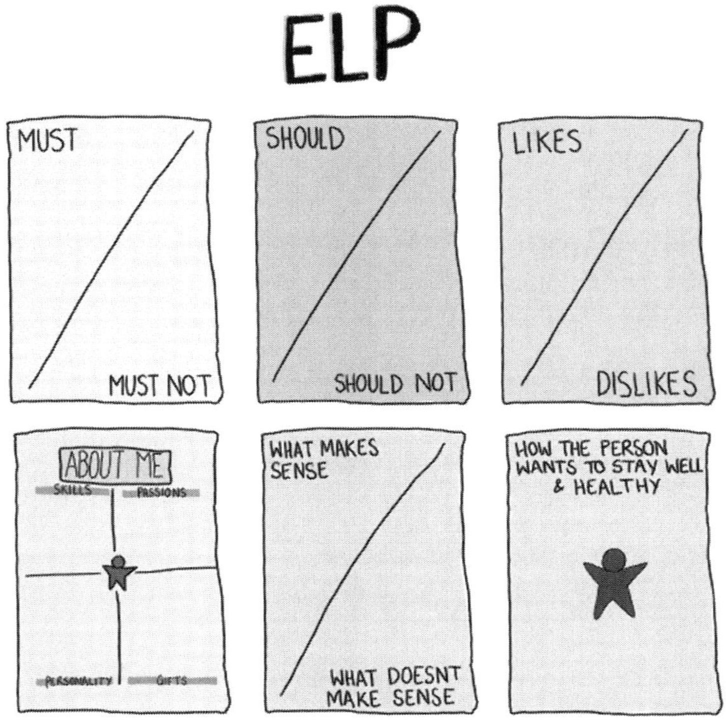
ELP
MUST
MUST NOT
SHOULD
SHOULD NOT
LIKES
DISLIKES
ABOUT ME
SKILLS
PASSIONS
PERSONALITY
GIFTS
WHAT MAKES SENSE
WHAT DOESNT MAKE SENSE
HOW THE PERSON WANTS TO STAY WELL & HEALTHY

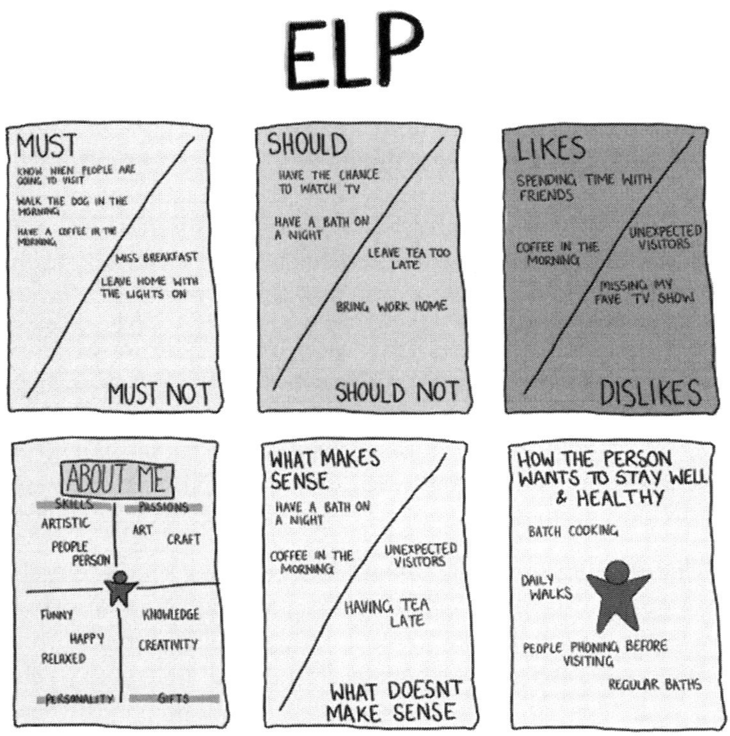
ELP
MUST
KNOW WHEN PEOPLE ARE GOING TO VISIT
WALK THE DOG IN THE MORNING
HAVE A COFFEE IN THE MORNING
MISS BREAKFAST
LEAVE HOME WITH THE LIGHTS ON
MUST NOT
SHOULD
HAVE THE CHANCE TO WATCH TV
HAVE A BATH ON A NIGHT
LEAVE TEA TOO LATE
BRING WORK HOME
SHOULD NOT
LIKES
SPENDING TIME WITH FRIENDS
COFFEE IN THE MORNING
UNEXPECTED VISITORS
MISSING MY FAVE TV SHOW
DISLIKES
ABOUT ME
SKILLS
ARTISTIC
PEOPLE PERSON
PASSIONS
ART
CRAFT
FUNNY
HAPPY
RELAXED
KNOWLEDGE
CREATIVITY
PERSONALITY
GIFTS
WHAT MAKES SENSE
HAVE A BATH ON A NIGHT
COFFEE IN THE MORNING
UNEXPECTED VISITORS
HAVING TEA LATE
WHAT DOESNT MAKE SENSE
HOW THE PERSON WANTS TO STAY WELL & HEALTHY
BATCH COOKING
DAILY WALKS
PEOPLE PHONING BEFORE VISITING
REGULAR BATHS

Personal futures planning

Personal futures planning was developed by Beth Mount (2000a,b). This approach encourages the focus person to meet with the people who are important to them to plan for the future. Personal futures planning is a series of maps that gather information about the focus person and their:

- background – their history and the past events that have significance;
- people – the people who are important to them in a paid or unpaid capacity;
- places – the places that are important to the person for leisure, hobbies and health;
- preferences – what is important to the person regarding how they like things to be done;
- images of the future – what a good future looks like for the person.

There are additional maps that can be added as optional extras to a personal futures plan and these include:

- communication – sharing information about how the person communicates;
- capacities – capturing areas where the person can do things for themselves, including making decisions;
- contributions – recognising the way the person can make a positive contribution to other people's lives and the community;
- responsibilities – demonstrating the areas of the person's life where they have some responsibility, such as work, family or community.

Once the individual maps have been explored and drawn up, a picture of what is important to the focus person in each of the maps would have been developed. A conversation can then take place regarding how these maps reflect the focus person's life in the present and what needs to happen to make what is important to the focus person now and in the future a reality. Actions can then be identified to move forward in creating positive change for the focus person and the people close to them.

Personal futures planning calls on people, who are also able and willing to meet on a regular basis to look at how things are progressing for the focus person, to be part of the continued planning process. These meetings create the opportunity to address issues and opportunities and to work together to consider how to move forward.

Other approaches for planning meetings

The following approaches can also be utilised during the planning meetings.

- A question board – this captures questions that the planning process has generated that cannot be answered in the planning meeting and would also capture ideas to address these questions after the planning session.

- An ideas poster – this records ideas that are shared during the planning meeting, which the planning group can then refer to when the action plan is developed.
- Deciding 'when will we meet again?' – to keep the plan alive it is important that the planning group think about when they will get back together to discuss progress and consider how to overcome barriers and the next steps for progress.
- Action planning - It can be useful to record agreed actions; what needs to be done, how the action is going to be achieved, who is doing what and when things need to be done.

It has to be emphasised here that these are short introductions to planning processes that require a great deal of insight, understanding and sensitivity to be facilitated well. This introduction is intended to capture your interest, as the reader. If this has been successfully achieved more can be learnt about person-centred planning through the sources listed in the Bibliography at the end of the book.

The tools and approaches covered in this chapter serve a clear purpose to:

- raise awareness and understanding;
- develop good relationships between the person and everyone involved in their life, especially those providing care and support;
- notice changes that are taking place for the person and the people around them;
- achieve consistent and high-quality care and support;
- be prepared for future changes and how to respond to these changes;
- have a clear sense of purpose and direction;
- be able to clearly identify actions that need to be taken to achieve positive outcomes;
- be able to identify where some of the solutions can be found and the people who could be involved in making things happen.

Person-centred planning can help to create the momentum for change that is needed to achieve a good life for the focus person and those around. Sometimes it creates the space needed to notice and discuss what actions are needed to support the person to maintain what is in place for them, especially if this is working well and the people around them.

Action planning

It can be useful to record agreed actions; what needs to be done, how the action is going to be achieved, who is doing what and when things need to be done.

Key lessons learnt

- There are a number of skills and approaches that can be utilised to support the achievement of personalisation in dementia care. These skills and approaches can be utilised by the dementia care triad + 1 and the wider community to make the dementia journey an easier experience for the person with dementia.
- The skills and tools presented can be utilised in a creative and dynamic way to achieve the best outcome for the person with dementia and all the people that make up the dementia care triad + 1.
- The skills and tools introduced in this chapter have been practised for over 50 years; they are tried and tested and have been proven to work in a whole range of settings. They continue to be supported and embraced as good models of working together to make a real difference in enabling the voices of people to be heard; promoting positive interactions, respect and dignity; and protecting people's right to make decisions about their own lives.
- Having a detailed understanding of the person gathered through in-depth and advanced planning will help to ensure that the person's preferences and wishes are respected at each stage of the dementia journey. This will lead to care and support or professional input being appropriate and personalised in approach.
- Putting the tools and skills introduced in this chapter into practice will help everyone involved develop a detailed understanding of the person with dementia.
- The skills and tools presented in this chapter also represent a method of gathering, sorting and presenting information which can create a reference point for anyone involved in caring for or supporting the person.

Questions to aid reflection

1) Consider the time it would take to utilise the skills and tools presented in this chapter. When would be the best time in the dementia journey to introduce these?
2) What difference could these skills and tools make to someone's quality of life?
3) What difference could utilising these skills and tools make the people who are paid to provide care and support or any professional involved?

4) It is important to consider all potential outcomes of any actions and intervention initiated and to be prepared to respond effectively when there is an indication that something is about to go 'wrong'. In preparation, it is always good to consider any potential risks of initiating the use of these skills and tools and likewise the risk of not using these skills and tools. What could these risks be, and how would you respond?

5) What difficulties could be faced in developing an understanding of the person with dementia during the later stages of dementia?

6) How could these skills and tools be introduced during the later stages of the dementia journey?

7) What would need to happen to develop the confidence to utilise the skills and tools presented in this chapter?

7 Understanding behaviour and communication

This chapter covers:

- A description of behaviour as a form of communication
- An understanding of how to work alongside someone to reach an understanding of what someone is communicating through their behaviour
- Understanding behaviour as a response and an insight into a number of areas that could be influencing the person's behaviour
- A problem-solving and solution-focused approach
- An introduction to research that emphasises the importance of communication in the provision of care and support
- The importance of hearing the voice of the person with dementia
- The approaches and skills required to aid good approaches to communication
- A reminder of the principles of the Mental Capacity Act.

What is behaviour?

People with dementia may begin to behave differently in various stages of their dementia journey and how a person responds and behaves may depend on the form of dementia they have been diagnosed with. Please see Chapter 3 for more information on the dementia journey and different forms of the condition.

The person may develop different types of behaviours that are out of character. The most common types of behaviour include restlessness, repetitive behaviour, shouting, aggression, screaming, walking about a lot more, disturbed sleeping and waking during the night.

Living with dementia can be the cause of a person's behaviour. '*I think it's important that people realise that it is hard living with dementia – there's a big emotional impact*' (Harry, Social Care Institute for Excellence (SCIE), 2020). Dementia can cause confusion for the person and what otherwise would be deemed as familiar surroundings become frightening and unfamiliar. People with dementia often feel a sense of grief, loss, frustration, anger and hopelessness which can all be emotional states that directly influence how the person responds or behaves in given circumstances. A person's behaviour can be extreme and can be completely out of character, and these behaviours can be seen by many as negative.

Behaviour that can be deemed negatively or pose a challenge includes any '*actions that detract from the well-being of the individual due to the physical or psychological distress they cause*' (James, 2011). Behaviours that challenge can have a significant impact on the lives of people with dementia, and the lives of those around them. These behaviours can lead to distress and confusion.

The person's behaviour may be:

- a direct result of the symptom of dementia, especially in the case of Lewy bodies;
- a result of the difficulties related to dementia, for instance, language, disorientation or memory loss;
- a response to how the person is feeling due their experiences and interactions with others;
- a demonstration of boredom or frustration, especially if the person's social interaction and engagement in enjoyable activities has declined;
- related to physical pain the person is experiencing but is unable to express;
- a reaction to a threat even if this is a perceived threat.

If there has been a sudden change in the person's behaviour, particularly where the person becomes clearly confused and distressed, this is often the result of a physical health problem. A visit to the GP would rule out or identify any potential physical problems, side effects of medication or changes to mental health.

Explaining all aspects of a person's behaviour as an outcome of dementia may not be accurate as it is possible that the behaviour is a way of communicating an unmet need.

> *The times when I have felt aggressive it was because of the frustration of living with Alzheimer's – it was about how I felt, not a symptom. Let me give you an example. I have limited mobility – bad hip joint and can't walk easily – and that makes me angry and annoyed sometimes. But no one would say that was a symptom of a*

broken hip would they? They do that with dementia all the time too though don't they, and it can be incredibly frustrating.

(Roy, Social Care Institute for Excellence (SCIE), 2020)

Plato recognised that '*Human behavior flows from three main sources: desire, emotion and knowledge*'. Through their behaviour the person may be expressing unhappiness, frustration or confusion with an aspect of what is taking place around them. This could be based on what is actually happening around them or their perception of what is taking place around them.

Sundowning

The term 'sundowning' is particular to dementia and refers to a behaviour that occurs at a particular time of day, usually late afternoon and early evening. At this time people with dementia can become more agitated, confused and aggressive. This can be caused by a lack of sleep or disturbed sleep, a loss of a familiar routine, lots of noise, a response to medication or medication wearing off.

Communication

Within person-centred approaches to psychology, Abraham Maslow identified the feelings of security and affection as some of the main foundations for positive behaviour: '*The fact is that people are good, Give people affection and security, and they will give affection and be secure in their feelings and their behaviour*'. Making a commitment to discover what the person with dementia is communicating and acting upon this constitutes a positive way to respond to behaviours that are otherwise regarded negatively.

The first step in this journey is to see the world and the situation from the person's perspective. Adopting this mindset can support the identification of what is happening around or for the person, what is causing the upset and what solutions would address this. Through a commitment to this approach, people involved in the person's life can begin to learn what experiences, interactions and environmental factors influence a good or a negative emotional state for the person.

Solution circle

Once an appreciation of the person's perspective has been developed, there may be some long-standing issues identified. Finding a solution to these issues can be supported by a solution circle. This is a facilitated process which helps to identify new solutions to an issue or situation. There are four stages to this approach: firstly, the sharing of the issue; secondly, the sharing of ideas to resolve the problem; thirdly, identifying which ideas to try; and lastly, action planning. More details about solution circles can be found in Chapter 6 on page 163.

Learning logs

It can take time to fully understand a person's communication that is being shared through their behaviour. It may require adopting approaches of how to respond to the person's behaviour on the basis of what is believed to be what the person needs or wants at the time. It will take time to try these approaches and learn from them, adapting or changing the approach, with the intention of finding what works best for the person.

Learning logs are a way of recording this information; what the person did, who was there, what worked well, what didn't work well and finally, from what has been learnt, what needs to keep being done and what needs to be done differently.

This approach can help to identify how the person is communicating via their behaviour about their health, well-being, environment, the people around them and the way people are communicating with them.

Learning logs are similar to the 'Working/Not Working' exercise (introduced on page 155 of Chapter 6), but while 'Working/Not Working' focuses on what is going well and what is not working well for all members of the dementia care triad+1, learning logs focus solely on what is working well and what is not working well for the person with dementia and how they are communicating this.

Challenging and difficult times

It is recognised that everyone experiences challenging times and difficulties, including family members of those with dementia and those providing care and support.

> *The other day my sister lost her temper with me when I couldn't remember something – she's usually so good – and it was really really horrible – I cried and cried after she had gone, it was horrendous. It must be so hard for her to put up with me with a smile all the time.*
>
> (Sandy, Social Care Institute for Excellence (SCIE), 2020)

People with dementia and their families will experience difficult times as they come to terms with how their circumstances are changing their experience of day-to-day life and the long term plans they have in place. The changes happening in their lives will be beyond their control and they will be unwanted changes.

These experiences and changing circumstances can result in emotional responses:

- fear;
- anger;
- confusion;

- loss;
- grief;
- frustration;
- tiredness;
- stress;
- guilt.

> *What I really hate is having to ask for help – it makes me really angry with myself – and I get cross with others probably because I hate having to ask. It's hard when it feels like someone else is getting in the way of your independence. If I went down the road of asking for help from social services and all the official bodies, I'd lose some of the power to be able to do it myself – I wouldn't have the motivation – it would be, 'Well I'll ask someone to do it for me'.*
>
> (Roy, Social Care Institute for Excellence (SCIE), 2020)

Finding time to talk

Creating an opportunity to talk about emotions and experiences openly and without fear of judgement or ridicule may be helpful to:

- create a safe space for people to express their feelings;
- to support one another to find ways to recognise and address these feelings;
- to be open about how someone is feelings and their emotions in a way that doesn't have a negative impact;
- work together to identify what is the root cause to these feelings and look to see if there is anything that can be changed or done to overcome this.

It can be difficult to initiate a conversation about emotions and experiences. These conversations may be avoided due to concerns about; how people may respond, creating an awkward situation or making the circumstances worse.

There may be many reasons for a person to not be able to talk about feelings, or circumstances that have been created to prevent them from talking about feelings, some of which include:

- the person has become preoccupied with other activities and distractions, in essence filling their time to be able to take their mind off things and therefore they do not have the time to think about it in a constructive way or to talk about it;
- the person has difficulty in finding the words, or the right words, to express themselves;

- the person has concerns about what other people will think or how they will respond;
- the person has concerns about burdening other people or bringing additional worries or concerns into other people's lives.

When a person finds themselves in these circumstances, they may inadvertently, or intentionally, begin to express the way they are feeling through their behaviour.

Challenging behaviour?

The language used to describe a person's behaviour must also be carefully considered:

- 'difficult behaviours';
- 'challenging behaviour';
- 'behaviours that challenge'.

These statements promote the impression that the person is the root cause of the difficulty as it is their behaviour that is posing the challenge. However, in reality, it is most likely the person's behaviour is a response to an unmet need or want, or a representation of a disconnection between the person and those around them.

The use of this type of terminology when describing a person's behaviour lends to creating a negative reputation about them. The use of negative terminology such as 'challenging behaviour' can actually add to the problem as the person is likely to then feel worse about themselves, which will then continue to be communicated via their behaviour, further adding to the reputation they are acquiring of being 'challenging'.

Challenging circumstances

It is a good idea to develop an appreciation that it may not be the person who has 'challenging behaviour' but the circumstances the person finds themselves in are challenging for them.

> *People need to understand that you're frightened and alone. You start out on the pathway and often you're on your own. You can't understand why things are happening. Understanding the details of the problem removes the fear.*
>
> (Peter H, Social Care Institute for Excellence (SCIE), 2020)

To work in a manner that encourages a personalised approach, the person with dementia, their circumstances and the insights into their day-to-day experience that the person is providing through their behaviour need to be considered.

To achieve a person-centred response the following can to be explored:

- What is the person telling the people around them through their behaviour?

- What is happening around that person or to that person that is causing them to react in this way?
- Is there something happening to the person that we are not yet aware of, such as pain and discomfort?
- Is the person's needs being met in a way that makes sense to them and in a respectful manner that upholds their dignity?

Evidence based practice has demonstrated that when a person-centred approach is developed and delivered within dementia care and support there is a substantial reduction in negative experiences and therefore in instances of 'challenging behaviour' while simultaneously reducing pharmaceutical interventions (drugs) (McMaster University, 2019; Fazio et al, 2018).

When a person-centred approach is adopted and time is given to watch, listen and learn, we can begin to appreciate what the person is communicating:

- Has there been a change to their day-to-day routine that may be causing upset? For instance, a change in the people they are spending time with or a change in the things they are doing?
- Are the person's day-to-day routines dictated by the practices and routines of the care setting or of another person rather than built around their preferences and what matters to them?
- Has the person experienced something recently that could have caused upset that has not been resolved?

A conscientious effort to learn what the person is communicating through their behaviour can help to resolve some of the issues the person is experiencing while also supporting people to understand the person's feelings and the emotional support they need.

If the person's day-to-day life is working well for them and they have a good network of care and support around them, this is often reflected in how they are feeling, which, in turn, will reflect in the way they are with themselves and the people around them.

Learning about how someone is communicating through their behaviour

When someone is struggling to communicate this is often seen in their behaviour; unexpected and out of character changes in their behaviour. The people around the person, those that form the dementia care triad+1, can capture what they are beginning to learn and understand through a communication map as described later in this chapter. This approach helps to map out what is happening in a person's behaviour and what those supporting the person believe that are aiming to communicate. The communication map also encourages exploration around what response the person needs at that time.

A communication map encourages continued learning through trying different approaches consistently over a period of time until the right response is found.

Discovering what the person is communicating

Working through some explorative questions can help to gain an insight into what is happening to the person and pinpoint the root cause of any upset they are experiencing. Below is a list of questions that can aid the exploration:

- What is it that is happening around the person or to the person that is causing upset or discomfort?
- Was there anything that happened recently that could have caused them upset?
- Is there something that the person is wanting to know that they have not yet been told?
- Are they feeling insecure about anything, do they need reassurance?
- Is the person comfortable or are they experiencing discomfort?
- Is the person in any pain, is there anything that could indicate a secondary health issue? Weight loss or gain? Change of skin tone?
- Has there been a change to their daily routine?
- Are their preferences, those captured in the future planning work, being honoured?
- Is something that matters to the person being missed?
- Has there been any significant changes in their relationships?

What can be learnt from working through exploratory questions can lead to identifying what can be changed or put in place to better support the person.

It is then possible for people providing any care or support to respond to what they have learnt, leading to the person with dementia recognising that they are understood and that they continue to have choice and control in their life.

This could be demonstrated through, involving the person in changing the environment to better suit them, creating the opportunity to spend quality time with someone who the person wants to see or changing day-to-day routines so someone can get up and ready for the day in a way that suits them or to include the activities that are important to the person.

A problem-solving and solution-focused approach

Taking a problem-solving approach can help to identify the cause of the behaviour or what the person is communicating and to find a positive solution.

A problem-solving approach covers three steps:

1. Define the problem.

   What is happening at the moment to the person that is causing concern?

   What element of the person's behaviour is a cause of concern?

   Is the impact of the person's behaviour significantly affecting them?

   Is the impact of the person's behaviour significantly affecting other people?

   Is the reaction from other people also causing a problem?

2. Look at the situation and circumstances.

   When does the person behave in this way?

   Is there a pattern around when the person's behaviour occurs?

   Where does the person's behaviour take place?

   Is there a pattern relating to the place when the person behaves in this way?

   Who is present when the person behaves in this way?

   Is this behaviour occurring when certain people are present? If so, which people? Are any patterns in the person's behaviour noticeable?

   What else have we noticed about the person when they behave in this way?

3. Think about the solution.

   Can the person express how they felt at the time?

   Is there an approach that has not yet been tried that could support the person?

   Is there something that could be tried to aid communication?

   Is there a change needed in the approach to how the person is cared for or supported?

   How can the ideas of what to try be communicated with the rest of the dementia care triad?

Forward planning

Thinking ahead and planning for what good care and support would look like for the person in the current and later stages of dementia can help to reduce the likelihood of any negative experiences.

Planning ahead in this way can support the aims around preventative practice in the sense of aiming to avoid the situation where the person is communicating their upset and frustration, of any given situation, through their behaviour.

The approach to responding to behaviour covered in this chapter is in line with a person-centred approach. Other considerations when supporting someone who is behaving in a manner that is having a negative impact on themselves and others include:

- ensuring the person's daily routine is based on their preferences and it is clearly communicated;
- introducing an activity that soothes the person when they are agitated, for instance, hand massage, aromatherapy, music or light therapy;
- making sure that the person has the opportunity to spend quality time with people, sharing a task together or doing something together that both parties equally enjoy;
- supporting and encouraging the person to keep active doing something that they enjoy, such as going for a walk, going swimming or dancing;
- creating opportunities for the person to have a change of scenery and to spend time somewhere they enjoy.

Utilising the skills

Utilising the skills introduced in Chapter 4 when thinking about behaviour:

- Skills Box 1 – Skills that promote respect and dignity.

  The skill titled 'Recognition' on page 146 of Chapter 6 plays a vital role in appreciating behaviour.

- Skills Box 2 – Skills that help people with dementia make choices.

  'Good Day and Bad Day' exercise – helps to inform people providing care and support as to what needs to be in place for the person to be able to experience good days and how to avoid situations and experiences that would create a bad day.

  Communication map – captures the detail of what a person is communicating and how they communicate it. It is also a method to capture the detail of how to best approach communicating with them and how to let them know what

The 'Communication' section below introduces skills and approaches that enable the voice of people with dementia to be heard.

Taking care of the carers

When a person's behaviour significantly changes, families, carers and people providing support in a paid capacity may find it useful to have some strategies to avoid negative situations.

Here are some ideas that might help in these situations:

- Try to distract the person, see what is in the immediate environment and what would capture their attention. If there is something there, use this as an opportunity to gently distract the person.
- Have something on you that is of interest to the person which can be useful as a gentle way to distract the person or re-focus their attention – a picture or a book, for instance.
- Become familiar with what could cause the person to react and behave in an agitated or unusual way; nosy places, busy places, certain smells or sounds, and avoid these places whenever possible.
- Consider the potential cause of the behaviour, is the person tired, hungry, in pain, frustrated or bored? If this could be the root cause of how the person is responding, think about what can be done to alleviate the cause.
- If the person is rude, do not attempt to correct them. Remember that the person is living their reality and perspective of the world. To correct them or try to change their current reality could lead to more confusion or agitation. Again, think about how the person could be distracted and employ this strategy.
- If the person has become aggressive, provide them some space to help them calm down and anything that is known to help them reduce their heightened state. Remain safe to avoid being harmed at this time and do not respond with aggression.
- Remain as calm as possible, try to not get angry and upset. Remember that the person is not behaving this way on purpose.
- Consider in each situation, is the person's behaviour really a problem? Try to remain rational in the situation and the response.
- Carers should make sure they take some time out and have some rest to be able to recuperate from a situation that they have found difficult to manage. To have an opportunity to talk to people from the dementia care triad+1 about it, they may also have some useful suggestions.

Here are some insights from a family carer, Janet, about the lessons she's learnt to help her cope with caring for her husband Martin who lives with dementia.

Lessons I have learnt (the painful way!)

- Be positive.
- Share the diagnosis with your family and friends as soon as you can. This brought me great relief that I could stop compensating.

- Remove everything from your life which causes you stress (work, early morning appointments, hospital visits etc).
- Carry on with all the things you enjoy for as long as you can.
- Try not to get angry with each other; it creates more stress for you both.
- Find a good carer(s) ASAP. It spreads the load and allowed Martin and his ladies time to become good friends.
- Look for the joy (there is some, trust me).

Family

- Caring is an all-consuming onerous task. It remains an overriding responsibility and cannot be denied, delegated or ignored but the emotional and physical support from family is of immeasurable value. We are very lucky.

Friends

- Amazingly and thankfully, all our friends have stuck by us (so far!). Friends keep you sane, they make you laugh, they give you perspective. We have some very lovely friends.

Where are we now?

- Martin remains fit and mobile. He sleeps well and his appetite, though small, is still healthy. His memories are of his early days. His speech is coherent but frequently nonsensical. He has no recollection of names or faces. He has no concept of time or place. Although very happy for the most part, Martin can sometimes be frustrated and angry early in the morning, particularly when getting washed and dressed.

The joy

- As time passes our world shrinks. But it is a world filled with love. Hugs and kisses are the best medicine. Laughter is always better than tears. Each day starts with a cuddle. Martin's smile still lights up the room.

> **Janet and Martin** *live in North Oxfordshire. They have recently taken the big step of employing a live in carer. Janet says it is 'to help Martin and I to continue to be able to get the best of each other' (Young Dementia UK, n.d.).*

Questions to aid reflection

1) Based on the information provided so far in this chapter, how would you approach behaviour differently in the future?

2) Upon reflection, are there any experiences you have had of managing a person's unexpected behaviour that you would now respond to differently?

3) How could you share the information provided in this chapter to others supporting people with dementia?

4) What impact would sharing this information have on people who are confronted with unexpected behaviour shown by the people they care for?

Effective communication: tools and approaches to use to support people with dementia

The approaches that are pertinent for developing and understanding behaviour and aiding communication include:

- removing unwanted distractions so that those involved in the conversations or interaction are better able to focus and concentrate on the conversation;
- introducing items that aid communication, for instance, pictures or objects that hold meaning for the person;
- giving communication the time it needs, this shouldn't be rushed as what is learnt during conversation is fundamental to achieving a good understanding and therefore providing a good support and care.

Good communication is key in achieving good outcomes for all people within the dementia care triad+1: people with dementia, informal carers, health and social care professionals and the community.

Information needs to be shared with the person with dementia in a manner that enables them to be involved in the discussion and exercise control over the decisions that are being made about their future, including their care and support.

People supporting the person with dementia need to explore all approaches to communication to identify the approach that works best and enables the person to maintain control over their decisions, make future-based decisions and continue to exercise control over day-to-day choices.

This may involve exercising some creativity and a willingness to develop new ways of approaching communication to find an approach that works for the person.

There are a number of established approaches to communication which can be explored, including objects of reference, symbols and Talking Mats, which are all introduced later in this chapter.

Practice example: Philip found it difficult to respond to direct questions and would easily become distracted by the activities going on around him. When asked his opinion about something, he found it difficult to express what he liked and what he didn't like, and this could lead to him feeling frustrated. We wanted to find a way to communicate with Philip in a manner that worked for him and didn't create frustration. We had tried using pictures to explore what he would like, we had tried symbols and we had attempted looking on the internet.

When we thought we had exhausted all the options, one of the person-centred planning facilitators suggested we meet in the local town where Philip had lived most of his adult life.

The meeting was arranged in a local café that Philip used to go to on a regular basis when he lived in the area. On the way to the café, the person with Philip noticed how much he was looking around, looking into shop windows and how much he seemed to enjoy being back in the town.

In the small group meeting Philip decided that, rather than spend a long time in the café, it would be good to make the most of the opportunity to revisit some places that he used to go to on a regular basis, such as the post office, greengrocers, charity shops and the local pub.

So much was learnt on this visit about the friendships Philip had in the area, the shops he really liked, the things he looked for in these shops, the items that captured his attention.

Sometimes good communication does not require talking or discussing but simply watching, observing and learning.

Communication is critical to ensuring that the person with dementia can maintain a quality of life and ensure that their wishes and needs are understood fully and responded to. A person's identity is maintained through good communication as it enables the person to share their preferences and wishes for all aspects of their life.

The Alzheimer's Society has produced some useful information and advice regarding good communication on their 'Communicating and Dementia' webpage (Alzheimer's Society, n.d.a; Alzheimer's Society, n.d.b). These approaches can support the person with dementia and the people around them to engage in positive two-way communication.

Good tips for good communication

Communication takes place in a variety of ways: small conversations throughout the day or detailed and meaningful conversation which has a specific purpose. Here are some tips that help to facilitate healthy two-way communication:

- Make sure that the person with dementia can see you clearly.
- Make eye contact, as this helps the person with dementia focus on you.
- Minimise background noises such as the radio, TV or other people's conversations.

When communicating, speak clearly and calmly in short sentences, use everyday language, avoid jargon and maintain a steady pace, allowing time between sentences for the person to process the information and to respond. Talk to the person in a positive, respectful and patient manner. Do not alter the tone of your voice, nor adopt a tone that would appear patronising.

At all times during group conversations, do not talk about the person as if they are not there and involve the person in the conversation whenever possible and appropriate to do so.

Making choices

When supporting the person to make a choice, be mindful of communicating with the person in a manner that they can engage with, for instance offer a manageable amount of options so as to avoid overload which can lead to confusion or frustration. Similarly, avoid asking too many direct questions in quick succession without giving the time for the person to answer the question.

Where there are a number of questions to address, ask the person these one at a time over a comfortable timeframe or over a number of conversations, phrasing them in such a way that allows for a 'yes' or 'no' answer where possible.

Explore further with conversations and open questions that encourage a more detailed response when this is possible.

When communicating for the purpose of learning and developing a greater understanding of the person and what is important to them, actively listen to the person's responses, including their spoken responses and those given through facial expressions, gestures and body language. To gain clarity and avoid misunderstanding, repeat back to the person what you believe you have understood and check with them to see if you are right.

Be mindful of body language, physical presence and physical contact when communicating with the person with dementia. The person could read body language, sudden movements or facial expressions negatively which may cause upset or distress. This will lead to communication becoming more difficult.

Never stand too close or stand over someone to communicate as this will feel intimidating. Instead, respect the person's personal space and drop below their eye level. This will help the person to feel more in control of the situation.

At times, communicating can be frustrating for the person with dementia and the people around them. If there are signs those frustrations are beginning to occur, take a break and come back to the conversation later when it is a better time.

Preparing for a conversation

Before entering any conversation, allow enough time to reflect on past conversations and what has been learnt from these regarding what creates a positive communication exchange. Take what has been learnt to be prepared and ready for the next opportunity to have a conversation and learn more about the person.

If a conversation with a person with dementia is approached or conducted with no preparation or consideration for creating a positive experience, the communication exchange can leave the person feeling frustrated and confused. As such, a conscious commitment should be made to ensure that all communication leads to a positive exchange that does not have a negative impact on the person with dementia.

Physical barriers to communication

The success of a communication exchange is not solely dependent on the words chosen, the tone of voice or the approach used. Physical factors can either aid or hinder communication for people with dementia. Think about the environment. Are there a lot of distractions? Are there other people using the same space? Is the space and the people in it busy and moving around the environment? Are there other conversations taking place at the same time? Is there music or a television playing in the background? What is the lighting like? Is it bright enough to be able to see well?

Think about how the person is feeling. Have they slept well? Are they hungry? Are they feeling well at the moment? Are they in any pain or discomfort? Was it a positive experience the last time you spent time together? Is there anything that needs to be addressed to rebuild the relationship or rapport with them?

Think about the timing of the conversation. Is this a good time for the person? Does this conversation or meeting change an important part of the person's routine? Is there something else that should be happening right now that the person is expecting? Will it cause confusion, or frustration, if this doesn't happen? Would they prefer to be doing something else?

Consideration of these factors and planning accordingly can make a significant and worthwhile difference and lead to a positive experience and good communication.

Hearing loss

Most people experience hearing loss over the age of seventy. This may be a factor that is affecting a person's ability to engage fully in verbal communication. The Alzheimer's Society has produced useful guidance about communicating with a person with dementia who may also be experiencing hearing loss (Alzheimer's Society, n.d.).

Communicating with a person who has hearing loss

- Speak slightly slower than usual but try to keep the natural rhythms of your speech.
- Do not shout or over-exaggerate words as this will distort your speech.
- Do not cover your mouth as this will interfere with lip-reading. The person should be able to see your face clearly – get onto the same level as them so that they are looking at your face straight on.
- Consider the physical environment – make sure the area is quiet and well-lit.
- Use visual clues – write your message down if the person is able to read and use objects or pictures to help them understand what you're trying to convey. For example, show the person the meals they can choose from.

Reflection

- If you were struggling to understand the message that was being conveyed to you, how would you like the person speaking to you to act?
- What type of environment might make it difficult for a person with dementia to participate in a conversation in a meaningful way?
- How do we engage in a conversation with someone with dementia that is respectful and avoids a patronising approach?

Involving the right people in communication

Family carers who hold a longstanding relationship with the person with dementia have a particularly important role to play in supporting communication. People who have a close and trusted relationship with the person with dementia are more likely to be able to facilitate, as defined by Tom Kitwood (1997) in his '12 Positive Interactions' as discussed in Chapter 1. The role of a facilitator requires a great deal of trust as the interpretation of a person's communication needs to be without any bias towards the facilitator's own preferences and wishes.

Communication within the dementia care triad+1

Good and regular communication between the people who form the person's support network is an important part of achieving the best approach to care and support.

To achieve the principles of good communication, as developed by the Care Service Improvement Partnership (CSIP), the following should be considered and put into practice.

- Always believe that communication is possible.
- Focus on the non-verbal signs as well as the verbal.
- Avoid making assumptions; check things out with the person.
- Make your communication a two-way process that engages the person.
- Avoid the use of jargon or complicated explanations.
- Keep your style of conversation 'down to earth'.
- Do not become patronising or sound childish.
- Avoid questions that contain the word 'why?' as these are 'justification' questions which can be unreasonable to expect a person to answer.
- Be a good listener; give the person your full attention and resist the temptation to finish their sentences or talk for them.
- Talk at a slower pace so that the person has the opportunity to understand what is being said.
- Maintain a calm and unhurried approach.
- Above all, don't be afraid to say: 'I don't understand'.

(Care Services Improvement Partnership (CSIP) National Older People's Mental Health Programme, 2007, p 19)

Reflection

- How would this approach to communication improve the relationships within the dementia care triad+1?
- Could practising these principles strengthen relationships in the wider community?
- Is there any additional principle that could strengthen those already presented by the CSIP?

The principles set out by CSIP would address some of the common issues that occur within health and social care where communication is often at the root of the problem. The CSIP communication principles would avoid actions and decisions that are based on assumptions and opinions and would promote a well-informed approach founded on the information that has been shared by the person with dementia and their family, friends, carers and support workers.

Recognising that the ability to communicate changes over time

In the early stages of dementia, if an early diagnosis has been given, the person may find it possible to share their views and opinions, should they be given the right opportunity to do so. The abilities of people with dementia to engage with communication may vary day-to-day and, as people reach the later stages of dementia, their ability to communicate may rely heavily on body language, gestures and facial expressions. All contributions to the communication exchange need to be recognised and valued and those involved have a responsibility to make sure the interaction is a positive experience where people feel valued and respected.

Practice example: Mr M was diagnosed with dementia eight years ago and he is now in the later stages of the condition. Mr M has lost all his strength in his body, is often in bed and is cared for 24 hours a day. He remains living in the family home and he has support workers/care workers with him each day. When Mr M is happy he lays still, his eyes look soft and his face is relaxed. People caring for Mr M know how to read the signs that he is happy. At other times, he can be agitated, and his family and support workers have learnt that when he is restless in bed he is too warm, when his face is tense he wants to move position and when his eyes are alert he is in pain.

During the middle to later stages of dementia, it may be increasingly difficult for the person to articulate their views. At this time, the person's views and opinions may continue to be gained by moving away from a reliance on words to communicate. The different communication methods are known as total communication.

Total communication

Total communication refers to an approach to communication that recognises all methods of communication:

- speech;
- lip-reading;
- spelling;
- gestures;
- facial expressions;
- formal signs;
- behaviour;
- body language.

Total communication supports the belief that all behaviour is a form of communication. Developing an awareness of each one of these methods, then exploring and finding the one, or combination of approaches, that works best will support the maintenance and development of strong and positive relationships.

Resources to support communication

There are numerous resources and approaches available to aid communication:

- **Symbols** – Using symbols to represent everyday objects, feelings and people, to aid decision-making and conversation.

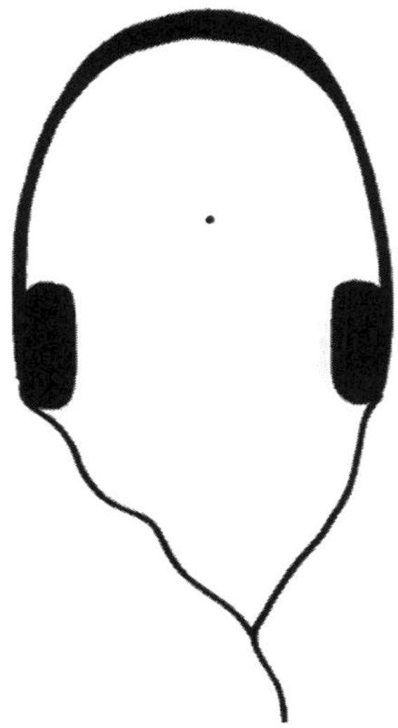

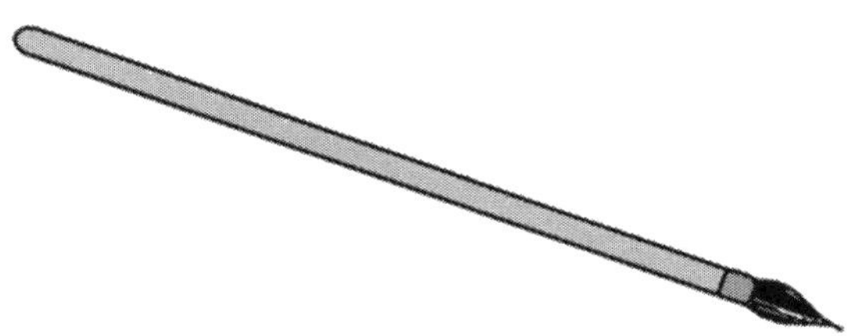

- **Talking Mats** – This tool utilises a combination of symbols to create a story or a question. The symbols are positioned on a mat in an order that represents the conversation or question, for instance, if someone has been swimming the story about going swimming will be organised on the mat to aid a conversation about the experience to establish important information such as: was it enjoyable? Would the person like to go again? Does anything about the experience need to change for it to work better for the person?

These images can be found through an organisation called Talking Mats (2013). They are based in Scotland and provide practical advice and guidance on communication. In a blog post describing training they provided to families of people with dementia, the family members participating in the training found that Talking Mats helped them see that their spouse was satisfied with many aspects of their life. The family members found this reassuring as many had made the assumption that the person with dementia was frustrated or discontent (Mackay, 2016).

In another blog post, Talking Mats shared the positive feedback from care workers, based at two residential care homes in Denmark, regarding the communication tool:

- *Talking Mats helps people to understand their options and thereby motivates* [them] *to social activities, eating, physical exercise, etc.*
- *Talking Mats increases the possibility of active participation in caregiving plans*
- *The Talking Mats conversations support a closer relation between* [the] *elderly and care giver*

(Matthews, 2016)

- **Pictures** – Images that are relevant to the person with dementia can aid communication. It is important to choose the images carefully to ensure that they will produce a positive reaction for the person and not one of anxiety and confusion. Having an understanding of the person's interests, passions and the people and times that have been important to them can help in selecting the right pictures.

  Pictures to Share (n.d.) is a community interest company working with people with dementia who have, through their work, revealed the power of an image and storytelling to engage a person with dementia. They advocate that this lies not only in the visual and neurological accessibility of the image, but also when the image offers the following:

  - beautiful and vivid colours or subjects;
  - strong photographic or painting style;
  - human or animal subjects looking directly out at the viewer;
  - a strong sense of narrative that encourages storytelling;
  - a strong line or sense of texture that will encourage tactile exploration;

- showing of positive emotions such as happiness;
- an element of humour that does not demand sophisticated interpretation.

Images to be avoided include anything that could be disturbing for someone with dementia, such as people in an aggressive or distressed state, or showing vulnerable people or animals at risk. These can lead to feelings of anxiety or distress that people with dementia may be unable to rationalise.

- **Objects of reference** – Objects that are relevant to the person or to the subject being communicated are useful to aid conversation. It is good to use objects consistently each time the same topic is discussed, and to think creatively about how to use smaller items to represent bigger objects or objects to represent an activity or emotion. For example, referring to a key ring to represent leaving the house or a small towel to represent the choice to have a shower. Objects of reference over time become a form of two-way communication where the person uses the object to express to someone what they want when they are not able to use the words to express this. Therefore, the objects that have been used to aid communication need to be kept in an accessible place for the person with dementia as well as people providing care, support or companionship.
- **Timelines** – Timelines are a useful way to support someone to remember, or become less anxious about, their daily routines or to prepare for an event happening in the near future.

An individual can become confused about the following elements of events and routines:

- the order for daily tasks and routines, for example, when getting ready in the morning;
- on the run up to a holiday or a short break; the person may get confused about when this will be taking place, when they are leaving, how they are getting there, who they are going with, where they are going and for what reasons they are going;
- when expecting a visit from family or from home care, the person can become confused about when their loved ones or home care staff are intending to arrive, who is coming, what they are visiting for.

A timeline is a reference point to remind a person of what will be taking place, when it will be happening and some of the finer details to support the person's understanding.

The visual timelines form a representation of a routine or a visual countdown to when an event is taking place, whether this be a small event such as going shopping or a bigger event such as a holiday or a house move.

Timelines provide a greater sense of control in a person's day-to-day life, while reducing confusion and anxiety.

Here are some examples of timelines which demonstrate how they can be implemented in practice:

– A countdown in days to when a person is going to visit a family member, go somewhere for a break or a holiday or when an event is happening. Using a calendar of dates which are clearly marked when past is a good way of having a visual timeline for this purpose.

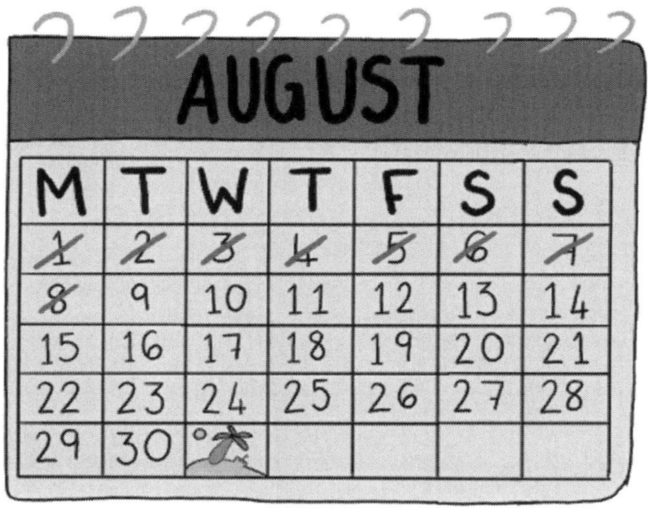

– A daily task broken down into manageable steps, such as the example shown below that gives a person's morning routine. These routines will be particular to the individual. Therefore, each person's timeline would look unique.

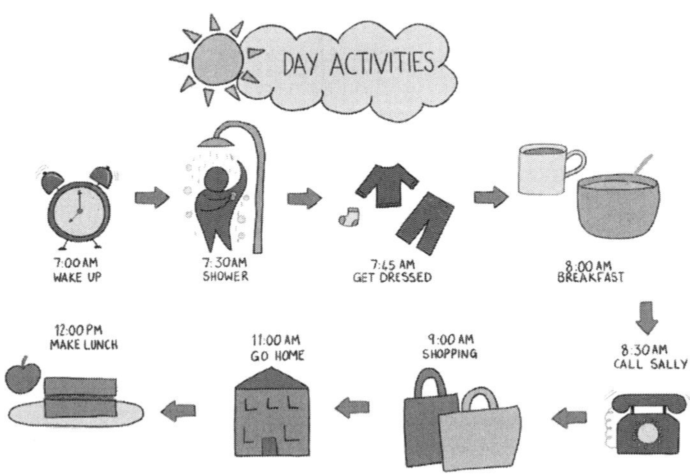

- **iPad and touchscreen technology** – Embracing technology can be a supportive means of communicating with people with dementia as well as opening up new avenues to record people's lives, achievements and to support decision-making.

  A report study by the University of Worcester in 2011 (Upton et al, 2011) showcased the many benefits of the use of touchscreen technology within a care service setting. These benefits included:

  - supported reminiscence;
  - aiding recall;
  - increasing interpersonal interaction;
  - intergenerational communication;
  - staff–resident relationships;
  - improving quality of life;
  - ease of use;
  - positive impact on the wider care environment.

  > *There is now a wide array of apps available for iPads and touchscreen devices that are intended to aid communication. Using the terminology 'communication tool' in the App Store on the device will lead to a list of potential apps to be utilised, for instance, 'Know Me – Communicating Personhood" by Know Me Inc. (Know Me Inc., 2021)*

  Many speech and language therapists are now trained in touchscreen technology and the applications available to aid communication and can therefore provide valuable advice. Some speech and language therapy departments are also able to loan the equipment to trial before deciding whether the investment of purchasing a device will be worthwhile.

- **Communication maps** – A communication map captures two-way communication:

  1. how a person is communicating;
  2. how to communicate with the person.

  A communication map provides an insight into how a person is expressing themselves and communicating with others, as well as strategies to successfully communicate with them in a manner that they will understand.

  The information added to a communication map is gathered from the individual, the people who are important to them and the people who have a good understanding of how they communicate, including those within the dementia care triad+1. This tool is especially useful when a person has stopped using words and is relying heavily on the people around them to be able to interpret their body language, behaviour, gestures, sounds and other non-verbal forms of communication.

Communication maps are intended to be used when:

– there are a number of people caring or supporting the person and a consistent, but not robotic, approach would be beneficial across the team;

– when there is an effort to identify what the person is communicating.

The completion of a communication map can provide a focus to those involved and assist the process of learning about how the person is communicating. While developing it those involved may realise that they had previously made assumptions about what the person is communicating and, through adopting this approach, these assumptions can be tested and reviewed. Therefore, a completed communication map helps to fine tune the understanding held by those supporting and caring for the person with dementia.

Communication maps need to be reviewed regularly and amended to make sure the content reflects the current communication adopted by and understanding of the person with dementia. Regular reviews also help to ensure that anyone following the information provided in the communication map will achieve the best possible results when communicating with the person.

HOW I COMMUNICATE

WHEN JOE BLOGGS DOES THIS	WE THINK IT MEANS/IT DOES MEAN	WE SHOULD RESPOND BY?	IF WE DO NOT LISTEN OR RESPOND THIS WILL HAPPEN	WHAT COULD MAKE THE SITUATION WORSE?
SMILES	HAPPY, LIKES WHAT IS GOING ON AROUND HIM	CARRYING ON THE MOOD IN A POSITIVE WAY		IF THE MOOD IN THE ROOM CHANGED
CRIES	UPSET, ANGRY	TRYING TO CHEER JOE UP WITH MUSIC.	JOE WILL GET MORE UPSET AND DISTRESSED	CARERS/PEOPLE IGNORING JOE.

HOW TO COMMUNICATE WITH ME

WHEN WE NEED TO TELL THE FOCUS PERSON THIS, OR LET THEM KNOW THIS...	WE SHOULD SAY OR DO THIS...	WE KNOW THE PERSON UNDERSTANDS WHEN THEY DO OR SAY...	AND WE SHOULD RESPOND BY...
THEIR LUNCH IS READY	"YOUR LUNCH IS READY, ARE YOU READY TO EAT?"	SMILE THEY ARE READY TO START THE MEALTIME ROUTINE. WHEN THEY SHOUT, THEY DO NOT WANT TO START THEIR MEAL.	GETTING THE FOCUS PERSON READY FOR THEIR MEAL. PUT THEIR MEAL SOMEWHERE APPROPRIATE TO REHEAT LATER

- **Decision-making tables** – While it is important to recognise that people with dementia may have an impaired ability to make decisions, it is also essential to realise that their decision-making ability will vary. This will largely depend on them as an individual, their circumstances, how they are feeling at the time of making a decision and the stage of the dementia journey that they have reached. At all times, it must be assumed that the person has the capacity to make decisions, as stated in the principles of the Mental Capacity Act 2005 (Mental Capacity Act 2005). It is the responsibility of those supporting the person to utilise a range of methods of communication to engage with the person to enable them to be involved in the decision-making process. More information about mental capacity can be found in Chapter 2.

  A decision-making table helps to capture the important decisions in a person's life and how these decisions are made.

  The level of 'importance' of the decision is judged by the impact this decision has on the person's quality of life, no matter how big or small the choice is. This could include decisions about where the person chooses to live, what specialist health treatment they wish to receive and it also can capture day-to-day decisions such as what the person wants to wear and what they choose to eat.

  Decision-making tables help to record:

  – the decisions the person wants to be in control of;

  – how a person wants to make these decisions;

  – what support they need to make the decisions;

  – whom they would like to make the decision on their behalf if, and when, they are not able to do so.

DECISION MAKING AGREEMENT

IMPORTANT DECISIONS IN MY LIFE	HOW I MUST BE INVOLVED	WHO WILL MAKE THE FINAL DECISION
WHAT I HAVE TO EAT	I MUST BE SHOWN OPTIONS TO HELP ME MAKE A DECISION	I WILL
WHAT MEDICATION I TAKE	I MUST ATTEND ALL MEDICAL APPOINTMENTS. WHEN I AM NOT HAVING A GOOD TIME I WILL NOT ENGAGE IN THESE DECISIONS	MY BROTHER

A completed decision-making table can ensure that:

– the person with dementia maintains as much control as possible;

– the person's preferences are known;

- everyone involved is clear on the important decisions and how these need to be made;
- everyone is clear about their role in supporting the person to make a decision.

A decision-making table can continue to support a person through their dementia journey. The content of a decision-making table should be checked at regular intervals to ensure the information in the table is still accurate and representative of the person and their circumstances. The person is fully involved in checking the content and discussions about this at every stage of the journey.

- **Timelines of change** – This is a useful summary of significant changes, achievements and events. The information recorded on a timeline of change can be helpful in aiding conversation with the person to be able to identify topics to talk about. A record of the person's recent events can also help to observe changes in the person's memory and ability to recollect.

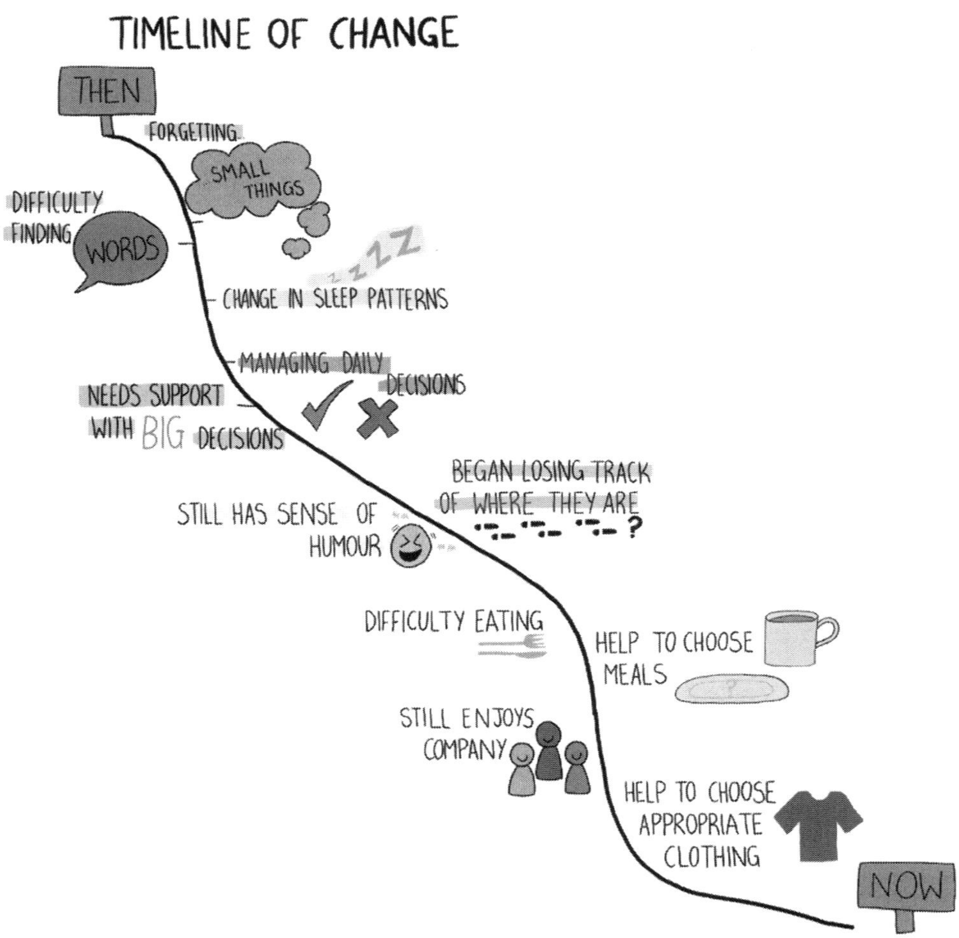

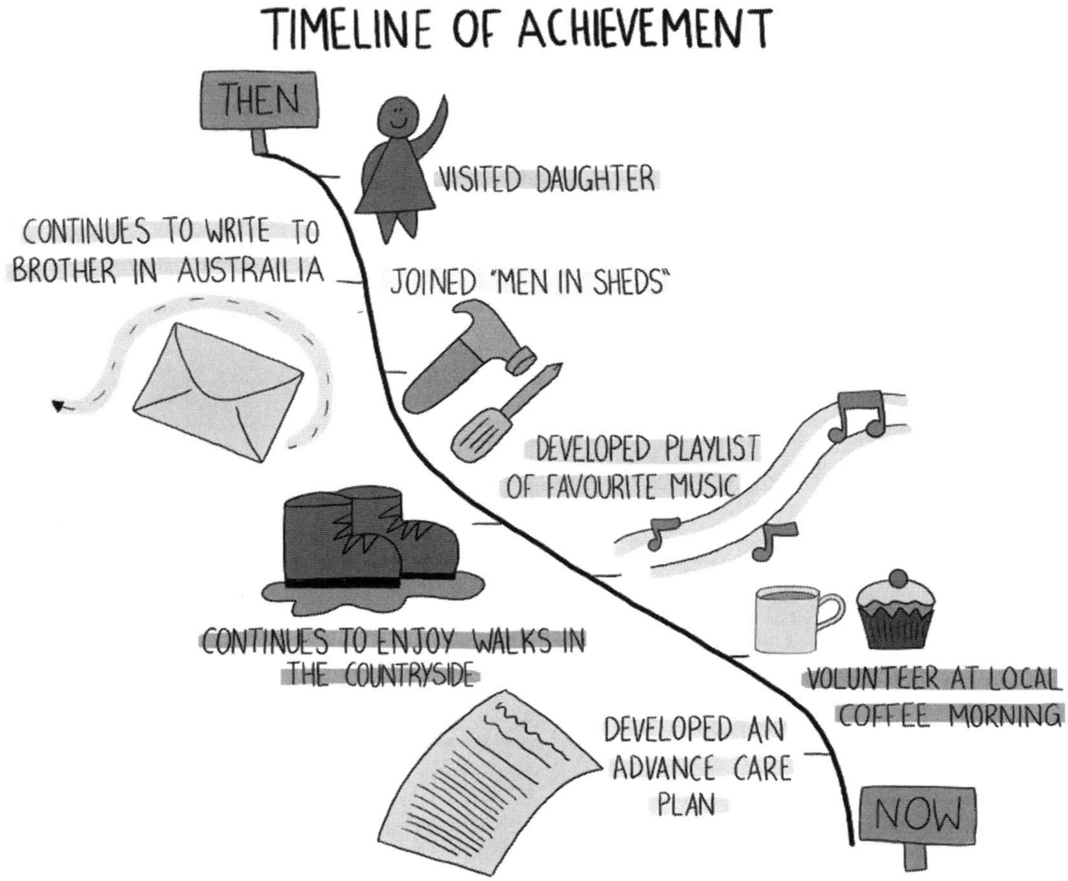

Having a voice

The importance of hearing the views and opinions of people with dementia was highlighted when, in 1996, Malcom Goldsmith wrote *Hearing the Voice of People with Dementia: Opportunities and Obstacles*, a seminal book in the study of dementia. The book advocated that people with dementia had a voice and that, in listening to this voice and responding to what had been learnt, their care and support could be provided in a manner that improved quality of life. Later writers, such as Christine Bryden (2015) and Lucy Whitman (2015), have explored this idea further, providing insight into the positive difference made to a person's day-to-day experience if those around them truly listened to them.

True and real involvement

People with dementia should be actively involved in any decisions that are to be made about their life, their care and their support.

This can be challenging in the later stages of dementia as the person may no longer be using words to communicate, they may find it difficult to comprehend what is happening around them and to be involved in conversations. Even in these circumstances, the principle still stands that the person should be involved. So, the challenge of ensuring that the person with dementia is involved in decisions made about them is the responsibility of those organising the discussions. To find a way to overcome the barriers, consider what would support the person's involvement and plan for this to be available.

Reflection

- What could you do to prepare for a discussion to ensure the person is involved and part of the decision-making?
- As someone who is looking to provide good care and support, what would you demonstrate in practice to support the person to be involved in the discussion and to assist them in making their own decisions?
- Considering what has already been covered in this book, what could you utilise to support a positive outcome?
- Is there any time when the person with dementia should not be involved on ethical and moral grounds?

Skills that enable the voice of people with dementia to be heard

Developing skills that will help people with dementia make their views known and their voice heard is an important element of providing good support. This includes the interaction that occurs between the person with dementia and another person, a linear interaction, as well as within larger groups interactions – such as the interaction between those in the dementia care triad+1.

Developing positive approaches to communication, which has been established as a two-way process and a means of exchanging ideas, feelings and memories, can support everyone involved to feel heard and understood. Everyone involved should be given the opportunity to express their views and to share their opinions. It must be remembered that the person with dementia may need to be supported to make their views and opinions known using the techniques introduced in this chapter and in Chapter 4.

In a conversation focused on the right care and support, the person's opinions and views should take precedence wherever possible and the views and opinions of others ought not to overshadow the views of the person with dementia. Paid-for carers and professionals also have an important role in making sure the person with dementia and family carers have an opportunity to share their views about the sort of care and support the person with dementia wants, and how, or if, what the person wants fits in with what the primary family carers themselves want.

To facilitate these conversations the following areas need to be considered.

Removing unwanted stimuli

This form of enabling communication occurs when the family carer or the health and social care professional reduces the number of stimuli that are impeding the person's ability to communicate.

Practice example: Mr E, who has dementia, was not responding to what was being said in the meeting because the sight of his daughter gardening through the patio doors was distracting him. However, Mrs E and the Community Mental Health Nurse (CMHN) tried to get him involved in the conversation. The CMHN suggested changing positions with Mr E so that he was not distracted by the activity in the garden. Mr E agreed and became more actively involved in the conversation once he was able to focus on the conversation.

Creating the stimuli that aids communication

If it is clear that a certain stimulus encourages a person to communicate, try to make sure that this stimulus is available at the time you want to communicate with the individual. This can assist the person in relaxing, being in a happy state and talking openly.

Practice example: Mr W had a fun-filled and lively lifestyle; he loved spending time with his children and was always singing, dancing and going to see shows. His daughter remembers how he used to dance and sing as they walked along the street together. These days Mr W is often in his 'own world' and does not recognise his daughter. The nurse in the home where he lived helped to organise some music on an MP3 player with a set of headphones for Mr W to listen to music that he enjoys. When Mr W listens to this music his posture changes, he recognises people and engages fluently in conversation, expressing himself and his emotions.

This approach has been documented in the film *Alive Inside* (please see the Further Reading section at the end of the chapter).

Getting in the right position

The spatial position in which people place themselves affects the ability of the person with dementia to communicate. It is important to be aware of what positioning will aid the flow of communication and to organise the space to enable this to happen.

Practice example: Mrs D invited CMHN to sit next to Mr D, who has dementia. However, Mrs D took her seat on the other side of the room from them. Throughout the conversation

Mr D continually looked to Mrs D for support and assistance before responding to the conversation or to questions. The CMHN noticed this and realised that Mr D was not feeling comfortable about the conversation. The CMHN then suggested a change in seating arrangement. The CMHN exchanged seats with Mrs D and moved a chair closer so that the three of them sat at an equal distance from each other. Mr D appeared more relaxed with this and contributed more fluently to the conversation and Mr D was able to hear clearly what was being said and therefore was able to get more involved.

Giving communication the time it needs

When a person is having trouble with communicating it is important not to rush them. Giving people the time to express themselves is important in making sure that they are understood, including their needs or wants.

Confirming that the support and care they are receiving is working well for them depends on friends', family members' and paid-for carers' ability to understand the person.

Practice example: Mrs C can take a long time to think about what she wants to say and to find the right words when she is replying to people. Mrs C's support worker had noticed that people in Mrs C's life were answering the questions for her when there were long gaps between a question being asked of Mrs C and her response. The support worker felt that people were answering for Mrs C as a way to help her, that some people felt uncomfortable with the length of silence and that other people were answering as they had reached the conclusion that Mrs C was no longer able to answer the questions. The support worker was concerned that Mrs C was losing her opportunity to express herself and that the other people in her life were losing their chance to fully understand Mrs C and what she wanted. Mrs C's support worker talked to the group about this and encouraged everyone to give Mrs C the time to answer and, by doing this, the group began to appreciate that some of the answers that had been given on Mrs C's behalf by others were not quite what Mrs C wanted.

Providing opportunities to talk

Life can get incredibly busy, with appointments, household tasks and family commitments. People who are living in a service setting, for example, in a supported living scheme or a care home, can find themselves in an environment with other people and staff members focused on their daily routines and tasks. In whichever setting a person with dementia finds themselves, making time to talk is vital, whether the conversation happens via having a chat over a cup of tea or through spending time with the person during one of their favourite activities.

Structured or timetabled time for conversations, such as review meetings, should not become the only times for meaningful conversation. Instead, opportunities for a conversation should be captured as they occur.

Practice example: Miss D lives in a care home with 39 other residents and to be able to manage everything that needs to be done within the home everyone living there has to follow set routines. Everyone gets up at a set time, has breakfast at the same time and continues to follow the routines applied in the care home setting until people go to bed in the evening.

There are eight care assistants/nurses on duty at any one time and they are often busy providing personal care to people, record keeping, tidying and making appointments for people. There is very little chance to sit and have a chat. Miss D is often sat watching television and gets very little chance to do anything else.

Apart from knowing that Miss D has a favourite set of nightwear, what she likes to eat and her favourite flower, the carnation, the people working at the care home know very little else about her and especially how she is feeling each day. This is a very lonely existence for Miss D even though she is surrounded by so many people.

The home where Miss D is a resident recognised that they needed to know much more about the people they supported and cared for to be able to offer an increased quality of life for the residents. Time was made to get to know the residents and to listen to what mattered to them, their stories and their day-to-day preferences. The family and friends of the residents were also invited into these conversations based on whom each individual resident wished to invite.

Based on what was learnt through these conversations, the routines in the home were changed to be able to meet each person's preferences, the options for food and mealtimes became more flexible as well as opportunities to get involved in activities inside and outside the home that were set up based on people's interests, skills and hobbies.

Good communication and personalisation

A report published by the King's Fund (McCrone et al, 2008), titled 'Paying the Price: The Cost of Mental Health Care in England to 2026', highlighted the important role communication plays in delivering quality person-centred care and support. This report was published at the same time as a report from the Commission for Social Care Inspection (CSCI) that found some inadequacies in communication with people with dementia in some care homes. The findings demonstrated that residents with higher levels of communication impairment spent the least time engaged in any meaningful activities and inspectors observed a number of instances when staff were insensitive to people's emotional needs and feelings. The report stated that urgent action was needed to make care homes a positive care option for people with dementia and that '*Care home managers need to provide leadership, home ethos, staff support and training to ensure excellent personalised care*' (CSCI et al, 2008, p 49).

Good communication between the individual, their family, paid support and the health and social care professionals involved is essential to achieving a good outcome, based on the perspective of the person with dementia.

Without good communication, misunderstandings will occur with the potential to lead to a breakdown of understanding and good relationships, which has the possibility of leading to the person not receiving the care and support they need in a manner that works best for them.

Key lessons learnt

Behaviour is a form of communication; to understand a person's behaviour is to get to the root of what the person is communicating.

It is important to remember that the reasons underpinning a person's behaviour could be explained by a number of factors:

- an expression of how they are feeling;
- a response to the medication the person is taking;
- an expression of confusion or delirium if the person's surroundings or environment has changed;
- a representation of the physical changes that are taking place within the person;
- a representation of pain and discomfort.

The importance in providing a positive experience for the person with dementia is investing time and energy in understanding the meaning behind their behaviour and in responding to this rather than the behaviour itself.

8 Developing and embedding person-centred cultures

This chapter covers:

- **The implementation of personal budget and direct payments**
- **The barriers experienced by those wishing to access a personal budget or a direct payment**
- **Recognising the person's perspective and working with the person to achieve the best outcome**
- **Mental capacity and direct payments, and how to support direct payment delivery in a situation where someone lacks capacity**
- **Direct payment responsibilities and how these can be managed**
- **Preparing a well-considered care and support plan**
- **Recognising the need to continually focus on the person**
- **The future of personalisation for older people.**

Strategic direction

The central government leads the way in publishing national strategy documents in relation to dementia care, such as the Prime Minister's Challenge on Dementia 2020 (2015). Some of these documents have informed the development of the Personalisation Agenda: '*We want to see greater provision of innovative and high quality dementia care at home, delivered in a way that is personalised and appropriate to the specific needs of the person with dementia, their family and carers*' (Department of Health, 2015).

The responsibility for implementing the actions set out in the national dementia strategies falls on the Department of Health alongside local authorities, clinical commissioning groups (CCGs), service providers and third sector, community-based organisations.

Ongoing commitment to the coordination of dementia-friendly communities, alongside the development of partnerships with those implementing the personalisation agenda, would strengthen the intended positive outcomes of any published strategy. Working together with the shared commitment of improving the lived experience of people with dementia would assist in the progression of the strategies and agendas. Collective working enables the sharing of experience, knowledge and resources available.

How many people have been reached with direct payments?

The ASCOF (Adult Social Care Outcomes Framework) for 2018–19 reported that:

- 17.6% of adults aged 65 and over, in England, accessing long-term support at the year-end 31st March 2019 were receiving Direct Payments
- 90.3% of adults aged 65 and over in England accessing long-term community support at year-end 31st March 2019 were accessing Self Directed Support.

(NHS Digital, 2019)

Although the number of adults aged over 65 taking the option of self-directed support and direct payments appears at a healthy level in these figures, a report by the National Adult Social Care Intelligence Service (NASCIS) in 2014 stated that: '*local authority data shows that ten or fewer older people with dementia have a direct payment in 70 councils*' (Alzheimer's Society, 2020). The low uptake in direct payments for people with dementia in 2014 raises some concerns. What are the reasons why so few people are accessing a direct payment, especially when this option has been available to people accessing social care support since the Community Care (Direct Payments) Act 1996.

Since their implementation, direct payments have provided people with greater choice and control. For example, in her book *Where Memories Go: Why Dementia Changes Everything* by Sally Magnusson (2014) explains the experience she and her two sisters had as a family caring for their mum with dementia. Within this story they explained how having access to a direct payment supported them as a family and enabled them to employ people to care for their mum within the home.

To achieve a personalised approach and self-directed support, it is of the utmost importance that people understand the full picture of what is available to them. This includes an awareness that the option for a personal budget, if funded by the local authority, or a personal health budget, if funded by the local health authority, exists and that these can be managed as a direct payment.

Often individuals and families are not made aware of this option as highlighted in the Dispatches programme 'How to Avoid the Dementia Tax' (2017). The programme also addressed the issues people face in accessing a care assessment and understanding the contribution they have to make towards their own support and care when funded via their local authority.

The Alzheimer's Society (2010, cited in Feltoe and Orellana, 2013, p 9) reported that a key barrier to older people accessing a personal budget was: '*a personal budgets system that has not yet adapted to the needs of people with dementia and their carers, and is overly complex and burdensome*'.

An example of this is the assessment process. Often people experience long waits for their assessment by the local authority which is required to determine a person's eligibility for health and social care support. For example,

> *In Cambridgeshire, people told their local Healthwatch that waiting times vary hugely across the country with older people in particular waiting increasingly long times for their assessments, in some cases waiting up to 47 weeks.*
>
> (healthwatch, 2016)

Often how quickly a person receives the support they require post-assessment depends on the circumstances of them and their family and that of the service providers in their area. Yates et al (2019) state that: '*Receipt of support soon after diagnosis can facilitate better adjustment and ongoing management of dementia*'.

If someone who has been referred for health and social care support waits a long time for the input from a social worker for an assessment, their circumstances may have changed significantly within that time frame. It may have reached the stage where the person needs support putting in place quickly which wouldn't leave enough time to explore what would work best for the person, the options available to them and their preferences around self-directed support. If support is put in place quickly the social worker will be referring to the services already available within the person's area and identifying the services which have capacity to work with that person. This means the social worker moves away from the potential of a broad range of options to a very narrow picture of what is available.

It is, however, possible to respond to the immediate support needs of the person with an intermediary arrangement with a local care or support provider in order to overcome the immediate crisis situation and then continue the discussions with the person about how they would like to live, what good support and care would look like for them and the options available to them with the intention to move towards this over a period of time.

Further information about the implementation of personalisation for people with dementia can be found in the 2013 Think Local Act Personal report, 'Improving Personal Budgets for Older People' (Routledge and Carr, 2013). This report highlights what helps and hinders those living with dementia in accessing a direct payment. It emphasises the need for people to have access to good information, advice and guidance throughout the direct payment/personal budget process to support them to make decisions at each stage.

Personal budgets form part of a person's individual budget, where the individual budget includes other sources of income available to the person, such as wages, pensions, welfare income. Personal budgets working well for older people and their carers has been a prominent issue since the original Individual Budgets Evaluation Network (IBSEN) research on individual budgets (Glendinning et al, 2008). This research suggested that during the early stages of the development of individualised funding there was low satisfaction and it presented recommendations to improve delivery for older people. The recommendations included:

- practicing an approach that supports Individual Budgets;
- making improvements and streamlining the process of accessing funding;
- taking a more a transparent approach to allocating resources; and
- developing monitoring and review systems that would be appropriate for Self-Directed Support.

The success of personal budgets also have to be measured within the current context of the health and social care system. The Health and Social Care Information Centre, now renamed NHS Digital, reported that the number of adults receiving social care services commissioned and/or provided by local authorities in 2019–20 were:

- 838,530 people aged 18–64 (1.5% of all adults aged 18–64);
- 548,450 people aged 65+.

The Health and Social Care Information Centre also reported a local authority expenditure on adult social services for those aged 65+ in 2019/2020 of £8.3 billion where the total spend for Adult Social Care was £15.4 billion in 2019–20.

Age UK reported that £160 million had been cut from the social care system by the year 2015 and the cuts have continued to be made to the present day. In real terms in the year the report was written,

> *Age UK's analysis shows there are now nearly 1.2 million people (1,183,900) aged 65+ who don't receive the help they need with essential daily living activities. This represents a 17.9 per cent increase on last year and a 48 percent increase since 2010.*
>
> (Age UK, 2017, p 4)

This trend suggests the social care system no longer meets the needs of people as it did ten years ago due to the sharp change in funding and resources available as a result of the austerity measures imposed throughout the country.

People with dementia and their families can however still expect to receive support, if they are assessed as being eligible. When a person is determined as not being eligible, the local authority has a duty to provide relevant and accurate information, advice and guidance as well as signposting to community-based organisations.

The support made available via the social care system must be personalised with the person deciding how they want it to be provided. This approach to supporting the person can be accompanied by, and work well alongside, the support available to them from within their networks and community.

The experience so far

Some older people have been accessing direct payments across the UK since 2000 and personal budgets since 2005, and many stories of positive experiences have emerged. The Personal Budgets Outcomes Evaluation Tool (POET) was developed by In Control and it has been utilised across the social care sector. Here are some key findings:

- The majority of older people said Personal Budgets had a positive impact on their lives
- 70% or more of older people reported Personal Budgets have resulted in a good level of dignity within the support they receive, experiencing quality of life and feeling safe and secure
- 60%-69% of older people reported having access to information to help with making decisions about the support they receive and being happy where they live
- 50%-59% of older people reported a positive impact of Personal Budgets on their relationships and everyday activity such as work, leisure and volunteering
- The majority of older people reported a positive impact of Personal Budgets in regard to their quality of life, health and feeling safe

(In Control, 2017)

The Association of Directors of Adult Social Services (ADASS) brought the issue of personal budgets and older people strongly to the attention of the sector and policy makers via 'The Case for Tomorrow', a discussion paper on the future of services for older people. Importantly, ADASS puts its concerns about personal budget delivery in the context of its wider aspirations for older people. It argues that the following need to be in place:

- Personalisation recognises that Personal Budget is a route to people achieving choice and control. For many people the choice about who provides the care is the most important as is being cared for by someone they have a rapport with
- Services are not keeping up to the demand of Personalised care and support. Personalisation does not reach the intended outcome if people have a limit in the options available to them. The Local Authority's role in developing and facilitating the market to enable Personalisation to work is still underdeveloped in many councils
- Direct Payments remain underused as older people are often assessed at a time of crisis and feel unable to manage the Direct Payment

- There has been a reported significant increase in the number of older people accessing Self Directed Support between the years 2009/2010 - 2010/2011 where the number of people quadrupled. This has been delivered via a Personal Budget that has been managed internally by the Local Authority
- Confusion around employer responsibilities continues to present challenges to people becoming the budget holder
- Council workers have reported an increase in bureaucracy since the introduction of Direct Payments, with an increased level of assessment and monitoring processes

(Association of Directors of Adult Services (ADASS), 2012, pp 2–4)

Personalisation, and personal budgets especially, will require transformational change in how people receive and access care and support for the implementation and outcomes to be successful. Personalisation continues to require a full transformation of the social care system. Change of this scale will inevitably entail difficulties and problems which, at times, can seem insurmountable. Experience to date has shown that the move towards achieving personalised outcomes results in a positive impact on the life experience of those supported through the social care system, such as the people with dementia. This means that there is a clear reason and purpose in overcoming the barriers and problems experienced in implementing this practice.

Barriers to achieving personalisation

There have been a number of barriers to achieving personalisation and personal budgets. For instance:

- Social workers have reported that there are internal structural issues such as paperwork and bureaucracy. (Jeremy Dunning, 2011 and Jeremy Dunning, 2011 both cited in Association of Directors of Adult Services (ADASS), 2012, pp 3–4)

People accessing social care services reported that they were not aware of the options available to them and had experienced a process of accessing the social care support that captured their circumstances and needs *and then* they were informed of the support available to them via the services available in their area. In this process they had not been informed of self-directed support, personalisation of personal budgets. It is important to recognise the barriers faced in the continued development and roll out of personalised practice and self-directed support so that the solutions to these can be found. Working with a solution focus enables everyone involved through the dementia care triad+1 – the person, their family, professionals, paid carers/support workers and the community – to continue to find ways to shift the barriers, overcome the challenges.

It is helpful to remember that people have achieved personalised and self-directed outcomes. It is possible as it has *already been achieved*.

The legal framework for health and social care supports this approach.

The guidance accompanying the legal framework also supports this approach.

When people are given the opportunity to think about how they would like to be supported and how they would like to be spending their time each day they think about things that would work well for them and not necessarily from a list of available services. The ideas and ways to be supported will be varied and determined by the person's wishes, relationships, interests and opportunities. When putting the ideas of how the person wants to be supported into practice, it may require a wider exploration of options than those that reside with the usual health and social care system. Involving people who would have the knowledge and ideas regarding where resources reside in the local area. This approach provides the opportunity to find new ways that people wish to be supported and cared for. It engages people from a wider network of potential support, it develops discussions that focus on what can be achieved, finding new ideas and solutions within the community.

Mental capacity and direct payments

More information about mental capacity and its relevance within personalisation can be found in Chapter 2, this includes the Mental Capacity Act principle which states that capacity has to be assumed (Mental Capacity Act 2005).

In practice, a person's capacity will need to be determined before a decision can be made about the person's ability to manage a direct payment. If, after a full and appropriate capacity assessment has been completed, a person is assessed as not having the capacity to decide to have, or manage a direct payment, another approach to accessing this would need to be considered.

Another person, a friend or a family member for instance, can act in a formal capacity to access and manage the direct payment on the person's behalf. Ideally this would be someone who has the appropriate legal powers in place, for instance, appointeeship, guardianship or power of attorney.

Direct payments and responsibilities

Many older people accessing direct payment, which includes people with dementia, have reported anxiety regarding the responsibility of managing the budget and managing their own support (Moran et al, 2012). Knowing how to record the income and expenditure of the budget, understanding what records need to be kept and employer responsibilities/ understanding employment law were the cause of these anxieties.

Managing a direct payment may seem less daunting to a person with a certain skill set, for instance, keeping up-to-date with paperwork, organising files and information, team management and keeping financial records. The freedom and flexibility that can be found through accessing a direct payment can be appealing. The positives that can be achieved with a direct payment lead some people to the conclusion that the extra responsibility is worth the outcomes that can be achieved.

When the elements of responsibility are considered alongside the intention of self-directed support a disparity becomes clear. Self-directed support gives the opportunity for people to have choice and control over their day-to-day lives and how they are supported. It is about having the chance to achieve a good quality of life which is recognised and built into how they are cared for and supported. It is not intended to bring more responsibility into a person's life or placing barriers in the way of people being able to achieve choice, control and quality of life. People who have received a personal budget as a direct payment have stated that it has provided greater flexibility, choice and control, although it has taken them time to fill in paperwork, to keep records and report back to the local authority (Lewis, 2005, p 4).

As part of the discussions about what a good life looks like and what good support would look like, there can also be a conversation about 'how will this be managed?' This question can then lead to the person having the opportunity to explore what support they wish to have in place to be able to manage the direct payment, support with the paperwork, the finances, the recruitment and management of a team and the monitoring.

Once the areas that the person wants support with have been identified this can be followed by a conversation to explore 'who would be available to or who would like to undertake these areas or function/responsibility?' The person themselves may be best placed to fulfil some of the responsibilities, with or without support. A family member may be able to help, especially if they have the time, experience and skills to do so. The option to utilise part of the budget available to the person to purchase in elements of this support should also be considered, for instance, the person may pay a neighbour to manage their paperwork or a local accountant to do the bookkeeping.

- What could be the reasons behind the low uptake of direct payments?
- What attitudes do you think the majority of people hold when it comes to considering how a person with dementia would manage a direct payment?
- What are the key principles of the Mental Capacity Act 2005 (Mental Capacity Act 2005) that could possibly be overlooked when it comes to a person with dementia managing a direct payment?

Employing people

If someone has opted for a direct payment to employ a team of people directly they would then be responsible for managing them. This may be an area of responsibility that is new to the person. There is a lot to consider when employing people; finding the right people, how to recruit them, having the right paperwork in place, offering the employees continued support and managing any employment related issues. Despite the extra responsibilities, many people who have employed support workers, personal assistants or carers directly have enjoyed many benefits from being supported in this way (Lewis, 2005, p 11).

Employing a person	Receiving care through an agency
The person with dementia can decide who to employ.	The agency will introduce the person to the people they have available, rarely will they employ someone specifically to work with the person.
The person with dementia can find someone who shares the same interests and has the skills and knowledge they need.	The person with dementia might be lucky and find someone who shares the same interests and who also has the specific skills and knowledge they need.
The person can plan ahead with their own recruitment to find someone who is available when they need them.	Often the person has to fit in with the rotas developed by the agency.
They can determine the training and qualifications that their support workers receive.	The agency will be regulated by the Care Quality Commission and therefore they will have to provide the staff with all the mandatory training, whether it is relevant or not. Sometimes agencies will also provide additional training
The person can have direct communications with the people they employ.	The person's communications with the support worker will be via the agency.
The person with dementia can be certain about who will be supporting them.	The agency may send people who the person has not met before and who do not know the person.

There is support available to people who employ their own care and support workers. Since 1996 local authorities have been providing direct payments to people who wish to employ their own staff and in this time the infrastructure support for this option has been built. Often there is a team of people within the local authority who are available to help, or this function has been contracted out to a local organisation. This help can include support with:

- recruitment;
- payroll;
- pension;
- training;
- ongoing advice and information regarding employment law.

There are also national organisations who provide free advice, guidance and resources. ACAS is a reliable source of support and skills for care and provides a wide range of resources to help people employ their own team of staff, including access to grants for training.

When the person with dementia is embarking on employing people, a number of things need to be in place:

- **Recruitment** – When recruiting people the advert can be designed in a way to attract the right people. It could include information about the person's interests, the skills and qualities they are looking for in their care and support workers. It can also request the practical things the person needs to have in place, that is, does the support worker or carer need to be a driver, what days and times of the week do they need to be available? The information could be gathered from completing the matching staff exercise covered in Chapter 6.

  Where the advert is placed is to the person's discretion and adverts could be pinned up in the places where it is likely to find a good support or care worker; if the person loves rugby why not put an advert up in the local rugby club's stadium to find someone who shares the same interest?

  Online approaches to recruitment can be explored, for instance, social media or the jobs section of online ads pages.

  A job description and person specification can be written to capture what the person specifically needs from the individual, rather than generic statements. The information for the job description and person specification could be gathered, again, using the matching staff exercise.

  The interview process can also be managed in a way that provides the opportunity for both the person and the candidate to decide if they would work together well. As well as asking interview questions, it could be arranged for the person with dementia and their potential support worker to spend time together sharing some time pursuing the person's interest, such as going to look at cars or going for a walk in the park.

- **Insurance** – It is important to have the right insurance in place; as an employer, the person living with dementia and/or their nominee would need employers' liability insurance. There are some specialist insurance companies that provide insurance specifically for people in receipt of a direct payment/personal budget. Local centres of independent living (sometimes called integration or inclusion living) can often provide information and guidance on specialist insurance companies. The insurance companies also provide access to employment law advice and support.

- **A payroll provider** – The person can provide the payroll themselves if they feel confident to do so, or a family member may do this on their behalf. There are organisations that can provide the payroll for people in receipt of a direct payment and most local accountants can provide payroll services.

- **Access to training** – Making sure employees have access to the training they need to do their job well is another key element of employing a team of support workers as part of the person's care and support. This may be training that the person and their family provide; detailed information about the person and how they want to be supported. The training may also be on topics such as safeguarding, person-centred practice and communication. It is important to recognise the training that is needed and ensure the cost of this is included in the support plan.

Finding what is possible

People with dementia and their families may find it valuable to research what is available and what is possible when accessing social care support before they reach a decision about what would be the best option for them. This could be achieved through:

- the professionals involved in their care and support providing information about what they know is available in their area;
- researching the internet to look for information about activities, associations and organisations in the local area;
- making contact with the local organisations, that is, Age UK or Alzheimer's Society, to seek their support on finding services that are available and to speak to them about the option of self-directed support;
- visiting the local library or community centre to find information about what is happening in the local area.

This research could be led by the person, their family, people who are paid to support them or the professionals involved in the person's care and support. Support networks available in a person's area can change over time and it is good to continue to research over time so as to be kept informed of these changes and new opportunities.

If on researching what is available in a person's local area it has not been possible to find something that would be right for the person, it is worth a conversation with the person and the people around them, referencing the dementia care triad+1, to explore whether it is possible to set something up that is specifically designed around the person and based on what they would like to achieve or how they would like to live.

A well-considered plan

Time is an important factor in the success of a direct payment arrangement; people need the time to consider their situation, what options are available to them, explore ideas, think about their community and find solutions.

While developing the ideas for the use of a direct payment consideration can also be given to any contingency and risk plans that form part of the person's support plan. Contingency plans would give consideration to what steps to take when something does not go to plan, for instance, if someone's support cannot make it to them due to ill health. The contingency plans can help to make sure appropriate consideration has been given to these circumstances so that the person can plan ahead and continue to be supported in a way that works well.

The risk plan considers when the person feels that they could be at risk and what measures to put in place to reduce the likelihood of this risk occurring or the severity of this risk if it does occur. The person, as with all the planning approaches introduced in this book, needs to be led by the carer, as far as possible, and by those that know the person well, that is, the dementia care triad+1.

Having a fully developed contingency and risk plan developed can lead to people feeling more secure about the arrangements they have in place and can prevent issues of crisis in the future. At times it can be challenging for a social worker or any other professional involved, to have the time required to support the person to explore the options available to them and gather and record the level of detail needed for an assessment, support plan and/or person-centred plan.

Personalisation and self-directed support opens up the opportunity for people to complete their own assessment and develop their own support plan if they wish to do so, which is underpinned in legislation within the Care Act 2014 (Care Act 2014) This means that the person, their family and other people in their life could be taking a lead in exploring and developing content of the assessment and the support plan where they feel able to do so and where they wish to take this on. There would need to be involvement from a social worker or clinical lead to ensure the information contained within the assessment and support plan is accurate and provides all the details required. This approach could lead to the person being able to develop and drive the content of their assessment and support plan while significantly decreasing the time requirements of a social worker or clinical lead.

Limitations on choice

People who have accessed health and social care support experience limited choices available to them; for example, those living in an area where there are a few care providers who have a monopoly over the service provision, or those who reside in rural areas experiencing trouble finding a provider that covers their area.

Some areas have limited providers and funding cuts have led to community-based initiatives closing down. The pandemic has also had an impact on the provision of vital community-based support. '*More than 60% of community groups have been forced to close or decrease their services, research by community charity Groundwork has found*' (Whitehead, 2020).

A focus on how to meet a person's outcomes on the basis of the services that are available could result in limited options, depending on where the person lives. Instead, developing an ability to think about what is possible can begin to open up the doorway for new and different opportunities. When what is possible is considered it may involve developing new ideas and initiatives based on what would work well for the person. These initiatives although originally developed for one person could be a positive option for other members of the local community. For instance, setting up a cafe so that someone has somewhere to meet friends close to their home can become a place for other members of the community forming a hub for local residents. Thinking and working in this way involves creative thinking, with a focus on achieving the outcomes that make sense for that person while also seeing the bigger picture of how this could be a positive addition for the local community.

How thinking about what is possible works in practice

Brenda is a keen arts and crafts person; she would like to continue to enjoy these pastimes and would like to find other people to share this interest with. She spent a bit of time with her daughter having a walk around the local area to look at the community notice boards but there was nothing about arts and crafts groups. They decided to pop into the local library and have a look on the internet. They found a group that met on a Wednesday in the community centre in the next village.

Brenda would want to go along to the group with someone; she does not want to travel alone. For the first few weeks, Brenda went with her daughter until she got to know someone in the group, Enid. As they got to know each other they learned that Enid drives past Brenda's house on her way to the community centre. A conversation is had and Enid starts to give Brenda a lift to the group. Brenda then attends with Enid and gradually gets to know the rest of the people who attend. She is really enjoying her time there and the group have started to sell some of the crafts to raise money for a local charity. As Brenda has settled into the group, she now feels comfortable getting a taxi there when Enid is on holiday; Brenda uses some of her budget to cover the cost of a taxi.

The aim of a personalised approach is for the person to still have choice and control in their lives and that they have the liberty to decide how and where they are supported and cared for.

Don't get stuck on the plan

The care and support plan provides the opportunity for the person to communicate and make a record of the support and care that would work well for them. Those from the dementia care triad+1 can then work in cooperation to support the realisation of the plan.

In the efforts to put the plan into practice, it is important to make sure the focus remains on what is important for the person. People's circumstances and choices do change;

sometimes these changes can happen frequently. After experiencing the care and support designed at the support planning stage, the person may change their mind about what they want and how they want to be supported or their circumstances might dictate that a change is needed.

It would be wrong to expect them to continue to be supported and cared for as determined by the information in their care and support plan. The core feature of personalisation is to ensure that the person continues to be heard and their preferences understood.

If change is necessary then steps can be taken to achieve this; for instance, if the person no longer enjoys going to the local community coffee morning and they would prefer to get some exercise and go for a walk, and there are no cost implications to this, then this could be changed as soon as it is feasible to do so without needing to look how to resource the cost of the change. However, if the change the person wants to make would result in them utilising their budget differently, this would need to be communicated with the social work team and finance team. This communication would be to seek agreement from the social worker that the existing budget can be used differently and to save any misunderstandings with the finance team at the time of auditing the direct payment. This is the case unless the person has found an organisation who can manage an individual service fund on their behalf, in which case the change could be arranged directly between the person and the service provider without the need to seek agreement from the social worker.

An individual service fund is a model of service provision where the Personal Budget amount determined to meet a person's social care or health outcomes is managed by an organisation of the persons choosing. This approach to managing a budget is mentioned within the Care Act 2014 which supports this option in the roll-out of social care funds. Within health, this option of how to manage a personal health budget is called a third-party budget.

An organisation managing an individual service fund or third-party budget on a person's behalf would:

- hold part or all of the budget available to the person;
- manage the budget appropriately, being able to account for all income and expenditure of that person's budget, including over and under spend;
- be able to respond to the persons changing needs by offering a flexible approach to the use of the budget which is decided between the person and the organisation;
- utilise the budget to cover the cost of paid support, items to be purchased or the cost of any sessions/activities the person is taking part in;
- be the employer of the persons care and support therefore placing the employment responsibility with the organisation, taking care of recruitment, training and ongoing development.

The key is to utilise the resources available to the person, including their budget from the local authority or CCG, to meet the person's outcomes and needs in the most flexible and responsive way possible. This approach should ensure that the person is supported in a manner that is preventative to any circumstances getting worse, while avoiding any unnecessary bureaucracy.

If the person's circumstances or needs have changed since their last assessment and care and support plan and these changes result in the person needing more care and support, the social work team or clinical team would conduct a review of the assessment to capture these changes. This would lead to a review of the budget available to the person to ensure this is suitable to continue to meet the person's needs.

The reviewed assessment and budget would then lead to a review of the person's care and support plan, which would be the opportunity to address what changes are needed in how the person then wishes to be supported.

The future of personalisation for older people

There is a future for personalisation in the UK for older people. This approach is recognised within the most recent legislation and guidance that will influence the future for health and social care in the UK (see Chapter 1 for more information).

Personalisation, to date, has made a positive difference for those people who have experienced this approach to meeting their health and social care needs:

- The person can continue to be in control of their lives.
- Their quality of life can be maintained and even enhanced.
- The family can have direct involvement in ensuring that the person is being supported well and is happy with their day-to-day life. This, in turn, can reduce their anxieties and also ensure that they are able to continue with their own life, responsibilities and commitments.
- Social workers and clinical leads can be confident that the person is being supported, their needs are being met, positive outcomes reached and that they are meeting their statutory duty in a positive and proactive way.
- The opportunity is there to develop a positive relationship and reduce the likelihood of the person and family becoming dependent on professional or statutory involvement as they develop their understanding and ability to utilise the resources available to best meet the person's needs.
- Commissioners and local authorities can develop a less structured and flexible way of ensuring that public money is utilised as it is intended, to meet the needs of those who require care and support and are eligible for local authority or health funding.

Recommendations

These recommendations are made to those who are actively involved in the development and delivery of personalisation and personalised practice, including personal budgets, personal health budget and direct payments.

Local authorities and clinical commissioning groups

There is a need for major changes within local authorities and CCGs in order to scale up personalisation so that the majority of people with dementia and their carers can have genuine control over their care and support.

Here are some recommendations to support local authorities and CCGs to move forward in a positive direction when supporting people living with dementia to achieve personalised outcomes.

- Develop access to impartial information so that people living with dementia and their families/carers are aware of the option of personal budgets, personal health budgets and direct payments. Include information about how budgets can be managed. This information needs to be available and shared with the person ahead of an assessment.
- Improve understanding among professionals about personal budgets, personal health budgets and direct payments and the positive benefits for people with dementia.
- Ensure the provision of access to timely diagnosis and person-centred early stage support.
- Resources within adult health and social care should be organised to enable personal budgets, personal health budgets and direct payments, with a fair and proportionate budget provided to each individual.
- Reduce any existing complexity regarding accessing personal budgets, personal health budgets and direct payments to ensure the process is easy to understand and quick to access.
- People with dementia and their family/carers should be actively involved in assessing their own need for care and support, and also be provided the opportunity to take the lead in completing the assessment.
- An outcomes-, strengths- and assets-based approach should be adopted when assessing the care and support needs of people with dementia. This requires that the outcomes that influence a person's well-being are taken into consideration and the strengths, skills, knowledge, talents and abilities of the person, as well as assets, relationships, opportunities and community connections are recognised.

- Provide clarity to people as to whether they are being supported by the older people's social work team or the mental health team.
- Enable people to design the care and support around them with a variety of options for managing the social care money to suit individual circumstances.
- Ensure financial assessments are clear and easy to understand. Make sure that there is a full understanding and appreciation of the person's circumstances regarding disability-related expenditure and that this is taken into account. Make sure the person and their family, where appropriate, are informed about the contributions they will need to make towards their own care and support before they start the support planning process, as discussed in Chapter 3.
- Increase access to support for people in receipt of direct payments. Help them to manage their budget and the people they will be recruiting.
- Work with an appropriate person to take on the management of the direct payment as a nominee on behalf of a person with dementia, when the person lacks capacity and there is no one with power of attorney or guardianship.
- People who have chosen a direct payment need to complete an audit to show the local authority or CCG how the money has been used; the local authority should ensure that the person knows about this requirement and clearly explains what is required. This process needs to be as easy to complete as possible.
- Provide support in a timely manner throughout the dementia journey to enable the person with dementia to have a good understanding and level of control and choice over how they are cared for or supported.
- Ensure that the person is given an indication of the budget available to them before they begin to develop their care and support plan, known as an indicative budget. This is crucial in ensuring that the person can plan within the realms of what is possible in the sense of the Budget available to them, while being able to take into consideration all the other potential resources available to them, that is, wages, Department of Work and Pensions income, savings, grants.
- Avoid the situation where a person develops a care and support plan without an indicative budget and this is submitted for consideration and the level of spend is deemed as too high. Make it clear from the beginning of the care and support planning process. Clarity and transparency are important.

Social workers

Social work teams and the social care departments within local authorities have a number of legislative and policy frameworks they have to work within. One of the most recent laws that will shape the future of social work is the Care Act 2014 (Care Act 2014) of which personalisation, personal budgets and direct payments play a central role. Therefore, there continues to be an emphasis on delivering the Personalisation Agenda, which was predominantly established in the Putting People First Concordat (Policy Navigator, 2007).

- Ensure that people are informed of the options available to them without demonstrating any personal bias or opinion, and support people to make their own decisions regarding what best suits them.
- If someone chooses a direct payment, make them aware of the support available in the local area to manage the direct payment and how someone could utilise part of their budget to cover the costs of this support if they choose to do so.
- Ensure that financial assessments are completed at the start of the process, directly after their eligibility has been determined via the care assessment, so people can be clear at the outset what their personal financial contribution will be before they begin to develop their care and support plan.
- Adopt a non-restrictive approach, listen to the solutions someone has found to meet their support and care requirements. Make sure that social work practice is in line with the principles set in the Care Act 2014 (*Care Act 2014.* s.1(2) (b)(e)(f)) and that the support plan is considered on the following criteria:
  - Are the costs in the support plan within budget?
  - Are the ideas around how the person wants to be supported legal?
  - Do the ideas also meet the assessed need and are any risks considered and planned for?
- Apply the Mental Capacity Act appropriately and assume capacity. Follow due process around capacity assessment and best interest approaches when this is in doubt (Mental Capacity Act 2005. s.1.(1)(1-6)).
- Enable the person and their family to take the lead in the development of their assessment and support plan if they wish to do so.

Health/Nursing

At some stage in the dementia journey, the person will need input from a health professional. This will especially be the case during the later/severe stages of dementia.

At this stage, the person and family should still continue to receive their care and support in a personalised way.

- Ensure that people who meet the eligibility for Continuing Healthcare know that they have a 'right to ask' for a personal health budget.

- Learn about what has worked well for the person in relation to the support they have received up until the point of health involvement. Work together to ensure that this approach continues for the person to maintain consistency and familiarity.
- Address areas that are not working well for the person at this moment in time and collectively find solutions to these problems. Chapter 4 provides practical advice on how to do this.
- If someone chooses a personal health budget and to manage this as a direct payment ensure that they are aware of *all* the support available to them to help them manage this arrangement from within the local CCG, local organisations, who are commissioned to provide this support, and local community organisations.
- Be knowledgeable about the support available within a person's local community and share this information in the most appropriate way possible.

For people accessing a personal budget

There is a change of focus away from the person's needs and areas of life where they are experiencing difficulties to a focus on what is possible and ideas around what great care and support would look like.

The care and support plan should be positive and liberating for the person and their family, as they begin to realise the level of choice and control that is possible. The person should be able to realise that they do not have to accept any approach to support and care that would not work well for them.

Equally, it can be overwhelming and fearful at times as the person with dementia and their family begin to learn about the complex health and social care systems, while also exploring the options available to them. At this time, it is important for people to be able to develop a clear idea of what would work well and to remain resolute on what they believe would work best, even if these ideas change over time. This can be achieved through the following ways:

- Look at a wide range of options available to the person. This includes people and places in the community, groups and associations in the local area, equipment or technology and the current services available.
- Rather than thinking about day care, perhaps think about places where the person would like to spend time; for instance, the café where other friends meet, the garden centre where they can indulge in an interest, a walk around the lake to get out of the house and have a chance to exercise. Consider places that capture the person's interest and imagination. There is growing evidence that keeping active and getting regular exercise can slow down the progression of dementia (Alty

et al, 2019). Eating well and keeping socially active also positively slow down the symptoms.

- When looking for support, consider personalising the recruitment process, based on the 'matching staff' exercise introduced in Chapter 6. Look for people on the basis of shared interests, a personality or character that would suit the person. Also consider the practical elements to make sure the arrangement will work well, such as the times the person would need to be available, or if they need to be able to drive.
- Ensure that time is made to have important discussions with the people the person is close to, talk about the future and what the person would like to happen. Think about developing a person-centred plan, an advanced care plan or an advanced directive, which are covered in Chapter 3. This is about the person and ensuring that people understand what they would like to happen. These conversations and discussions can help the people close to the person manage situations as they arise and it will also provide them with some emotional support and reassurance that they are supporting the person in a way that respects their wishes.
- Use some of the ways of recording discussions and decisions that have been introduced in Chapter 4.
- Access the information and advice that is available, and when needed, access advice and support that is impartial and independent of the social care and health system.
- Be positive and be in control; the person has the right to make decisions about how they are supported, make use of this right to ensure that their life is how they want it to be.
- Ask questions and make sure the person and the people supporting them understand as much as possible; the people who are involved from a professional capacity should want the person to understand their rights and what is available and possible for them.
- The person is the expert in their own life, they know how they want to live their life and this needs to be shared with others, such as family, paid care and support and professionals, those who form the dementia triad+1 to make this possible.

Families

Seeing a family member's life change, at times drastically, can be emotionally draining and at times it is difficult to adapt.

This is especially so for the family members who are closest to the person and are providing the support and care that the person needs. The dynamics of their relationship could begin to change significantly, and the person who was once a caregiver could become a care receiver.

Recognising when care and support is needed from outside the immediate family unit can pose the first hurdle as family members may try to remain self-sufficient in managing their situation.

Dementia care triad+1

One of the factors that prevent a person or a family from making a referral for support from the health and social care system is a concern about what will happen. Will they be listened to? Will they have any say over the support they receive? Will they have any control over what happens? Will they receive the support they need in a way that makes a positive difference?

The emphasis is now for the person to have a sense of control over how they live their life and the support and care that is provided.

Here are some questions to consider when measuring how much this has been achieved.

- Is the person taking the lead in discussions and decision-making?
- Does the person have support from other people which helps them to take the lead, without people taking over or taking control from them?
- Is the person's voice heard?
- Is the person answering the questions that are about them?
- Has there been the opportunity to fully understand the person's preferences, their likes and dislikes, the routines that are important to them and their future wishes?
- Is the support network around the person functioning from a place of full understanding about what the person wants and needs, or are assumptions being made about what would work best for them?
- Is the person receiving support from those that are from their own networks while they are going through their diagnosis, assessments and the development of their plans about ongoing care and support?
- Is the person being informed about the care and support available through social care and health commissioned provision, have they also had the opportunity to think about the support available within their community?
- Has everyone involved in the dementia care triad+1 had the opportunity to learn about dementia and do they understand the condition?

- Is the information learnt from discussions being recorded in a meaningful way such that members of the dementia care triad+1 can refer to this afterwards?

Community

Each person is part of a community; how they interact with this community is dependent on where they live, the relationships they have with the people around them, the interests they have and the places they go to pursue these interests.

If a community is to open and inclusive, members of that community can play a part in creating a welcoming place that takes care of one another.

Here are some suggestions of how this can be achieved.

- Build awareness of dementia, make sure there is access to information so people can read about it and create opportunities to share this knowledge and stories of personal experiences.
- Groups, associations and organisations who are providing a community service, for example, the local shop, library, doctor's practice, provide a welcoming environment with people running the space who are dementia aware.
- Encourage the use of the community spaces, community centres, sports grounds and schools, as a means of bringing people together and building relationships.
- Consider creating a 'dementia-friendly community. where the standards set with the BSI are recognised in how the community functions (BSI Group, n.d.). More information on this is available in Chapter 1.
- Encourage the development of more safe places, a national scheme that recognises places within the community that are safe for people to go to if they are feeling scared, vulnerable, confused or lost. More details about Safe Places National Network can be found in Appendix 1.

Achieving personalised services

Home care, residential care, support living, day services and community-based supports all have the potential to offer a personalised provision.

When a service is personalised, it will work with people on the premise of their choices and preferences, a respectful approach that upholds the person's identity, wishes and dignity.

For those providing and working within services, it is important to appreciate the difference between a service-led and person-led approach within that setting.

The difference between being person-led and service-led

Person-led	Service-led
Planning *with* the person	Planning *for* the person
Talking *with* the person	Talking *about* the person
Doing things *with* the person	*Following* a programme
Having a life and the person is living somewhere and in a way that they have chosen	The person is living where they 'fit' or where this is a 'space'
Start with *what matters* to the person	Start with *what's wrong* with the person
Health and safety is addressed to enable the person to achieve what they wish to accomplish in life	Health and safety determines what happens and restricts a person's choices or options
The team 'support', 'assist', 'help'	The team 'let', 'allow', 'place'
The team suggests and the person decides	The team sets the person's goals
Living plans – changing with the person as their circumstances and needs change	An approach where the person's life is determined by an outdated plan – 'updated annually'

Here are some considerations for service providers to aim towards in achieving a personalised provision.

The person being supported

- is understood, both in the present tense and what has made the person who they are today, their past and their important relationships;
- has access to the information they need to make decisions about the care and support available to them;
- has access to information that is presented to them in a manner that means they can engage with it, understand it and be fully involved in their care and support;
- has a range of options to choose from regarding the service they choose and who supports or cares for them in that service;
- is making choices about how they wish to live, day-to-day and in the future;
- has an opportunity to pursue, share and develop skills and interests within the service setting and in the community;

- has access to the right level of funding to meet their health and social care needs and if it is identified that funding levels are not appropriate the necessary action is taken to address this;
- has the option to become the purchaser of the care and support they receive via the route of a personal budget, personal health budget or direct payment.

For those providing the care and support

- Listen to the person who is being cared for and supported and respond to what has been learnt.
- Read the information that has been gathered and documented about the person's preferences and future wishes.
- Review the routines and protocols to ensure that the care and support provided meets the needs, preferences and choices of each person receiving the service.
- Create opportunities for the people accessing the service and those working within it to spend quality time together to celebrate successes, build trusting relationships and continue to learn about what makes sense to the person being supported and cared for.
- Look at what is recorded and the paperwork and assess whether it is all needed. Can it be reduced, merged or removed altogether so more time can be devoted to being with the people being cared for and supported rather than to complete paper-based tasks?
- Create a person-centred culture within the team and organisations. Creating opportunities to develop this culture is crucial in achieving personalised practice. Consider how this is reflected in the recruitment process, in how team members are supported through supervisions, in team meetings and in day-to-day conversations.
- Team meetings create opportunities for team members to get to know each other better and this is where the culture can really begin to be established. Consider utilising some of the person-centred approaches introduced in Chapter 4 within these team gatherings to achieve this.

Continued control and self-determination

Personalisation is not to be experienced as a one-off event, planning meeting or response. It is a collection of values and approaches that are embedded throughout a person's life and especially at the stage when a person accesses health and social care support. Achieving personalisation is creating a culture that ensures people continue to have control and self-determination in how they live their life and how they choose to be supported. This requires:

- getting to know the *person* and developing an appreciation of their identity and their perspective of what makes a good life.
- valuing *relationships* between the person, their family, friends, members of the community and professionals. This is accomplished when people are actively involved and engaged in conversations and actions that ensure that the person with dementia continues to live a good, healthy and safe life, while having the opportunity to share ideas and find their own solutions.
- ensuring the input from *paid and professional support* is timely and responsive, avoiding crisis situations and ensuring that the support provided is based on what the person has chosen.

People are dynamic with needs, aspirations, circumstances and preferences that can change. The key is having the time to connect and to have meaningful conversations to continue to learn and develop understanding.

Here are some questions that could be seen as great questions to bring into conversations:

- What really matters to you?
- What is significant about your story, your achievements and good memories?
- What makes a good day for you?
- What is important in your life and what does a good life look like for you?
- What would make the biggest difference to you right now?
- What would you like to happen now? And what next?

Here are some great questions regarding maintaining and enhancing meaningful relationships:

- Tell me about the people that matter to you?
- What is it about the connections with the people in your life that mean the most to you?
- Who inspires you?
- Who do you look forward to seeing?
- When do you know that there is potential for a great relationship with someone you have met?
- Do you know what support is available to you and your family?

Here are some questions that could be considered when health and social care professionals are evaluating and reflecting on the health and social care practice they have witnessed:

- Is the person being supported and cared for taking the lead?
- Are people listening to the stories and the details of what makes sense to the person and what their life is like?
- Are people effectively engaging in conversation with the person to ask, 'what does a good life look like for you?'
- Are people acting on what they have learnt about the person?
- Is the balance right between meeting the wants and needs of the person?
- Is it recognised that supporting a person to achieve their wants and aspirations may be an effective way of meeting the assessed needs and outcomes?
- Are people being resourceful and creative when considering how to find solutions?
- Is the support and care that the person is being offered based on the Medical Model/Professional Gift Model? (see Chapter 2)
- Are people thinking and functioning openly, taking everything into consideration and working with the principle 'what is possible?' and not just what is available?

Key lessons learnt

- Personalisation provides the opportunity to realise the aspirations of choice and control for those who are accessing social care support and poses the challenge of how this can be brought into the real-life day-to-day experience for people with dementia and their families.
- As personalisation has developed, practical techniques have emerged that encourage the conversation among those in the dementia care triad+1, namely the person, their family, paid professionals and members of the community, regarding what is wanted and needed from the perspective of the person with dementia.
- As with any significant change, there are challenges to overcome to achieve the intended vision and outcome for people. Through collective working, optimism and willingness to achieve the best for people, it is possible to overcome these challenges and learn from how that was achieved.

- Personalisation, personal budgets, personal health budgets, direct payments and self-directed support continue to be emerging approaches that are developing and refining as lessons are learnt from implementation. As a community of practice, it will continue to be a journey of learning through which innovative new ways of achieving what really works for a person, from planning through to delivery will emerge.

Conclusion

We are in a time when the delivery of health and social care is aligned with law, strategy and policy. There is a clear message throughout these areas that align with personalisation, person-centred outcomes and people accessing health and social care experiencing a greater sense of control and choice, being about determining their own outcomes on a basis of what makes sense to them.

However, the areas of practice and delivery still require some further development and encouragement to reach these objectives.

This could be achieved through

- actively changing older and out-of-date working practices;
- changing the mindsets of people involved in the delivery of health and social care;
- considering how time is used to the best effect;
- setting a clear intention and purpose within practice.

When delivering change within culture and working practices it is often best to start with the question 'Why?'. This is where we find the purpose and intention. My hope is that the content of this book has been able to give you some clear insight into the purpose and intention. Once a strong sense of this has been achieved and a good foundation has been laid it is possible to then consider 'How'.

When considering the 'How' this book has been rich in a diverse range of options on approaches and tools. It is important to not rush into using all these tools and approaches but to give everyone some thinking time between the 'Why' and 'How' to consider which of these tools and approaches would be the most effective for the people involved, the circumstances and the outcomes everyone from the dementia care triad+1 is working towards.

As a strong believer in being part of a community of practice that can offer encouragement and support, it would be really great to hear how reading this book and implementing the ideas within have made a difference. Stories of change are the greatest source of encouragement and inspiration, generating a belief that what we are all aiming for is achievable.

Appendix 1 Useful organisations

Here is a list of useful organisations. Some provide helpful and inspirational insight into approaches to supporting people living with dementia, and others will be available to help people through the complex social care and health systems.

ACAS – Advisory, Conciliation and Arbitration Service
ACAS provides information, advice, training, conciliation and other services for employers and employees to help prevent or resolve workplace problems.
Website: www.acas.org.uk
Tel: 0300 123 1100

Alive Inside
Transforming the lives of people living with dementia through music.
Website: www.aliveinside.org
Tel: (212) 533-8116
Email: info@aliveinside.org

Alzheimer's Research UK
Alzheimer's Research UK states: *'Our vision is a world where people are free from the fear, harm and heartbreak of dementia"*
Website: www.alzheimersresearchuk.org
Telephone: 0300 111 5333
Email: reception@alzheimersresearchuk.org

Alzheimer's Society
A leading charity representing people with dementia and their families.
Website: www.alzheimers.org.uk
Dementia Contact support line: 0333 150 3456
Email: enquiries@alzheimers.org.uk

Care Quality Commission
The CQC monitors, inspects and regulates health and social care services. They publish what they find, including ratings to help people choose care.
Website: www.cqc.org.uk
Telephone: 03000 616161

Carers Trust
Providing support to carers across the UK.
Website: www.carers.org
Tel: 0300 772 9600
Email: info@carers.org

Carers UK
Making life better for carers.
Website: www.carersuk.org
Carers UK Tel: 020 7378 4999
Carers Wales Tel: 029 2081 1370
Carers Scotland Tel: 0141 445 3070
Carers Northern Ireland Tel: 02890 439 843
Email: info@carersuk.org

Centre for Welfare Reform
This organisation wants to help build a society where making things better is everyone's business.
Website: www.centreforwelfarereform.org/
Tel: 0114 258 6965
Email: admin@centreforwelfarereform.org

Chartered Society of Physiotherapy
The professional, educational and trade union body for chartered physiotherapists, physiotherapy students and assistants. Provides contact details of private physiotherapists in your area.
Website: www.csp.org.uk
Tel: 020 7306 6666
Email: enquiries@csp.org.uk

Citizens Advice Bureau (CAB)
Your local CAB can provide information and advice in confidence or point you in the right direction. To find your nearest CAB, look in the phone book, ask at your local library or look on the website.
Website: www.citizensadvice.org.uk
www.adviceguide.org.uk (online information portal)
Advice Link (England) Tel: 0800 144 8848

College of Occupational Therapists
Provides details of independent occupational therapists in your local area.
Website: www.cot.co.uk
Tel: 020 3141 4600
Email: hello@rcot.co.uk

Dementia Action Alliance
Dementia Action Alliance represents organisations across the UK who are committed to transforming the lives of people living with dementia and their carers.

Website: www.dementiaaction.org.uk
Email: ndaa@alzheimers.org.uk

Dementia UK
Providing specialists one-to-one support and expert advice and providing admiral nurses who work hand-in-hand with families, helping them cope with the fear, uncertainty and the difficult everyday reality of dementia.
Website: www.dementiauk.org
Tel: 0300 365 5500
Email: info@dementiauk.org

Forget Me Not Book
Forget Me Not Dementia is a resource hub of publications aiming to provide updates and training for support workers and staff. They are fully committed to improving the lives of people living with dementia.
Website: https://www.forgetmenotdementia.co.uk/
Email: chris@forgetmenotdementia.co.uk
Tel: 01223 207855

Imagineer Development UK CIC
A passionate and creative locally rooted community interest company in the north of England, with a strong national reach and respected reputation for helping organisations, individuals and families to live fulfilling lives, contributing to a fairer society. Offers support brokerage, brokerage management, support planning and graphic facilitation services, along with consultancy and training.
Website: https://www.imagineer.org.uk/
Tel: 07572 322200
Email: info@imagineer.org.uk

In Control
A national charity working for an inclusive society where everyone has the support they need to live a good life and make a valued contribution.
Website: www.in-control.org.uk
Tel: 0121 474 5900
Email: admin@in-control.org.uk

Inclusion Network
Working towards an inclusive society, inspiring and providing practical ideas to encourage inclusion.
Website: https://inclusion.com/
Tel: (416) 658-5363
Email: inclusionpress@inclusion.com

NHS Choices
NHS website that allows you to search for health services near you.
Website: www.nhs.uk

NICE – National Institution for Health and Clinical Excellence
NICE provides national guidance and advice to improve health and social care.
Website: https://www.nice.org.uk/
Tel: 0300 323 0140
Email: nice@nice.org.uk

Royal College of Speech and Language Therapists
The professional body for speech and language therapists and support workers. Promotes excellence in practice and influences health, education and social care policies.
Website: www.rcslt.org
Tel: 020 7378 1200
Email: info@rcslt.org

Safe Places National Network
A safe place helps vulnerable people if they feel scared or at risk while they are out in the community and need support right away.
Website: https://www.safeplaces.org.uk/
Email: info@safeplaces.org.uk

Skills for Care
The employer-led workforce development body for adult social care in England. It has a dedicated section of its website to provide advice and guidance to people who are employing their own support.
Website: www.skillsforcare.org.uk
Tel: 0113 241 1275
Email: information.team@skillsforcare.org.uk

Society of Chiropodists and Podiatrists
The professional body and trade union for registered podiatrists. Provides patient information on common foot problems and details of private practice podiatrists.
Website: https://cop.org.uk/
Tel: 020 7234 8620

Talking Mats
A social enterprise whose vision is to improve the lives of people with communication difficulties.
Website: www.talkingmats.com
Tel: 01786 479511
Email: info@talkingmats.com

Appendix 2 Templates

About Me – https://www.imagineer.org.uk/product/about-me-template/

About Me!

Focus Person Name:		Date Completed:	
Who helped you complete this form?			

GUIDANCE NOTES:

This is a nice way to start a meeting positively.
The focus person should initially quickly decorate the person in the middle of the profile to represent themselves.

In each section as all the attendees of the meeting should write one or two words in each section of the profile.

Or as a group Ice Breaker, you could print one profile for each person in the meeting and everyone writes a couple of notes on each person's profile. This can boost conversations, relationships and team morale.

EXAMPLE:

ADMIRE FUNNY CARING HELPFUL PATIENT CALM	SKILLS THAT THEY HAVE COMPUTER SKILLS TECHNOLOGY GREAT AT DRAWING
ITS ALWAYS FUN THEY MAKE ME SMILE WHAT YOU ENJOY ABOUT SPENDING TIME TOGETHER	GOING TO THE PARK AND FEEDING THE DUCKS FOND MEMORIES

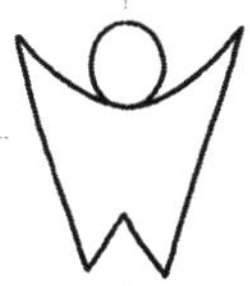

YOUR TURN:

On the next page complete your own About Me profile

ADMIRE

SKILLS THAT THEY HAVE

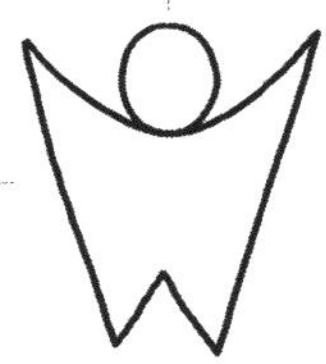

WHAT YOU ENJOY ABOUT SPENDING TIME TOGETHER

FOND MEMORIES

Doughnut Sort – https://www.imagineer.org.uk/product/doughnut-sort-template/

Doughnut Sort

Focus Person Name:		Date Completed:	
Who helped you complete this form?			

GUIDANCE NOTES:

The principle of the Doughnut Sort was designed by Charles Handy (2002) to support organisations to become good at achieving outcomes and organising their main resource, which in the majority of cases, is the people that work within the organisation.

Following the Doughnut Sort creates a clear sense of each person's role, responsibility and purpose within the organisation or the community of people who are working together to achieve a common goal.

The Doughnut Sort has been utilised within the context of community, health and social care as a way to identify and define the roles and core responsibilities of all the people involved in the care and support a person receives.

This would include people from within the Dementia Care Triad: people in a paid capacity, family members and the person with dementia, alongside people who have a meaningful relationship with the person and members of the community.

As the Doughnut Sort creates clarity regarding the role and responsibilities of each person involved, it can in turn help to improve the achievement of the desired outcomes and improve the effectiveness of the contributions people have to make towards these outcomes. This approach can increase the sense of satisfaction and purposefulness people feel within the role they play for the person with dementia.

The Doughnut provides a method to achieve a balance between what a person has to do within their role, the areas where they have scope to indulge in thinking and acting creatively and where their involvement would be valuable, and finally, the jobs and tasks where they need not have any involvement.

How to complete a Doughnut Sort:

If you can imagine an American style doughnut with jam in the middle.

1. The jam in the centre represents the tasks and responsibilities a person has to do within their job or role to fulfil it successfully. The tasks mentioned in the "jam" of the doughnut would be a person's core responsibilities and what they are expected to do well. These are the areas where people may need to follow guidance and instruction to achieve a good outcome. The guidance and instruction may be provided by the person with dementia, their immediate family or professionals involved in the care of the person.
2. The jam is not the whole of the Doughnut and the surrounding doughy areas represent the opportunities people have to make a difference, be creative and go beyond the bounds of duty to live up to their full potential. This would include opportunities for people to use judgement, creativity and to try out new things to see what could work. These are areas where people can use their imagination when working alongside the person with dementia to help to find new ways of doing things that work well for the person.
3. Areas that are not people's responsibility are signified by the area outside the Doughnut. This would determine the areas, responsibilities or tasks people should not be involved in as it is not their area of knowledge, skill or passion. Someone else who is better placed would have already agreed to take on these responsibilities.

Using the Doughnut Sort helps to build a better understanding of the roles people have to play and when they will be involved. It helps to build a stronger and connected network of people who are making sure, together, that all aspects of the support and care the person with dementia requires will be provided for. It can also provide clarity when there are a number of individuals and/or organisations involved.

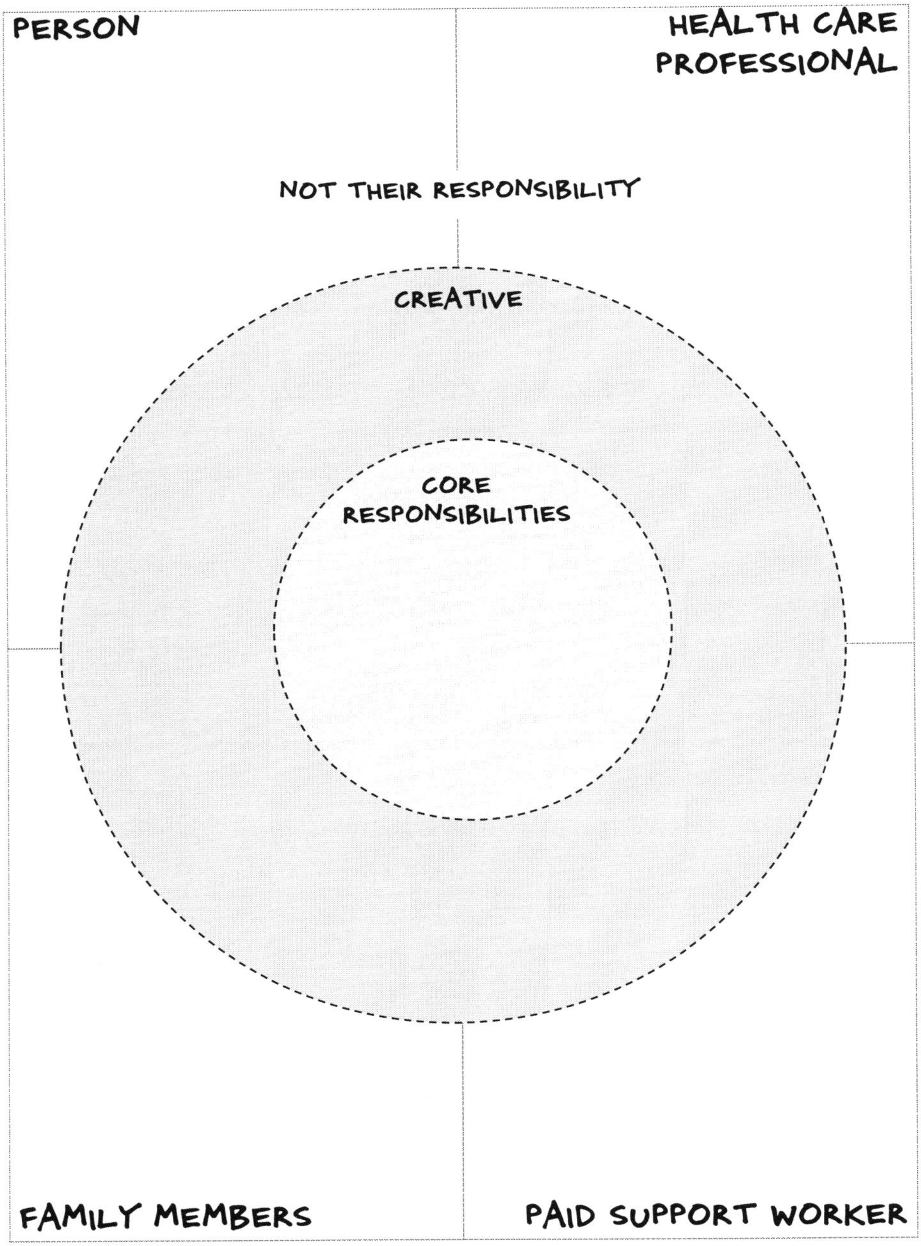
PERSON
HEALTH CARE PROFESSIONAL
NOT THEIR RESPONSIBILITY
CREATIVE
CORE RESPONSIBILITIES
FAMILY MEMBERS
PAID SUPPORT WORKER

Relationship Map – https://www.imagineer.org.uk/product/relationship-map-template/

Relationship Mapping

Focus Person Name:		Date Completed:	
Who helped you complete this form?			

GUIDANCE NOTES:

Using this template, you can write on the map the people in your life and how close your relationship is with the person. The map is split in to three different pieces:

1. Family
2. Friends
3. Paid People – This recognises people who are part of the persons network who are there because they are paid (PA's, GP's. Nurses and Social Workers. It could include the milkman)

This is a good template to do to identify the key people in your life.

The closer to the image of the person that a connection is placed on the relationship map signifies the importance of the relationship to the focus person.

EXAMPLE:

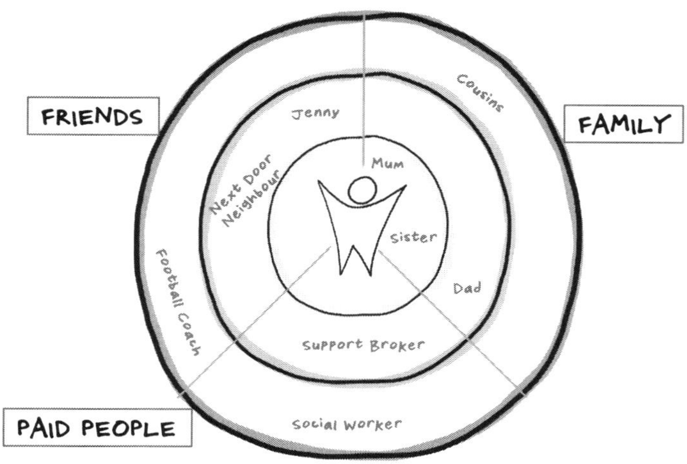

YOUR TURN:

On the next page complete your own Relationship map!

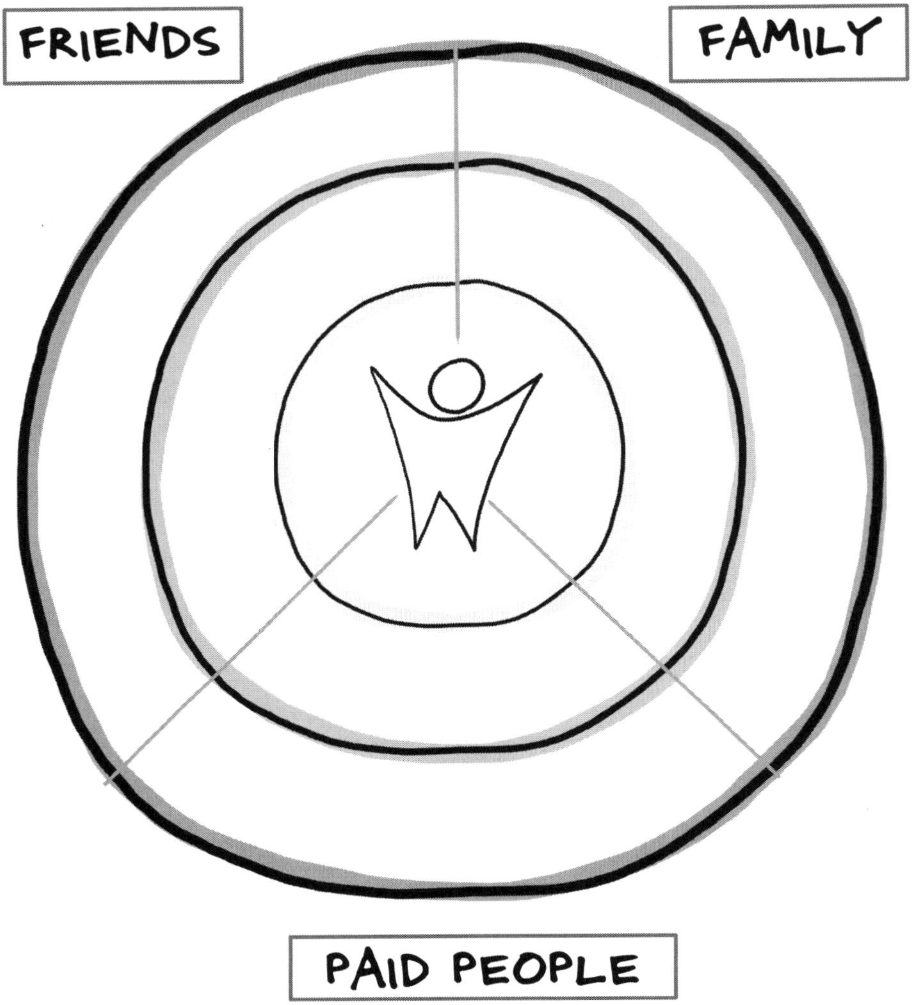
FRIENDS
FAMILY
PAID PEOPLE

Negotiables and Non Negotiable – https://www.imagineer.org.uk/product/negotiables-and-non-negotiables-template/

Negotiables and Non Negotiables

Focus Person Name:		Date Completed:	
Who helped you complete this form?			

GUIDANCE NOTES:

Utilising this approach helps to capture the "Negotiables and Non-Negotiables" within a person's life to identify what must be there for life to make sense to the person; what is essential and non-negotiable. The approach also captures what would be good to have in place if possible, although not absolutely essential, these areas are negotiable.

Developing an insight into what is negotiable or non-negotiable for the person provides the detail required to inform those around the person, including those providing support or care, about what works well for the person and how to strive towards achieving a good quality of life.

This approach recognises that the small things really matter and make a difference to achieving a quality of life and happiness. Paying attention to the finer detail of a person's daily experience and respecting the preferences they have can make the difference between a good day and great support and a bad day and support that does not fully recognise or respect the person.

To gather this information requires engagement in a conversation that enables the person with dementia to share what really matters to them. To hold conversations with people that know and understand the person well. Listening intently and actively to what the person and people around them are sharing establishes an understanding of what has been learnt from the conversation. When the information has been gathered it can be sorted under the headings of "Non-Negotiable" and "Negotiable".

If the person with dementia is not able to fully engage with a conversation it is possible to achieve this insight through gaining the information from the people who know the person well, this would include the people who would sit within the person's Circle of Intimacy and Circle of Friendship (see the information about Circles of Support in chapter 6). It is still important to involve the person with dementia in the conversation wherever possible and to engage them in a meaningful way and recognise their contribution to the conversation through listening to and observing the person's reactions.

The level of information gathered as a result of the conversations should provide the level of detail needed by those caring or supporting a person to know how to be able to fulfil their roles well. For instance, if this approach was utilised as a way to understand person's preferred morning routine it could include asking and exploring the following questions:

- What makes a good start to the day?
- What is the person's preference around how they get ready for their day?
- What is missing at the moment that is important to the person?
- How could the person's experience be better than it is now?
- Is there anything about now that needs to be maintained into the future?

The attention to the smaller details can often be overlooked. Honouring simple everyday preferences makes a difference to how a person feels: their wellbeing, self-esteem and sense of security. The following story illustrates this point:

'While on clinical placement on a general medical ward in my first year of training, I helped to care for an older patient, whom I will call William.

'The nursing staff had described William as confused and 'wondersome'. He seemed anxious and was touching his face constantly. Frequently, he could be found walking towards the bathroom in his dressing gown, so the nursing staff would help him back to his bed.

'My dementia training at university, along with my role as a 'dementia friends champion', led me to believe that William was not wandering without cause, and that there was something of interest to him in the bathroom.

'After talking to him, it became apparent that all he wanted was a shave. William was accustomed to shaving every Sunday but had not shaved in weeks. He had been wearing his dressing gown to go to the bathroom, which had a shaving brush and a safety razor in the pocket but had not yet managed to have a shave.

'William was not aware that he was able to shave, or that the staff could help him, so I found some shaving foam and walked with him to the bathroom. I helped him to foam his face, and then left him to have a shave, checking in on him regularly to make sure he was okay.

'Although William was with dementia, he was not at risk of falling or a danger to himself with the razor. He was clear on what his needs were, and I helped him to meet them. For the rest of the day William was calm and chatty, and there was no wandering or anxiety.

'This experience reaffirmed the importance of treating patients as individuals and supporting their choices so that they can be cared for with compassion, dignity and respect. I also have a better understanding of how my actions affect others and am committed to developing my nursing practice with the patient at the centre of all care decisions.'

(Perez-Merino, 2014)

From this story it is clear that a "Non-Negotiable" for William is to be able to have a shave on a Sunday morning. It would also be a "Non-Negotiable" that William receives support in the bathroom to get set up and ready to have a shave. The "Negotiable" would be discovered through having further conversations with William or observing his responses to situations or options given to him. The "Negotiables" may include the brand of shaving foam he uses or the time that he has a shave on a Sunday morning.

Investing time and energy in conversations to learn about the preferences of the person with dementia results in a greater level of understanding. The information gathered through these conversations can assist in the person being cared for and supported in a way that makes sense to them. Gaining this level of insight amongst the people supporting the person with dementia can avoid a misunderstanding, frustration and potential relationship breakdowns.

EXAMPLE:

NEGOTIABLES THINGS THAT SHOULD HAPPEN WHEN POSSIBLE	NON NEGOTIABLES THINGS THAT MUST HAPPEN
WHEN I HAVE A BATH	TO WALK THE DOG BEFORE I LEAVE THE HOUSE IN THE MORNING
THE TIME I GO TO BED	THE TIME I TAKE MY MEDICATION
WHERE I HAVE BREAKFAST	WRITING TO MY BROTHER ON A REGULAR BASIS
THE TIME I HAVE DINNER	

YOUR TURN: **On the next page complete your own "Negotiables and Non Negotiables" template.**

NEGOTIABLES THINGS THAT SHOULD HAPPEN WHEN POSSIBLE	NON NEGOTIABLES THINGS THAT MUST HAPPEN

Working and Not Working – https://www.imagineer.org.uk/product/working-and-not-working-template/

Working and Not Working

Focus Person Name:		Date Completed:	
Who helped you complete this form?			

GUIDANCE NOTES:

Using this template, you can really look at what is working and what is not working in a persons day to day life.

This could be looking at all aspects of their life. Once it has been shown what is working and what is not working you could then follow this up with an Action Plan to work on the "Not Working" section.

EXAMPLE:

✔ WORKING	NOT ✘ WORKING
I LIKE TRAVELLING TO SCHOOL ON MY OWN, I LIKE HOW INDEPENDENT I AM BECOMING	I DO NOT LIKE TRAVELLING ON BUSY BUSES ITS TOO LOUD AND IT MAKES ME ANXIOUS

YOUR TURN:

On the next page complete your own "What's Working and Not Working" template.

FOLLOW UP Complete an "Action Plan" after your "Working and Not Working" template to ensure that you can make the "Likes" possible and avoid the "Dislikes".

WORKING	NOT WORKING

Good Day and Bad Day – https://www.imagineer.org.uk/product/good-and-bad-day-template/

Good & Bad Days

Focus Person Name:		Date Completed:	
Who helped you complete this form?			

GUIDANCE NOTES:

Using this template, you can really look at what a good day and a bad day is for someone.
You start from the very beginning of their day from waking up to going to bed.
Asking the individual questions like:

- What would be the best way for you to wake up happy?
- What would your perfect morning routine be?
- What is the best way for you to get ready and motivated for the day ahead?

Then you ask similar questions about what would make their day a bad day.
This exercise is all about listening to the person and making sure that they are heard and understood.

The person may be acting in or feeling a certain way because their day has been spoiled by something earlier on in the morning. This may then affect their whole day.

EXAMPLE:

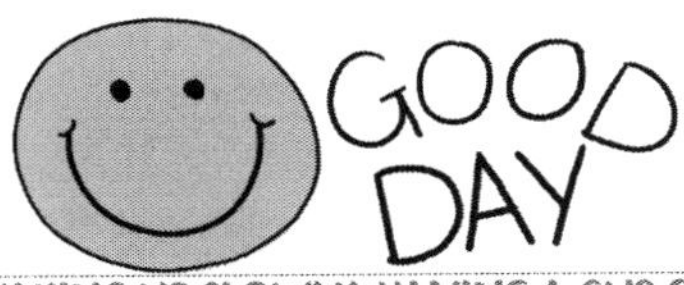

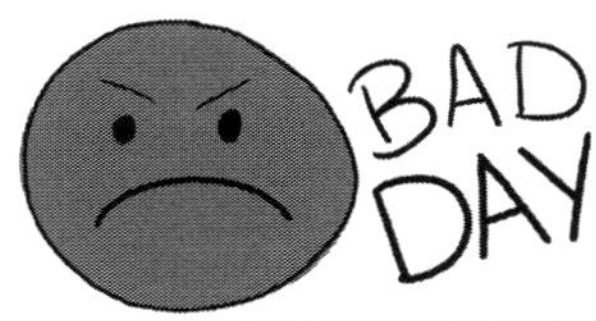

GOOD DAY	BAD DAY
WAKING UP SLOWLY, HAVING A CUP OF COFFEE AND HAVING A LITTLE SIT ON MY BED.	BEING RUSHED AWAKE, NOT HAVING TIME TO WAKE UP PROPERLY BEFORE MY ROUTINE STARTS.
HAVING MY CHOICE OF BREAKFAST, BRUSHING MY TEETH THEN CHOOSING MY OWN OUTFIT FOR THE DAY.	NOT HAVING CHOICE OF BREAKFAST, SOMEONE ELSE CHOOSING WHAT I WEAR AND SOMETIMES THE CLOTHES DON'T MATCH AND I LOOK SILLY.

YOUR TURN: On the next page complete your own "Good and Bad Day" template.

FOLLOW UP

Complete an "Action Plan" after your "Good and Bad Day" template to ensure that you avoid things on the "Bad Day" side and make the "Good Day" things possible.

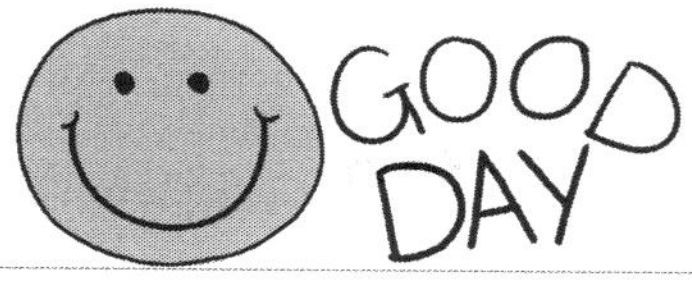
GOOD
DAY

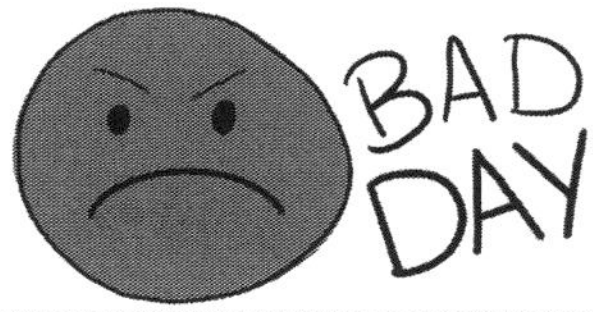
BAD
DAY

Appreciations – https://www.imagineer.org.uk/product/appreciations-template/

Appreciations

Focus Person Name:		Date Completed:	
Who helped you complete this form?			

GUIDANCE NOTES:

Developing Appreciations identifies the qualities and characteristics that other people value and admire about the person. Appreciations help people to recognise the person's uniqueness and to acknowledge and appreciate their:

- gifts - the aspects of a person's personality and character that draw people to them, the things that people remember about a person and what inspires people to spend more time with them
- qualities - what people admire about a person, their achievements and uniqueness
- talents - the things that the person shows an ability in, perhaps they have a natural talent?
- skills - the abilities that someone has learnt or received training or education in

Appreciations enable people, and those around them, to recognise, and have recognised, their positive qualities. Creating a focus on these qualities can shift the dynamic of any conversations and interaction to a space of positivity. It can be enlightening for the person, and those around them, to hear how they are regarded by others.

Appreciations can be gathered individually from people in the person's life and then collated and shared. Alternatively, the start of a meeting can be dedicated to gathering Appreciations from those attending.
A round of Appreciations at the start of a meeting can form a positive opening, for any form of meeting, which is being held with a focus on the person with dementia. This is a facilitated process where each person present at the meeting is asked to share something positive about the person who the meeting is for; something they like and admire about them.

To record people's contributions a piece of paper is placed on a wall or on a flip chart stand, with the person's name at the centre and the headings: "gifts", "qualities", "talents" and "skills" written around the person's name. The Facilitator would then ask each person present to contribute something to be added to the poster.

This exercise does not take long to facilitate and helps to set the tone for the rest of the meeting or planning session bringing a positive perspective for everyone involved which encourages people to consider the rest of the content of the meeting from a positive perspective which proves useful when encouraging people to find ideas and solutions.

Appreciation can challenge people who have previously focused on the negative perspective of the person or their situation. It encourages people to develop a positive outlook, regarding what the person can do, and what they do have to offer others.

EXAMPLE:

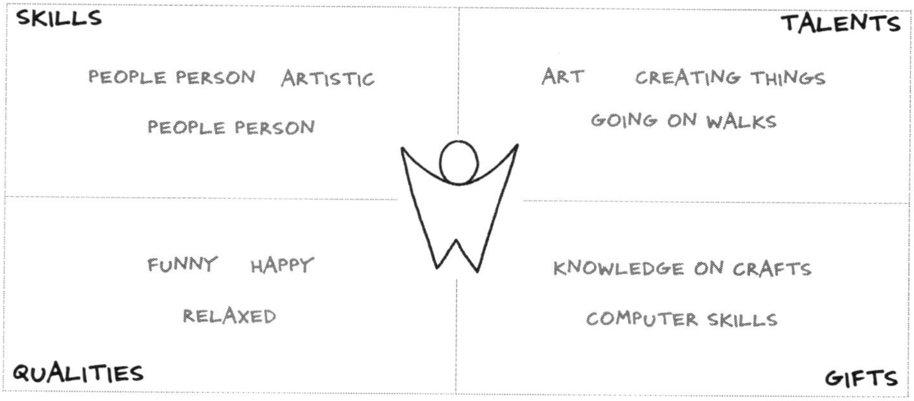

YOUR TURN:

On the next page complete your own Appreciations.

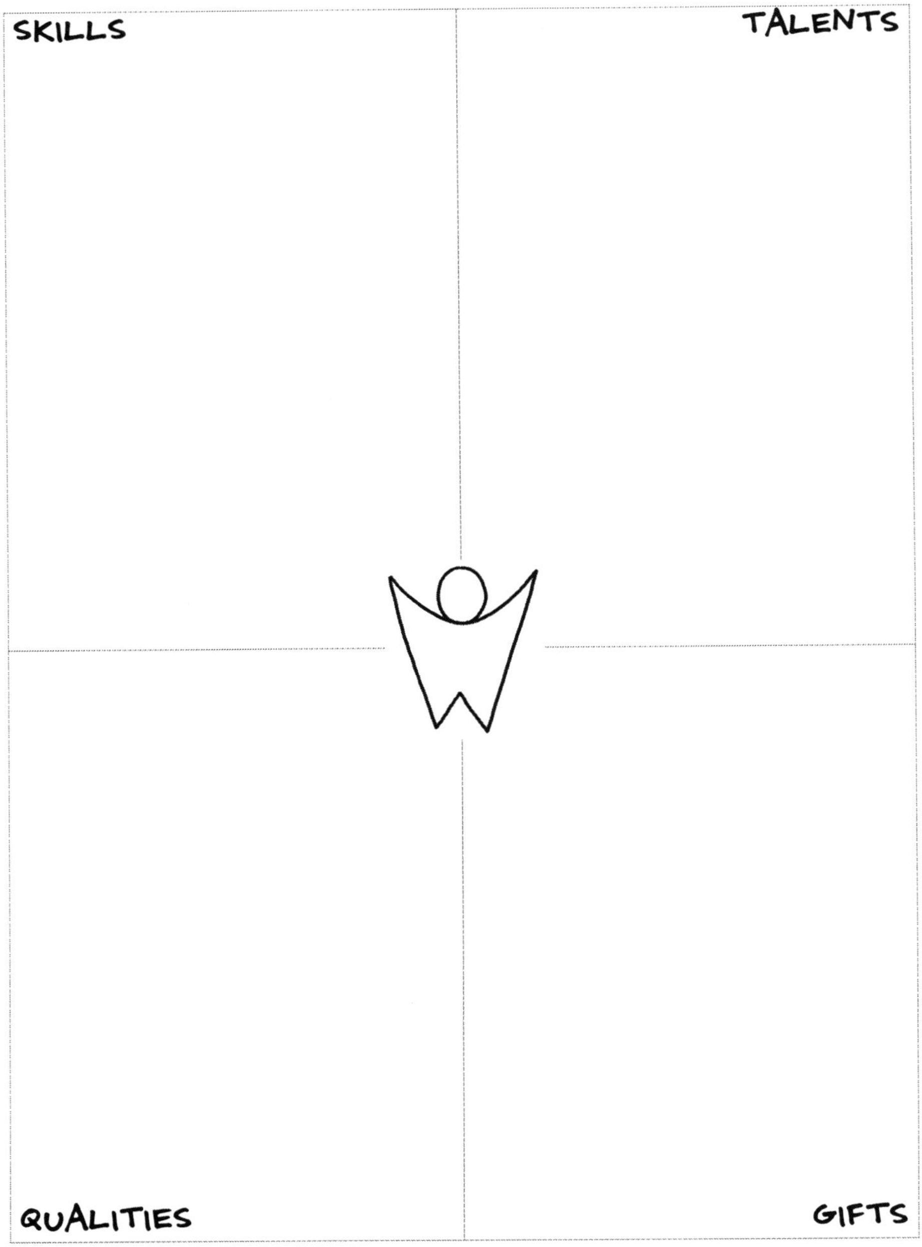
SKILLS
TALENTS
QUALITIES
GIFTS

Matching Staff

Matching Staff Approaches

Focus Person Name:		Date Completed:	
Who helped you complete this form?			

It is important that people are well supported and that those providing support, in any capacity, are a good match for the person being supported.

Producing a Matching Staff Profile identifies the skills, personality, characteristics, shared interests and practicalities that would be good for any supporter or carer, paid or unpaid, to have to create a good match and relationship between them and the person with dementia.

Completing a Matching Staff Profile encourages the person with dementia, and those around them, to think about what qualities they would like those providing care and support to have.

It is a good idea to complete a Matching Staff Profile prior to recruiting care and support, whether this is via an agency, employing directly or via natural support in the community.

The information gathered on a Matching Staff Profile can help in the creation of the advert, job description and the questions for and the way to conduct the interview process.

Investing the time to create a Matching Staff profile can help to ensure that:

- the person has a good quality of life
- the person enjoys spending time with those that are providing care or support

- a long lasting and enduring relationship is built between the person and those providing support or care.
- there is a good match in the relationship that goes beyond the action of care and support and into a realm of shared interests, passions and more meaningful connectedness
- the care or support worker and the person with dementia enjoy spending time together.

The detail needed to complete a Matching Staff Profile can be gathered from conversations about what good care or support would look like. This would include a conversation about:

- skills – what skills do the people providing care or support need to have? Do they need to be good at cooking particular meals and involving the person in the preparation, do they need to be confident in using health related equipment in a way that maintains respect and dignity, do they need to have skills in communication and a creative approach to communication to support the development of their relationship with the person they are caring for and supporting?
- interests – what interests does the person with dementia have and which of these interests would be good to have in common with the person who is providing care or support? Having a shared interest can help to build a relationships as interests can be pursued and shared together.
- personality & characteristics – what type of character and personality traits are needed when finding the right people to care and support. What is going to increase the chances of the person with dementia getting on with the people who will be caring for and supporting them? Discussing and thinking about the people the person has around them now and their past relationships helps to identify what makes the difference between someone they enjoy spending time with and

someone they do not. Are there certain characteristics that work well for the person, for example does the person tend to get on better with someone who is softly spoken and calm or do they get on better with someone who is bubbly and loud, or does this change depending on how the person feels?

- practicalities – what practical requirements does the person have of their carers and supporters? It is important to consider if there are certain needs that must be met. This would include times of the day or days of the week that the person needs care or support, does the person need someone who can drive and who has access to a vehicle, do they need someone who can use computers or someone trained in specific areas such as communication.

The information learnt from these conversations can be added to Matching Staff Profiles, here is an example of a completed profile

Skills and Knowledge	None Negotiables
Personality	Interests and Passions

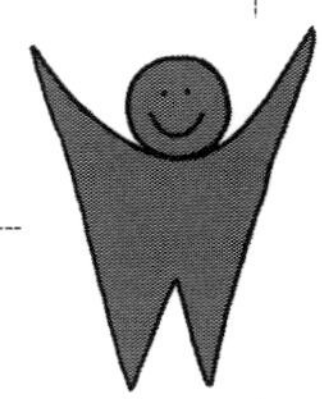

Summary for Job Description:

My Care and Support Profile – https://www.imagineer.org.uk/product/my-care-and-support-template/

My Care and Support

Focus Person Name:		Date Completed:	
Who helped you complete this form?			

GUIDANCE NOTES:

This opens the opportunity to discuss in detail how the person would like their care and support needs to be met:

- How I would like to be woken up
- How I would like to get dressed
- How I would like to stay in touch with family and friends

EXAMPLE:

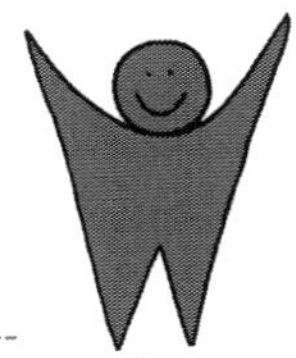

THE CARE & SUPPORT I WANT AND NEED!	HOW I WOULD LIKE IT FACILITATED!
I NEED MOTIVATION TO WAKE UP	I WOULD LIKE TO BE WOKEN UP WITH A CUP OF COFFEE
I NEED SUPPORT TO CHOOSE MY CLOTHES OUT	TO CHOOSE MY CLOTHES THE NIGHT BEFORE AND PUT THEM ON THE RADIATOR TO KEEP WARM FOR WHEN I GET DRESSED

YOUR TURN:

On the next page complete your own "Care and Support" template

FOLLOW UP Complete an "Action Plan" after your "Care and Support" template to ensure that there is an accurate thorough action plan in place.

THE CARE & SUPPORT I WANT AND NEED!

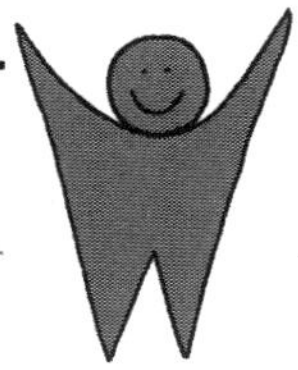

HOW I WOULD LIKE IT FACILITATED!

Treasure Chest – https://www.imagineer.org.uk/product/treasure-chest-template/

Treasure Chest

Focus Person Name:		Date Completed:	
Who helped you complete this form?			

GUIDANCE NOTES:

The "Treasure Chest" approach to connecting people was developed by an organisation called New Possibilities, who now specialise in Graphic Facilitation and previously were leaders in Person Centred Planning.

The "Treasure Chest" exercise brings people together to discover what opportunities and resources exist for the person within their network of friends and family. The exercise opens the idea that a person's quality of life can be improved through developing closer connections with people around them and the wider community. The "Treasure Chest" captures information about skills, interests, passions, and what people would love to learn. The information for the "Treasure Chest" is usually gathered at a meeting and all the people present contribute to its development.

The "Treasure Chest" can be developed at any time; it is particularly useful when completed alongside a Person Centred Plan, when people feel ready to start addressing the question "what needs to happen in order to make this plan happen?" The commitment to the person and their Person Centred Plan is likely to have increased as the plan was being developed and everyone involved may have found a new enthusiasm to help the person move towards achieving the aspirations set out in the plan. Following a Person Centred Plan with the "Treasure Chest" exercise builds on this enthusiasm and commitment.

Whether this is completed as a standalone exercise or as part of a Person Centred Plan, as people contribute to each section of the "Treasure Chest" it helps them to recognise what they have to offer and strengthens the connections that already exist.

When developing a "Treasure Chest", it helps to have a big sheet of paper divided into four sections with the following headings for each section:

- useful people to know.
- passions, interests, and hobbies
- skills and knowledge
- something you have always wanted to learn.

Someone can then take the lead in asking people in the group questions to help to complete each section of the paper. It is good for the person leading the meeting to have some useful examples to share to get the process started and to encourage other people to contribute, for instance:

- useful people to know – "I know a man who delivers free papers", "I know people who goes to line dancing classes" or "I know a solicitor".
- passions, interests, and hobbies – "I am passionate about baking/dancing/live theatre/shopping".
- skills and knowledge – "I have driving skills, "I can knit" or "I'm a good cook".
- something you have always wanted to learn – "I would like to learn a new language/to play a guitar/to tango".

The person leading the discussion will capture all the contributions from people or ask people to come and write their contributions onto the sheet of paper. Writing all the contributions onto the "Treasure Chest" makes it possible to appreciate the depth and range of resources available within a person's network. The connections between people will begin to emerge, which enables the development of stronger, more connected relationships and a sense of community. The extended networks of people can then emerge when people begin to identify the good people to know and how to link people together. This can include friends-of-friends, broadening the potential connections available to the person.

A completed "Treasure Chest" supports people to recognise how they can play a meaningful role in supporting the focus person to lead a life they are happy with, which (in turn) strengthens their relationship. A "Treasure Chest" activity is never truly complete as new connections can always be explored, but a "Treasure Chest" full of rich information creates the opportunity to find ideas regarding what is possible to be shared and discussed amongst the group- for example "I love dancing and if **Mary** would like to have the opportunity to dance on a regular basis, we could go together" or "I could make a connection for **Mary** with someone I know."

Follow a Treasure Chest with the completion of an Action Plan which we have a separate template for to capture the actions to move the ideas forward.

EXAMPLE:

USEFUL PEOPLE TO KNOW:

TERRY – HE IS A PAINTER AND DECORATOR.

JOANNE – SHE LOVES TO COOK AND BAKE.

BOB – HE IS GOOD AT DIY PROJECTS

PASSIONS AND OBSESSIONS:

GARDENING ART

MUSIC WALKING THE OUTDOORS

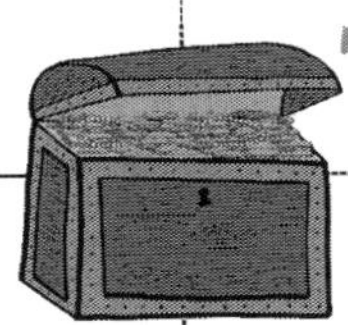

CLEANING

ORGANISATION

COMPUTER SKILLS

SKILLS AND KNOWLEDGE:

BAKING AND COOKING

LEARNING TO MAKE THINGS MYSELF (JOINERY/DIY PROJECTS)

NEW SKILLS YOU WOULD LIKE TO LEARN:

YOUR TURN:

On the next page complete your own "Treasure Chest" template

USEFUL PEOPLE TO KNOW:

PASSIONS AND OBSESSIONS:

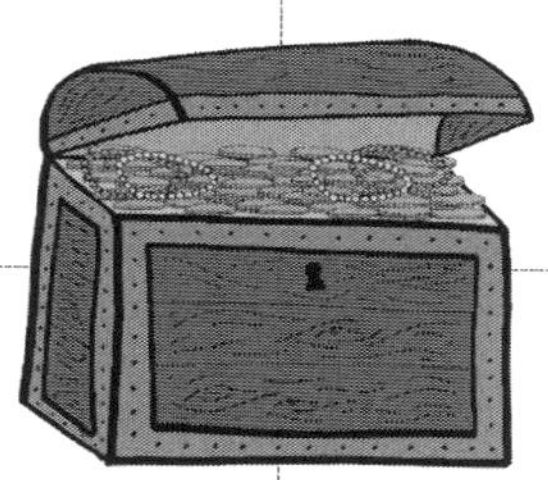

SKILLS AND KNOWLEDGE:

NEW SKILLS YOU WOULD LIKE TO LEARN:

Solutions Circle – https://www.imagineer.org.uk/product/solution-circle-template/

Solution Circle

Focus Person Name:		Date Completed:	
Who helped you complete this form?			

GUIDANCE NOTES:

A Solution Circle is a facilitated process that helps the people involved to identify new solutions to issues and challenges they are facing.

This is intended to be a short and focused facilitated process that is usually less than half an hour.

A Solution Circle can prove effective in addressing long-standing problems, especially areas that are preventing a person from achieving a good quality of life.

The Focus Person of the Solution Circle is the person who presents the problem or issue that they are experiencing. At the end of the process the Focus Person can select the idea, or ideas, that have been generated through the process which they would like to take forward.

Completing a Solution Circle holds the underpinning principle that the people who take part have the potential to help regardless of their background, experience, or the role they play in the person's life.

When planning to facilitate a Solution Circle it is best to involve five to nine people who can be present and actively engaged. Once you have the people find a space where it would be possible to hold the Solution Circle gathering. Choose somewhere that provides enough space for the people attending to be comfortable, with no distractions and a place that has somewhere to record the conversation in a clear visual way, either on a flip chart, whiteboard, or a room with blank wall space where big sheets of paper can be stuck to the wall. (From experience use an adhesive that does not leave marks – low tack masking tape is a good option)

There are four main roles that need to be fulfilled during the development of the Solution Circle, these include:

- Problem Presenter - also known as the Focus Person
- Process Facilitator - who will manage the people involved and be a timekeeper
- Note Taker or Graphic Recorder - who will clearly record all the information shared for everyone involved to see
- and everyone else – the people who will be supporting the Focus Person, actively engaging, listening, and contributing thoughts and ideas

Here are the steps to develop a Solution Circle, with a recommended six minutes being given to each step.

Step One: The Problem Presenter will start the process by outlining the problem they are experiencing; they will have six minutes of uninterrupted time to do this. At this stage, the job of the Process Facilitator is to make sure the Problem Presenter does not run over time and to prevent interruptions. During this first stage the Recorder will take notes and everyone else listens. If the Problem Presenter finishes saying what they have to share before the six minutes passes the group stays silent until the six minutes elapses. It is really important to honour the six minutes of uninterrupted time.

Step Two: Now the Process Facilitator will open up the session to the rest of the group and ask them to get involved by sharing their ideas and thoughts. It is important that everything is recorded and that the focus remains on sharing the ideas; this is not the time to ask questions, give advice or analyse any of the ideas and it is up to the Process Facilitator to keep everyone focused and to make sure that everyone gets a chance to contribute, ensuring that no one dominates the flow of the conversation. The Note Taker will make a record of all the ideas shared, making sure they use the actual words given by the others present and not placing their interpretation onto the notes taken. During this step the role of the Problem Presenter is to listen to the contributions being made by everyone else present and not to interrupt. Six minutes is dedicated to this step in the Solution Circle.

Step Three: The group enters into a dialogue which is led by the Problem Presenter. This step gives the group time to explore the ideas and further clarify the problem. The Process Facilitator needs to listen to the conversation to make sure that the content is covering the positive points only and to guide the group away from negativity and anything that relates to what cannot be done. Six minutes is also dedicated to this step in the Solution Circle.

Step Four: During this final step the Problem Presenter will identify the ideas that have stood out to them as having potential and the ones that would like to put into action after the meeting. The Problem Presenter and the group decide on what actions to set that are doable within the next three days and at least one action that can be initiated within 24 hours. It is critical to set actions that can be achieved within a short timeframe, such as researching information on the internet or making a phone call. Unless something is achieved soon after a planning meeting of this kind, people lose momentum and get "stuck". When concluding the Solution Circle, a person from the group volunteers to contact the Problem Presenter within 3 days to check if they have completed their first action. To bring the Solution Circle to a close the group does a round of words to describe the experience and the Recorder hands the finished record to the Problem Presenter. This final step is also completed within 6 minutes

A Solution Circle does not guarantee the perfect solution, but it usually gets people "unstuck" from the problem and helps the Problem Presenter / Focus Person to start to think about how to address it, with the momentum to keep going until the solution is found (Forest and Pearpoint, 1996).

YOUR TURN: On the next page complete your "Solution Circle"

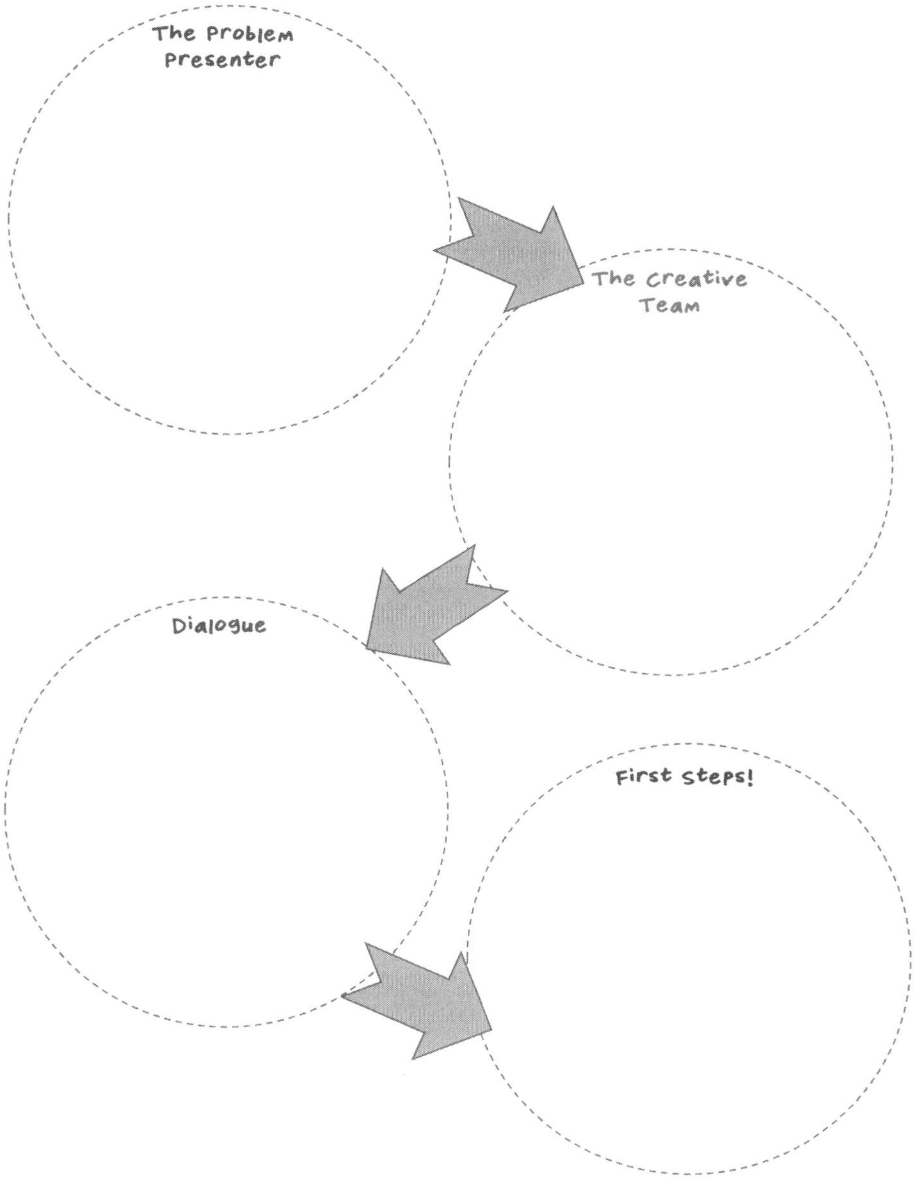
The Problem Presenter
The Creative Team
Dialogue
First steps!

Action Plan – https://www.imagineer.org.uk/product/action-plan-template/

Action Plan

Focus Person Name:		Date Completed:	
Who helped you complete this form?			

GUIDANCE NOTES:

Using this template, you can create an effective Action Plan.

- What is the task/action?
- Who will be completing this task/action?
- How will this task/action be completed?
- This task/action will be completed by when?

It is useful as it gives people a chance to talk through how they will approach and complete a task with the group before they take this on and therefor will be better prepared.

EXAMPLE:

WHAT? (WHAT IS THE ACTION)	WHO? (WHO WILL COMPLETE THIS ACTION)	HOW? (HOW WILL THIS ACTION BE COMPLETED)	BY WHEN? (WHEN IS THIS GOING TO BE COMPLETED)
TO CREATE MONTHLY CLEANING ROTAS	JO BLOGS WITH MUM	ON THE COMPUTER USING WORD	THE DRAFT TO BE COMPLETE AND SENT OUT IN 2 WEEKS

YOUR TURN:

On the next page complete your own Action Plan

FOLLOW UP

You could follow the Action plan up with our Review template.

WHAT? (WHAT IS THE ACTION)	WHO? (WHO WILL COMPLETE THIS ACTION)	HOW? (HOW WILL THIS ACTION BE COMPLETED)	BY WHEN? (WHEN IS THIS GOING TO BE COMPLETED)

REVIEW TO BE COMPLETED:

Bibliography

Able Magazine (n.d.) We're All Going on a Respite Holiday. [online] Available at: https://ablemagazine.co.uk/going-respite-holiday/ (accessed 12 June 2020).

Adams, T and Gardiner, P (2005) Communication and Interaction within Dementia Care Triads: Developing a Theory for Relationship-Centred Care. *Dementia*, [Article] 4 (2). Abstract only. Available through: Gale Academic OneFile. [online] Available at: https://go.gale.com/ps/anonymous?id=GALE%7CA140962504&sid=googleScholar&v=2.1&it=r&linkaccess=abs&issn=14713012&p=AONE&sw=w (accessed 9 May 2020).

Adults with Incapacity (Scotland) Act 2000. (c.4) Edinburgh: HMSO.

Advocacy Focus (2020) What Is Advocacy? [online] Available at: https://www.advocacyfocus.org.uk/understanding-advocacy (accessed 24 June 2020).

Advonet (2018) What Is Advocacy? [online] Available at: https://advonet.org.uk/how-we-can-help-you/what-is-advocacy/ (accessed 28 June 2020).

Age UK (2017) Briefing: Health and Care of Older People in England 2017. [pdf] *Age UK*. Available at: www.ageuk.org.uk/documents/EN-GB/For-professionals/Research/The_Health_and_Care_of_Older_People_in_England_2016.pdf?epslanguage=en-GB?dtrk=true (accessed 17 January 2021).

Alive Inside Foundation (2016) Alive Inside. [online] Available at: www.aliveinside.us (accessed 20 July 2020).

All-Party Parliamentary Group on Dementia (2014) *Building on the National Dementia Strategy: Change, Progress and Priorities*. [pdf] London: All-Party Parliamentary Group. Available at: www.alzheimers.org.uk/download/downloads/id/2249/building_on_the_national_dementia_strategy_change_progress_and_priorities.pdf (accessed 18 January 2018).

Alty, J, Farrow, M and Lawler, K (2019) How to Understand it Exercise and Dementia Prevention. *Practical Neurology,* [e-journal] 20 (3). Abstract only. Available through: British Medical Journal website. [online] Available at: https://pn.bmj.com/content/20/3/234 (accessed 29 January 2021).

Alzheimer's Association (2020) What Is Alzheimer's Disease? [online] Available at: https://www.alz.org/alzheimers-dementia/what-is-alzheimers (accessed 26 June 2020).

Alzheimer's Disease International (2016) *Dementia Friendly Communities Key Principles.* [pdf] London: Alzheimer's Disease International. Available at: www.alzint.org/u/dfc-principles.pdf (accessed 11 January 2021).

Alzheimer's Disease International (n.d.) *Dementia Friendly Communities (DFCs) New Domains and Global Examples*. [pdf] London: Alzheimer's Disease International. [online] Available at:

www.alzheimers.org.nz/getattachment/News-Info/Dementia-worldwide/dementia-friendly-communities-pdf.pdf/ (accessed 15 March 2021).

Alzheimer's Scotland (n.d.) Dementia Friendly Communities. [online] Available at: https://www.alzscot.org/our-work/dementia-friendly-communities (accessed 13 January 2021).

Alzheimer's Society (2007) *Home from Home. A Report Highlighting Opportunities for Improving Standards of Dementia Care in Care Homes.* [pdf] London: Alzheimer's Society. Available at: https://www.alzheimers.org.uk/sites/default/files/migrate/downloads/home_from_home_full_report.pdf? (accessed 6 July 2020).

Alzheimer's Society (2011) *Support. Stay. Save. Care and Support of People with Dementia in Their Own Homes*. [pdf] London: Alzheimer's Society. Available at: https://cdn.ps.emap.com/wp-content/uploads/sites/2/2011/01/Support_Stay_Save_Report.pdf (accessed 13 January 2021).

Alzheimer's Society (2014) 2014 APPG Report. [online] Available at: https://www.alzheimers.org.uk/about-us/policy-and-influencing/2014-appg-report (accessed 25 May 2020).

Alzheimer's Society (2014) Alzheimer's Society's View on Involving People with Dementia. [online] Available at: https://www.alzheimers.org.uk/about-us/policy-and-influencing/what-we-think/involving-people-dementia (accessed 22 July 2020).

Alzheimer's Society (2014) *Changes in Behaviour Factsheet 525LP.* [pdf] Alzheimer's Society. Available at: https://www.alzheimers.org.uk/sites/default/files/pdf/changes_in_behaviour.pdf (accessed 25 December 2020).

Alzheimer's Society (2014 – 2015). *Foundation Criteria for the Dementia-Friendly Communities Recognition Process*. [pdf] London: Alzheimer's Society. Available at: https://www.alzheimers.org.uk/sites/default/files/2018-06/DFC%20Foundation%20criteria_Fs%20Albert_4.pdf (accessed 11 January 2021).

Alzheimer's Society (2014) *What is Vascular Dementia?* [pdf] Alzheimer's Society. Available at: https://www.alzheimers.org.uk/sites/default/files/migrate/downloads/factsheet_what_is_vascular_dementia.pdf (accessed 26 June 2020).

Alzheimer's Society (2015) *The Progression of Alzheimer's Disease and Other Dementias Factsheet 458LP.* [pdf] Alzheimer's Society. Available at: https://www.alzheimers.org.uk/sites/default/files/2019-09/458lp-the-progression-of-alzheimers-disease-and-other-dementias-190521.pdf (accessed 8 June 2020).

Alzheimer's Society (2016) *Risk Factors for Dementia Facesheet 450LP.* [pdf] Alzheimer's Society. Available at: https://www.alzheimers.org.uk/sites/default/files/pdf/factsheet_risk_factors_for_dementia.pdf (accessed 8 June 2020).

Alzheimer's Society (2017) *This Is Me*. [pdf] Alzheimer's Society. Available at: https://www.alzheimers.org.uk/download/downloads/id/3423/this_is_me.pdf(accessed 3 July 2020).

Alzheimer's Society (2017) *What Is Dementia?* [pdf] Alzheimer's Society. Available at: https://www.alzheimers.org.uk/sites/default/files/pdf/what_is_dementia.pdf (accessed 1 June 2020).

Alzheimer's Society (2020) Alzheimer's Society's View on Personalisation. [online] (Last updated 31 July 2020) Available at: https://www.alzheimers.org.uk/about-us/policy-and-influencing/what-we-think/personalisation (accessed 20 January 2020).

Alzheimer's Society (2020) Diagnosing Dementia. [online] Available at: https://www.alzheimers.org.uk/about-dementia/types-dementia/diagnosing-dementia#:~:text=Dementia%20will%2

0usually%20be%20diagnosed,diseases%20of%20the%20nervous%20system (accessed 25 September 2020).

Alzheimer's Society (n.d.) Assessment Process and Tests. [online] Available at: https://www.alzheimers.org.uk/about-dementia/symptoms-and-diagnosis/diagnosis/assessment-process-tests#content-start (accessed 14 October 2020).

Alzheimer's Society (n.d.) Communication and Dementia. [online] Available at: https://www.alzheimers.org.uk/about-dementia/symptoms-and-diagnosis/symptoms/communicating-and-dementia (accessed 23 January 2021).

Alzheimer's Society (n.d.) Creating a Global Dementia Friendly Movement. [online] Available at: https://www.alzheimers.org.uk/about-us/policy-and-influencing/global-dementia-friends-network#:~:text=As%20of%20April%202020%2C%20there,number%20will%20continue%20to%20grow (accessed 17 March 2021).

Alzheimer's Society (n.d.) Facts for the Media. [online] Available at: https://www.alzheimers.org.uk/about-us/news-and-media/facts-media (accessed 6 March 2021).

Alzheimer's Society (n.d.) Mental Capacity Act. [online] Available at: https://www.alzheimers.org.uk/info/20032/legal_and_financial/127/mental_capacity_act (accessed 12 October 2020).

Alzheimer's Society (n.d.) The Mental Capacity Act and Dementia. [online] Available at: https://www.alzheimers.org.uk/get-support/daily-living/making-decisions-mental-capacity-act (accessed 30 September 2020).

Alzheimer's Society (n.d.) Tips for Communicating with a Person with Dementia. [online] Available at: https://www.alzheimers.org.uk/about-dementia/symptoms-and-diagnosis/symptoms/tips-for-communicating-dementia (accessed 23 January 2020).

Alzheimer's Society (n.d.) Sight and Hearing Loss with Dementia. [online] Available at: https://www.alzheimers.org.uk/about-dementia/symptoms-and-diagnosis/sight-hearing-loss (accessed 23 January 2020).

Arksey, H, Jackson, K, Croucher, K, Weatherly, H, Golder, S, Hare, P, Newbronner, E and Baldwin, S (2004) *Review of Respite Services and Short-Term Breaks for Carers for People with Dementia*. [pdf] London: National Co-ordinating Centre for NHS Service Delivery and Organisation (NCCSDO). Available at: https://www.york.ac.uk/inst/spru/pubs/pdf/respiteEx.pdf (accessed 28 June 2020).

Association of Directors of Adult Services (ADASS) (2012) *The Case for Tomorrow*. [pdf] Association of Directors of Adult Services (ADASS). Available at: https://www.adass.org.uk/adassmedia/stories/Policy%20Networks/Older%20People/Key%20Documents/TheCaseForTomorrow150312.pdf (accessed 17 January 2021).

Bamford, C, Arksey, H, Poole, M, Kirkley, C, Hughes, J, Corner, L and Bond, J (2009) *Person- and Carer-Centred Respite Care for People with Dementia: Developing Methods of Evaluating the Effectiveness of Different Models*. [pdf] Newcastle University: Institute of Health and Society. Available at: http://www.netscc.ac.uk/hsdr/files/project/SDO_FR_08-1511-113_V01.pdf (accessed 28 June 2020).

Bamford, C, Eccles, M, Steen, N and Robinson, L (2007) Can Primary Care Record Review Facilitate Earlier Diagnosis of Dementia? *Family Practice*. [online] Available at: https://academic.oup.com/fampra/article/24/2/108/468369 (accessed 10 June 2020).

Bartlett, R and O'Connor, D (2010) *Broadening the Dementia Debate: Towards Social Citizenship*. Bristol: Policy Press.

Batsch, N L, Mittelman, M S, and Alzheimer's Disease International (2012) *World Alzheimer Report 2012 Overcoming the Stigma of Dementia.* [pdf] London: Alzheimer's Disease International (ADI). Available at: https://www.alz.co.uk/research/WorldAlzheimerReport2012.pdf (accessed 23 May 2020).

Bettencourt, L A, Ostrom, A L, Brown, S W and Roundtree, R I (2002) Client Coproduction in Knowledge-Intensive Business Services. *California Management Review*, 44 (4): 100–128.

Boyle, D and Harris, M (2009) *The Challenge of Co-Production. How Equal Partnerships between Professionals and the Public Are Crucial to Improving Public Services*. London: Nesta. Available from https://media.nesta.org.uk/documents/the_challenge_of_co-production.pdf (accessed 25 May 2020).

Brooker, D (2004) What Is Person-Centred Care in Dementia? *Reviews in Clinical Gerontology*, [e-journal] 13 (3): 215–222. Available through: My Seniors Weebly website. [online] Available at: http://myseniors.weebly.com/uploads/2/1/8/5/21859032/what_is_person-centered_care.pdf (accessed 13 May 2020).

Brooker, D, May, H and Edwards, P (2009) *Enriched Care Planning for People with Dementia: A Good Practice for Delivering Person-Centred Care*. London: Jessica Kingsley Publishers.

Bryden, C (2015) *Nothing about Us, Without Us! 20 Years of Dementia Advocacy*. London: Jessica Kingsley Publishers.

BSI Group (n.d.) *Living with Dementia*. [pdf] BSI Group. Available at: https://www.bsigroup.com/LocalFiles/en-GB/consumer-guides/resources/BSI-Living-With-Dementia-Brochure-UK-EN.pdf (accessed 11 January 2021).

Burgener, S C and Dickerson-Putman, J (1999) Assessing Patients in the Early Stages of Irreversible Dementia. The Relevance of Patient Perspectives. *Journal of Gerontological Nursing,* [e-journal] 25 (2): 33–41. Abstract only. Available through: National Library of Medicine website. [online] Available at: https://pubmed.ncbi.nlm.nih.gov/10347435/ (accessed 18 July 2020).

Cabinet Office (2015) *Social Value Act Review*. [pdf] London: Cabinet Office. Available at: https://assets.publishing.service.gov.uk/government/uploads/system/uploads/attachment_data/file/403748/Social_Value_Act_review_report_150212.pdf (accessed 30 September 2020).

Cahn, E S (2000) *No More Throw-Away People: The Co-production Imperative*. 2nd ed. Washington: Essential Books Ltd.

Care Act 2014. (c.23). London: HMSO.

Care Quality Commission (CQC) (2014) *Cracks in the Pathway People's Experience of Dementia Care as They Move between Care Homes and Hospitals.* [pdf] Care Quality Commission. Available from: http://www.cqc.org.uk/sites/default/files/20141009_cracks_in_the_pathway_final_0.pdf (accessed 25 May 2020).

Care Quality Commission (CQC) (2015) Guidance for Providers on Meeting the Regulations. [online] Available at: https://www.cqc.org.uk/sites/default/files/20150210_guidance_for_providers_on_meeting_the_regulations_final_01.pdf (accessed 6 July 2020).

Care Quality Commission (CQC) (2017) Regulation 14: Meeting Nutritional and Hydration Needs. [online] (Last updated 29 May 2017) Available at: https://www.cqc.org.uk/guidance-providers/regulations-enforcement/regulation-14-meeting-nutritional-hydration-needs (accessed 12 July 2020).

Care Services Improvement Partnership (CSIP) National Older People's Mental Health Programme (2007) *Strengthening the Involvement of People with Dementia. A Resource for Implementation.* [pdf] York: Care Services Improvement Partnership (CSIP) National Older People's Mental Health Programme. Available at: https://dementiapartnerships.com/wp-content/uploads/sites/2/strengthening-involvement.pdf (accessed 15 July 2020).

Carers (Scotland) Act 2016. (asp.9). Edinburgh: Scottish Government.

Carers UK (2013) *The State of Caring 2013.* [pdf] Carers UK. Available at: https://www.carersuk.org/for-professionals/policy/policy-library/the-state-of-caring-2013 (accessed 19 June 2020).

Carers UK (2014) *Care Act 2014 Key Provisions for Carers.* [pdf] Carers UK. Available at: https://www.carersuk.org/for-professionals/policy/policy-library?task=download&file=policy_file&id=4730 (accessed 19 June 2020).

Carers UK (2014) *Caring and Family Finances Inquiry - UK Report - (Full Report).* [pdf] London: Carers UK. Available at: https://www.carersuk.org/for-professionals/policy/policy-library/caring-family-finances-inquiry (accessed 19 June 2020).

Carers UK (2014) *State of Caring 2014.* [pdf] London: Carers UK. Available at: https://www.carersuk.org/for-professionals/policy/policy-library/state-of-caring-2014 (accessed 19 June 2020).

Carers UK (2015) *Facts about Carers.* [pdf] Carers UK. Available at: https://www.carersuk.org/for-professionals/policy/policy-library/facts-about-carers-2015 (accessed 19 June 2020).

Carers UK (2019) *Facts about Carers.* [pdf] Carers UK. Available at: https://www.carersuk.org/images/Facts_about_Carers_2019.pdf (accessed 20 September 2020).

Centre for Ageing Better (n.d.) 'Soul-Destroying' Ageism in Recruitment Could Be Final Straw for Over 50s. [online] Available at: https://www.ageing-better.org.uk/ (accessed 9 March 2021).

Centre for Ageing Better (n.d.) *UK Network of Age-Friendly Communities*. [online] Available at: https://www.ageing-better.org.uk/uk-network-age-friendly-communities?gclid=Cj0KCQiAs5eCBhCBARIsAEhk4r47oSpiEFao997QzHrMtNUOHQwv6veYo5EvBn-EnAZTZwigztBvyw4aAj3cEALw_wcB (accessed 9 March 2021).

Chenoweth, L, King, M T, Jeon, Y, Brodaty, H, Stein-Parbury, J, Norman, R, Haas, M, and Luscombe, G (2009) Caring for Aged Dementia Care Resident Study (CADRES) of Person-Centred Care, Dementia-Care Mapping, and Usual Care in Dementia: A Cluster-Randomised Trial. *The Lancet Neurology*, 8 (4): 317–325.

Commission for Social Care Inspection (CSCI), Brooker, Surr and Scally (2008) *See Me, not Just the Dementia - Understanding People's Experiences of Living in a Care Home.* [pdf] London: Commission for Social Care Inspection (CSCI). Available at: https://bradscholars.brad.ac.uk/bitstream/handle/10454/6420/seemenotjustthedementia.pdf (accessed 23 May 2020).

Commission for the National Institute for Health and Clinical Excellence and Social Care Institute for Excellence (2007) *Dementia: A NICE-SCIE Guideline on Supporting People with Dementia and Their Carers in Health and Social Care*. [pdf] The British Psychological Society and Gaskell. Available at: https://www.scie.org.uk/publications/misc/dementia/dementia-fullguideline.pdf?res=true (accessed 23 May 2020).

Community Care (Direct Payments) Act 1996. (c.30). London: HMSO.

CommunityCare (2010) Research into the Use of Direct Payments by People with Dementia. [online] Available at: https://www.communitycare.co.uk/2010/09/01/research-into-the-use-of-direct-payments-by-people-with-dementia/ (accessed 2 May 2020).

Copestake, P, Sheikh, S, Johnston, S and Bollen, A (2014) Removing Barriers, Raising Disabled People's Living Standards. Available at: https://docplayer.net/16691383-Removing-barriers-raising-disabled-people-s-living-standards.html (accessed 23 May 2020).

Copland, E, Hodge, S, Clary, L and Cartwright, V, eds. (2018) *Memory Services National Accreditation Programme (MSNAP) Standards for Memory Services*. 6th ed. [pdf] London: Royal College of Psychiatrists. Available at: https://www.rcpsych.ac.uk/docs/default-source/improving-care/ccqi/quality-networks/memory-clinics-msnap/msnap-standards-6th-edition-2018.pdf?sfvrsn=d3a9bc94_2 (accessed 19 October 2020).

Davies, K (2005) *Creating a Circle of Support*. [online] Available at: https://www.iidc.indiana.edu/irca/articles/creating-a-circle-of-support (accessed 22 July 2020).

De Bellis, A, Bradley, S L, Wotherspoon, A, Walter, B, Guerin, P, Cecchin, M and Patterson, J (2009) *Come into My World.* [pdf] Adelaide: Flinders University of South Australia. Available at: http://nursing.flinders.edu.au/comeintomyworld/docs/Come%20Into%20My%20World%20-%20How%20to%20Interact%20with%20a%20Person%20who%20has%20Dementia.pdf (accessed 17 July 2020).

Deacon, A and Mann, K (1999) Agency, Modernity and Social Policy. *Journal of Social Policy*, 28 (3): 413–35.

Dementia Action Alliance (2010) *National Dementia Declaration for England.* [pdf] Dementia Action Alliance. Available at: https://www.dementiaaction.org.uk/assets/0001/1915/National_Dementia_Declaration_for_England.pdf (accessed 25 May 2020).

Dementia Alliance International (2017) Dementia Alliance International. [online] Available at: https://www.dementiaallianceinternational.org/ (accessed 29 June 2020).

Dementia Friends (2017) People Living with Dementia Face Social Isolation Now More Than ever. [online] Available at: https://www.dementiafriends.org.uk/ (accessed 5 May 2020).

Dementia Friends (n.d.) List of Dementia Friendly Communities. [online] Available at: https://www.dementiafriends.org.uk/WebArticle?page=dfc-public-listing#.X_y5xOj7TIU (accessed 11 January 2021).

Dementia Matters (2018) Mixed Dementia. [online] Available at: https://www.dementiamatters.net/mixed-dementia (accessed 8 June 2020).

Dementia Partnerships (n.d.) Step 3 Behaviours that Challenge Us. [online] Available at: https://dementiapartnerships.com/supported-well/learning-pathway/step-3/ (accessed 22 May 2020).

DementiaUK (2016) Memory Service. [online] Available at: https://www.dementiauk.org/faq/memory-service/ (accessed 17 October 2020).

Demos (2014) *"A Vision for Care Fit for the Twenty-First Century..." The Commission on Residential Care*. [pdf] London: Demos. Available at: https://www.demos.co.uk/files/Demos_CORC_report.pdf?1409673172 (accessed 3 July 2020).

Department for Constitutional Affairs (2007) *Mental Capacity Act 2005 Code of Practice.* [pdf] London: The Stationery Office. Available at: https://assets.publishing.service.gov.uk/government/uploads/system/uploads/attachment_data/file/497253/Mental-capacity-act-code-of-practice.pdf (accessed 30 September 2020).

Department for Education, Government Equalities Office and Office for Disability Issues (2015) Policy Paper 2010–2015 Government Policy: Equality. [online] (Last updated May 8 2015)

Available at: https://www.gov.uk/government/publications/2010-to-2015-government-policy-equality/2010-to-2015-government-policy-equality (accessed 23 May 2020).

Department of Health (2001) *Valuing People: A New Strategy for Learning Disability for the 21st Century.* (Cm 5086). London: TSO (The Stationery Office).

Department of Health (2009) *Living Well with Dementia: A National Dementia Strategy*. [pdf] Leeds: Department of Health. Available at: https://www.gov.uk/government/uploads/system/uploads/attachment_data/file/168220/dh_094051.pdf (accessed 14 October 2020).

Department of Health (2009) *Valuing People Now: A New Three-Year Strategy for People with Learning Disabilities.* [pdf] London: Department of Health. Available at: https://webarchive.nationalarchives.gov.uk/20110503151248/http://www.valuingpeoplenow.dh.gov.uk/sites/dhvpnweb.rroom.net/files/webfm/Valuing%20People%20Now%20Landing%20Page/Valuing%20People%20Now%20Strategy%20.pdf (accessed 18 May 2020).

Department of Health (2010) *Equity and Excellence. Liberating the NHS.* (Cmnd. 7881) London: TSO (The Stationery Office).

Department of Health (2010) Personalisation. [online] Available at: https://webarchive.nationalarchives.gov.uk/+/http://www.dh.gov.uk/en/SocialCare/Socialcarereform/Personalisation/index.htm (accessed 16 May 2020).

Department of Health (2010) *Quality Outcomes for People with Dementia: Building on the Work of the National Dementia Strategy*. [pdf] Department of Health. Available at: https://assets.publishing.service.gov.uk/government/uploads/system/uploads/attachment_data/file/213811/dh_119828.pdf (accessed 25 May 2020).

Department of Health (2012) *Caring for Our Future: Reforming Care and Support.* [pdf] Department of Health and Social Care. Available at: https://assets.publishing.service.gov.uk/government/uploads/system/uploads/attachment_data/file/136422/White-Paper-Caring-for-our-future-reforming-care-and-support-PDF-1580K.pdf (accessed 4 May 2020).

Department of Health (2013) *FACTSHEET 4 The Care Bill – Personalising Care and Support Planning.* [pdf] Department of Health. Available at: https://assets.publishing.service.gov.uk/government/uploads/system/uploads/attachment_data/file/268681/Factsheet_4_update.pdf (accessed 13 June 2020).

Department of Health (2014) *The Irish National Dementia Strategy.* [pdf] Department of Health. Available at: https://assets.gov.ie/10870/3276adf5273f4a9aa67e7f3a970d9cb1.pdf (accessed 4 May 2020).

Department of Health (2015) *Prime Minister's Challenge on Dementia 2020.* [pdf] Department of Health. Available at: https://www.gov.uk/government/uploads/system/uploads/attachment_data/file/414344/pm-dementia2020.pdf (accessed 25 May 2020).

Department of Health (2016) *Prime Minister's Challenge on Dementia 2020 Implementation Plan.* [pdf] Department of Health. Available at: https://assets.publishing.service.gov.uk/government/uploads/system/uploads/attachment_data/file/507981/PM_Dementia-main_acc.pdf (accessed 4 May 2020).

Department of Health and Social Care (2015) Policy Paper 2010 to 2015 Government Policy: Dementia. [online] (Last updated 8 May 2015) Available at: https://www.gov.uk/government/publications/2010-to-2015-government-policy-dementia/2010-to-2015-government-policy-dementia (accessed 10 January 2021).

Department of Health and Social Care (2016) Factsheet 3: Assessing Needs and Determining Eligibility. [online] (Last updated 19 April 2016) Available at: https://www.gov.uk/government/publications/care-act-2014-part-1-factsheets/care-act-factsheets#factsheet-3-assessing-needs-and-determining-eligibility (accessed 12 July 2020).

Department of Health and Social Care (2016) Factsheet 4: Personalising Care and Support Planning. [online] (Last updated 19 April 2016) Available at: https://www.gov.uk/government/publications/care-act-2014-part-1-factsheets/care-act-factsheets#factsheet-4-personalising-care-and-support-planning (accessed 12 July 2020).

Department of Health and Social Care (2016) Joint Declaration on Post-Diagnostic Dementia Care and Support. [online] Available at: https://www.gov.uk/government/publications/dementia-post-diagnostic-care-and-support/dementia-post-diagnostic-care-and-support (accessed 4 May 2020).

Department of Health and Social Care (2018) NHS Continuing Healthcare Decision Support Tool [online] Available at: https://www.gov.uk/government/publications/nhs-continuing-healthcare-decision-support-tool (accessed 11 November 2020).

Department of Health and Social Care (2019) *Dementia 2020 Challenge 2018: Review Phase 1.* [pdf] Department of Health and Social Care. Available at: https://assets.publishing.service.gov.uk/government/uploads/system/uploads/attachment_data/file/780777/dementia-2020-challenge-2018-review.pdf (accessed 4 May 2020).

Department of Health Putting People First Programme Personalisation (2010) *Putting People First: Personal Budgets for Older People – Making it Happen.* [pdf] Department of Health. Available at: https://www.choiceforum.org/docs/pb.pdf (accessed 25 May 2020).

Dinsdale, P (2013) Is Dudley Council Setting Out a New Model for Dementia Care? *The Guardian*, 10 June. [online] Available at: https://www.theguardian.com/social-care-network/2013/sep/10/dudley-council-example-dementia-care (accessed 25 September 2020).

Dubois, B, Padovani, A, Scheltens, P, Rossi, A and Dell'Agnello, G (2015) Timely Diagnosis for Alzheimer's Disease: A Literature Review on Benefits and Challenges. *Journal of Alzheimer's Disease*. [online] Available at: https://www.ncbi.nlm.nih.gov/pmc/articles/PMC4927869/ (accessed 10 June 2020).

Dudley Metropolitan Borough Council (2020) *Dementia Gateways*. [online] Available at: https://www.dudley.gov.uk/residents/care-and-health/adult-health-social-care/support-to-stay-independent/dementia-gateways/ (accessed 25 September 2020).

Duffy, S J (2004) In Control. *Journal of Integrated Care*, 12 (6).

Duffy, S J (2011) Citizenship & Professional Gift Models. [online] Available at: https://www.centreforwelfarereform.org/library/citizenship-professional-gift-models.html (accessed 25 May 2020).

Elsevier Mosby (2005) *Mosby's Dictionary of Complementary and Alternative Medicine*. St. Louis, MO: Elsevier Mosby.

Falvey, M A, Forest, M, Pearpoint, J, and Rosenberg, R L (2003) *All My Life's a Circle. Using the Tools: Circles, MAPs and PATHS*. Ontario: Inclusion Press.

Fazio, S, Pace, D, Flinner, J and Kallmyer, B (2018) The Fundamentals of Person-Centered Care for Individuals with Dementia. *The Gerontologist,* [e-journal] 58 (1): 10–19. [online] Available at: https://academic.oup.com/gerontologist/article/58/suppl_1/S10/4816735 (accessed 22 November 2020).

Feil, N (1993) *The Validation Breakthrough: Simple Techniques for Communicating with People with Alzheimer's-Type Dementia*. Michigan: Health Professions Press.

Feltoe, J and Orellana, K (2013) *Making Personal Budgets Work for Older People.* [pdf] London: Age UK. Available at: https://www.ageuk.org.uk/Documents/EN-GB/For-professionals/Care/Making_Personal_Budgets_work_for_older_people-Full_Report.pdf (accessed 17 January 2021).

Ferman, T J, Smith, G E and Melom, B (n.d.) Understanding Behavioral Changes in Dementia. [online] Available at: https://www.lbda.org/understanding-behavioral-changes-in-dementia/ (accessed 22 November 2020).

Forest, M and Pearpoint, J (1996) SOLUTION CIRCLE Getting Unstuck a Creative Problem Solving Tool. [online] Available at: https://inclusion.com/inclusion-resources/training-tools/solution-circle/ (accessed 3 August 2020).

Glendinning, C, Challis, D, Fernández, J-P, Jacobs, S, Jones, K, Knapp, M, Manthorpe, J, Moran, N, Netten, A, Stevens, M and Wilberforce, M (2008) *Evaluation of the Individual Budgets Pilot Programme Final Report.* [pdf] York: Individual Budgets Evaluation Network (IBSEN). Available at: https://www.york.ac.uk/inst/spru/pubs/pdf/IBSEN.pdf (accessed 17 January 2021).

Goldsmith, M (1996) *Hearing the Voice of People with Dementia: Opportunities and Obstacles.* London: Jessica Kingsley Publishers.

Green, G and Lakey, L (2013) *Building Dementia-Friendly Communities: A Priority for Everyone*. Alzheimer's Society. Available at: https://actonalz.org/sites/default/files/documents/Dementia_friendly_communities_full_report.pdf (accessed 15 July 2020).

Greenhalgh, L and Whitham, B (2016) *Hidden Charges in Care Homes Exploring Consumer Protections within the Care Home Market*. [pdf] London: Citizens Advice Bureau. Available at: https://www.citizensadvice.org.uk/Global/CitizensAdvice/Public%20services%20publications/Hidden%20charges%20in%20care%20homes.pdf (accessed 5 November 2016).

Hancock, G A, Woods, B, Challis, D and Orrell, M (2006) The Needs of Older People with Dementia in Residential Care. *International Journal of Geriatric Psychiatry*, [e-journal] 21 (1). Abstract only. Available through: Wiley Online Library [online] Available at: https://onlinelibrary.wiley.com/doi/abs/10.1002/gps.1421 (accessed 6 July 2020).

Handy, C (2002) *The Empty Raincoat: Making Sense of the Future*. London: Arrow.

Hatton, C, Centre for Disability Research, Lancaster University and Waters, J and In Control (2011) *The National Personal Budget Survey.* [pdf] Think Local Act Personal. Available at: http://www.in-control.org.uk/media/242956/national%20personal%20budget%20survey%20report%20june%202011.pdf (accessed 25 May 2020).

Health Innovation Network South London (2016) *What Is Person-Centred Care and Why Is it Important?* [pdf] Health Innovation Network South London. Available at: https://healthinnovationnetwork.com/system/ckeditor_assets/attachments/41/what_is_person-centred_care_and_why_is_it_important.pdf (accessed 5 May 2020).

healthwatch (2016) Are People Waiting Too Long to Be Assessed for Social Care Support? [online] Available at: https://www.healthwatch.co.uk/news/2016-07-19/are-people-waiting-too-long-be-assessed-social-care-support (accessed 17 January 2021).

Hirst, M (2014) *Transitions Into and Out of Unpaid Care.* [pdf] York: University of York. Available at: https://www.york.ac.uk/inst/spru/pubs/pdf/CUK2644.pdf (accessed 17 June 2020).

HM Government (2007) *Putting People First a Shared Vision and Commitment to the Transformation of Adult Social Care.* [pdf] London: HM Government. Available at: https://www.basw.co.uk/system/files/resources/basw_102631-4_0.pdf (accessed 9 March 2021).

How to Avoid the Dementia Tax (2017) Dispatches, Season 31 Episode 28 [TV Programme] Channel 4, 20 November 2017.

In Control (2017) *POET Personal Outcomes Evaluation Tool for Adults in Receipt of Social Care Support 2017 Report.* [pdf] Think Local Act Personal. Available at: http://s557941885.websitehome.co.uk/wp-content/uploads/2017/07/poetpb2017-emb-final.pdf (accessed 17 January 2021).

Inclusion (2019) Values of Inclusion – Heather Simmons. [online] Available at: https://inclusion.com/2019/values-of-inclusion-heather-simmons/ (accessed 12 June 2020).

Inclusive Solutions (2015) Inclusive Solutions. [online] Available at: https://inclusive-solutions.com/person-centred-planning/ (accessed 16 October 2020).

James, I A (2011) *Understanding Behaviour in Dementia that Challenges: A Guide to Assessment and Treatment*. London: Jessica Kingsley Publishers.

Kane, M and Terry, G (2015) *Dementia 2015: Aiming Higher to Transform Lives.* [pdf] Alzheimer's Society. Available at: https://www.alzheimers.org.uk/sites/default/files/migrate/downloads/dementia_2015_aiming_higher_to_transform_lives.pdf (accessed 25 May 2020).

Killeen, J (1996) *Advocacy and Dementia*. Edinburgh: Alzheimer Scotland Action on Dementia.

Kim, S K and Park, M (2017) Effectiveness of Person-Centered Care on People with Dementia: A Systematic Review and Meta-Analysis. *Clinical Interventions in Aging,* [e-journal] 12: 381–397. Available through: NCBI PMC US National Library of Medicine National Institutes of Health. [online] Available at: https://www.ncbi.nlm.nih.gov/pmc/articles/PMC5322939/ (accessed 20 May 2020).

Kitwood, T (1990) The Dialectics of Dementia: With Particular Reference to Alzheimer's Disease. *Ageing and Society*, 10 (2): 177–96.

Kitwood, T (1997) *Dementia Reconsidered: The Person Comes First*. Buckingham and Philadelphia: Open University Press.

Kitwood, T (1997) The Experience of Dementia. *Aging and Mental Health*, 1 (1): 13–22.

Kitwood, T and Bredin, K (1992) Towards a Theory of Dementia Care: Personhood and Well-Being. *Ageing and Society,* [e-journal] 12 (3): 269–287. Available through: Cambridge University Press website. [online] Available at: https://www.cambridge.org/core/journals/ageing-and-society/issue/C61595C3F017F66F053016D1B9C34ED9 (accessed 22 July 2020).

Know Me Inc. (2016) People with Communication Difficulties Can Have Trouble Quickly Conveying Important Information about Themselves. Know Me – Communicating Personhood. [online] (Last updated 23 June 2017). Available at: https://appadvice.com/app/know-me-communicating-personhood/1051805757 (accessed 24 January 2021).

Kumar, A, Singh, R R and Thressiakutty, A T (2015) Normalisation vs Social Role Valorization: Similar or Different? *International Journal of Special Education,* [e-journal] 30 (3). [online] Available at: https://www.researchgate.net/publication/283351346_Normalization_vs_Social_Role_Valorization_Similar_of_Different (accessed 24 May 2020).

Laing, R D (1971) *The Politics of the Family and Other Essays*. New York: Pantheon Books .

Leocadie, M-C, Roy, M-H and Rothan-Tondeur, M (2018) Barriers and Enablers in the Use of Respite Interventions by Caregivers of People with Dementia: An Integrative Review. *Archives of Public Health*. [online] Available at: https://www.ncbi.nlm.nih.gov/pmc/articles/PMC6249779/ (accessed 1 July 2020).

Leslie, M (2016) *Discussing Real-Life Examples I Could Use for This Book, Which Included Leslie's Mum's Care Situation*. [letter] (Personal, communication, n.d. 2016).

Levin, E, Moriarty, J and Gorbach, P (1994) *Better for the Break*. London: HMSO.

Lewis, S (2005) *Direct Payments: Answering Frequently Asked Questions.* [pdf] Social Care Institute for Excellence. Available at: https://www.scie.org.uk/publications/guides/guide10/files/guide10.pdf (accessed 31 January 2021).

Local Government Act 1999. (c.27). London: HMSO.

Mackay, M (2016) Talking Mats Training for Families Living with Dementia. [online] Available at: https://www.talkingmats.com/talking-mats-training-for-families-living-with-dementia/ (accessed 3 February 2021).

Magnusson, S. (2014) *Where Memories Go: Why Dementia Changes Everything*. London: Two Roads.

Maslow, A H (1943) A Theory of Human Motivation. *Psychological Review*, [e-journal] 50 (4). Available through: American Psychological Association (APA) PsycNet website. [online] Available at: https://doi.org/10.1037/h0054346 (accessed 16 May 2020).

Matthews, E A, Farrell, G A and Blackmore, A M (1996) Effects of an Environmental Manipulation Emphasizing Client-Centred Care on Agitation and Sleep in Dementia Sufferers in a Nursing Home. *JAN*, [e-journal] 24 (3): 439–37. Abstract only. Available through: Wiley Online Library. [online] Available at: https://onlinelibrary.wiley.com/doi/abs/10.1046/j.1365-2648.1996.02102.x (accessed 18 July 2020).

Matthews, R (2016) Using Talking Mats to Include People with Dementia in Their Care Plan. [online] Available at: https://www.talkingmats.com/using-talking-mats-to-include-people-with-dementia-in-their-care-plans/ (accessed 23 January 2021).

McCrae, R R and Costa, Jr, P T (2003) *Personality in Adulthood: A Five-Factor Theory Perspective*. 2nd ed. New York: Guildford Press.

McCrone, P, Dhanasir, S, Patel, A, Knapp, M and Lawton-Smith, S (2008) *Paying the Price: The Cost of Mental Health Care in England to 2026.* [pdf] London: The King's Fund. Available at: https://www.kingsfund.org.uk/sites/default/files/Paying-the-Price-the-cost-of-mental-health-care-England-2026-McCrone-Dhanasiri-Patel-Knapp-Lawton-Smith-Kings-Fund-May-2008_0.pdf (accessed 24 January 2021).

McMaster University (2019) 3 Simple Ways to Manage Challenging Behaviours Associated with Dementia. [online] (Last updated 20 December 2019) Available at: https://www.mcmasteroptimalaging.org/blog/detail/blog/2016/11/15/3-simple-ways-to-manage-challenging-behaviours-associated-with-dementia (accessed 22 November 2020).

Mental Capacity Act (Northern Ireland) 2016. (c.18). Belfast: HMSO.

Mental Health Capacity Act 2005. (c.9). London: HMSO.

Mental Health Foundation (2015) *Dementia, Rights, and the Social Model of Disability.* [pdf] London: Mental Health Foundation. Available at: https://www.mentalhealth.org.uk/sites/default/files/dementia-rights-policy-discussion.pdf (accessed 23 May 2020).

Mind (2018) Advocacy in Mental Health. [online] Available at: https://www.mind.org.uk/information-support/guides-to-support-and-services/advocacy/what-is-advocacy/ (accessed 24 June 2020).

Mitchell, G and Agnelli, J (2015) *Person-Centred Care for People with Dementia: Kitwood Reconsidered.* [pdf] Royal College of Nursing. Available at: https://www.researchgate.net/publication/283244999_Person-centred_care_for_people_with_dementia_Kitwood_reconsidered (accessed 17 May 2020).

Mount, Dr. B (2000) *Life Building, Opening Windows to Change Using Personal Futures Planning Personal Workbook*. New York: Capacity Works.

Mount, Dr. B (2000) *Person-Centred Planning: Finding Directions for Change Using Personal Futures Planning: A Sourcebook of Values, Ideals, and Methods to Encourage Person-Centered Development*. New York: Capacity Works.

Mount, Dr. B and O'Brien, C (2002) *Building New Worlds. A Sourcebook for Students with Disabilities in Transition from High School to Adult Life*. New York: Capacity Works.

Murphy, G and Gair, E (2013) *Communicating a Diagnosis of Dementia, Briefing Paper for Faculty for Psychology of Older People and Dementia Action Alliance*. [online] Available at: https://www.dementiaaction.org.uk/assets/0000/5805/BPS_FPOP_DAA_Communicating_Diagnosis_3.docx (accessed 22 September 2020).

National Disability Practitioners (NDP) (2016) *What Is a Person Centred Approach?* [pdf] National Disability Practitioners (NDP). Available at: https://www.ndp.org.au/images/factsheets/346/2016-10-person-centred-approach.pdf (accessed 17 October 2020).

National Institute for Health and Care Excellence (NICE) (2018) Dementia: Assessment, Management and Support for People Living with Dementia and Their Carers. [online] Available at: https://www.nice.org.uk/guidance/ng97/chapter/Person-centred-care (accessed 4 May 2020).

National Institute for Health and Care Excellence (NICE) (2019) *Dementia.* [pdf] National Institute for Health and Care Excellence (NICE). Available at: https://www.nice.org.uk/guidance/ng97/chapter/Person-centred-care (accessed 17 June 2020).

National Institute for Health and Care Excellence (NICE) (2020) News. [online] Available at: https://www.nice.org.uk/news (accessed 12 July 2018).

National Voices (2014) *Care and Support Planning Guide.* [pdf] National Voices. Available at: https://www.nationalvoices.org.uk/sites/default/files/public/publications/guide_to_care_and_support_planning_0.pdf (accessed 11 November 2020).

New Possibilities (n.d.) New Possibilities Approach. [online] Available at: https://www.newpossibilities.co.uk/ (accessed 29 July 2020).

NHS (2020) About Dementia. [online] (Last updated 25 June 2020) Available at: https://www.nhs.uk/conditions/dementia/about/ (accessed 10 January 2021).

NHS (2020) Advanced Decision (Living Will). [online] Available at: https://www.nhs.uk/conditions/end-of-life-care/advance-decision-to-refuse-treatment/ (accessed 25 November 2020).

NHS Choices (2015) Your Guide to Care and Support. [online] Available at: https://www.nhs.uk/conditions/social-care-and-support/ (accessed 8 January 2018).

NHS Digital (2013) Measures from the Adult Social Care Outcomes Framework - England, 2011–12, Final. [online] Available at: https://digital.nhs.uk/data-and-information/publications/statistical

/adult-social-care-outcomes-framework-ascof/archive/measures-from-the-adult-social-care-outcomes-framework—england-2011-12-final (accessed 7 June 2020).

NHS Digital (2015) Measures from the Adult Social Care Outcomes Framework, England –2014–15, Final Release. [online] Available at: https://digital.nhs.uk/data-and-information/publications/statistical/adult-social-care-outcomes-framework-ascof/archive/measures-from-the-adult-social-care-outcomes-framework-england—2014-15-final-release (accessed 13 June 2020).

NHS Digital (2015) Measures from the Adult Social Care Outcomes Framework, England –2014–15, Final Release. [online] Available at: https://digital.nhs.uk/data-and-information/publications/statistical/adult-social-care-outcomes-framework-ascof/archive/measures-from-the-adult-social-care-outcomes-framework-england—2014-15-final-release (accessed 17 January 2021). (Outlined in the "1C(1A) - rounded" and "1C(2A) 0 rounded" tabs of the "meas-from-asc-of-eng-1415-fin-dis-ang-anx" spreadsheet accessed by downloading the "ASCOF 2014–2015 data files" zip file under the "Resources" heading on the link above).

NHS Digital (2017) Measures from the Adult Social Care Outcomes Framework, England –2016–17. [online] Available at: https://digital.nhs.uk/data-and-information/publications/statistical/adult-social-care-outcomes-framework-ascof/archive/measures-from-the-adult-social-care-outcomes-framework-england—2016-17 (accessed 11 September 2020).

NHS Digital (2019) 1C - The Proportions of Users and Carers Receiving Self-Directed Support, and Self-Directed Support via Direct Payments. [online] Available at: https://digital.nhs.uk/data-and-information/publications/statistical/adult-social-care-outcomes-framework-ascof/current/indicator-files/1c—the-proportions-of-users-and-carers-receiving-self-directed-support-and-self-directed-support-via-direct-payments (accessed 17 January 2021). (Outlined in the "1C(1A): The proportion of people who use services who receive self-directed support" and "1C(2A): The proportion of people who use services who receive direct payments" tabs of the "1C- The proportions of users and carers receiving self-directed support, and self-directed support via direct payments" spreadsheet found under the "Resources" heading on the link above).

NHS Digital (2019) Measures from the Adult Social Care Outcomes Framework England, 2018–19. [online] Available at: https://digital.nhs.uk/data-and-information/publications/statistical/adult-social-care-outcomes-framework-ascof/current (accessed 12 June 2020).

NHS Digital (2020) CCG Outcomes Indicator Set - March 2020. [online] Available at: https://digital.nhs.uk/data-and-information/publications/statistical/ccg-outcomes-indicator-set/march-2020 (accessed 12 June 2020).

NHS Digital (2020) NHS Outcomes Framework Indicators - May 2020 Release. [online] Available at: https://digital.nhs.uk/data-and-information/publications/statistical/nhs-outcomes-framework/may-2020#data-sets (accessed 12 June 2020).

NHS England (2019) *Personalised Care Guidance on the Legal Rights to Have Personal Health Budgets and Personal Wheelchair Budgets Version 1.0: December 2019.* [pdf] NHS Improvement. Available at: https://www.england.nhs.uk/wp-content/uploads/2014/09/guidance-on-the-legal-rights-to-personal-health-budgets.pdf (accessed 25 May 2020).

NHS England (2020) *Dementia Assessment and Referral Data Collection – February 2020.* [pdf] NHS England. Available at: https://www.england.nhs.uk/statistics/wp-content/uploads/sites/2/2020/05/Dementia-Statistical-Summary-February-2020-PDF-126KB.pdf (accessed 12 July 2020).

NHS England and NHS Improvement (2019) *Personalised Care. Guidance on the Legal Rights to Have Personal Health Budgets and Personal Wheelchair Budgets.* [pdf] NHS England and NHS

Improvement. Available at: https://www.england.nhs.uk/wp-content/uploads/2014/09/guidance-on-the-legal-rights-to-personal-health-budgets.pdf (accessed 12 July 2020).

Nolan, M R, Brown, J, Davies, S, Nolan, J and Keady, J (2006) *The Senses Framework: Improving Care for Older People through a Relationship-Centred Approach. Getting Research into Practice (GRiP) Report No 2.* [pdf] Sheffield Hallam University. Available at: https://core.ac.uk/download/pdf/99946.pdf (accessed 10 May 2020).

Nolan, M R, Davies, S, Brown, J, Keady, J and Nolan, J (2002) *Longitudinal Study of the Effectiveness of Educational Preparation to Meet the Needs of Older People and Carers: The AGEIN (Advancing Gerontological Education in Nursing) Project*. London: English National Board for Nursing, Midwifery and Health Visiting.

Nuffield Council of Bioethics (2009) *Dementia: Ethical Issues*. [pdf] London: Nuffield Council of Bioethics. Available at: https://www.nuffieldbioethics.org/publications/dementia (accessed 16 September 2020).

Nursing Homes Undercover (2016) Panorama, Series 64. [TV Programme]. BBC, BBC1, 25 November 2016, 20.30.

Nursing Times (2017) Assisting Patients with Eating and Drinking to Prevent Malnutrition. [online] Available at: https://www.nursingtimes.net/clinical-archive/nutrition/assisting-patients-with-eating-and-drinking-to-prevent-malnutrition-09-10-2017/ (accessed 12 July 2020).

O'Brien, C L and O'Brien, J, eds. (2002) *Implementing Person-Centered Planning: Voices of Experience (Vol. II)*. Toronto: Inclusion Press.

O'Brien, J, Pearpoint, J and Kahn, L (2010) *The PATH and MAPs Handbook. Person-Centred Ways to Build Community*. Toronto: Inclusion Press International.

Office for National Statistics (2013) *2011 Census Analysis: Unpaid Care in England and Wales, 2011 and Comparison with 2001*. [online] (Last updated 15 February 2013) Available at: https://www.ons.gov.uk/peoplepopulationandcommunity/healthandsocialcare/healthcaresystem/articles/2011censusanalysisunpaidcareinenglandandwales2011andcomparisonwith2001/2013-02-15#national-comparisons (accessed 17 June 2020).

Office of the Public Guardian (2020) Make, Register or End a Lasting Power of Attorney. [online] Available at: https://www.gov.uk/power-of-attorney/ (accessed 20 October 2020).

Older People's Advocacy Alliance (OPAAL) UK (n.d.) Advocating Change for Older People. [online] Available at: http://opaal.org.uk/ (accessed 29 June 2020).

Owen, T, Meyer, J, Cornell, M, Dudman, P, Ferreira, Z, Hamilton, S, Moore, J and Wallis, J (2012) *My Home Life: Promoting Quality of Life in Care Homes*. [pdf] York: Joseph Rowntree Foundation. Available at: http://www.myhomelife.org.uk/wp-content/uploads/2015/02/JRF-report-on-care-home-quality-of-life-full.pdf (accessed 10 December 2020).

Pearpoint, J (2002) *Hints for Graphic Facilitators*. Toronto: Inclusion Press.

Pearpoint, J, O'Brien, J and Forest, M (2001) *PATH A Workbook for Planning Positive and Possible Futures*. Toronto: Inclusion Press.

Pearpoint, J, Forest, M and Snow, J (1992) *The Inclusion Papers: Strategies to Make Inclusion Work. A Collection of Articles.* [pdf] Toronto: Inclusion Press. Available at: https://files.eric.ed.gov/fulltext/ED359677.pdf (accessed 12 June 2020).

Peate, I (2006) *Becoming a Nurse in the 21st Century*. Chichester: John Wiley & Sons Ltd.

Perez-Merino, R (2014) Starting Out - By Listening to Patient, I Understood His Needs and Enhanced His Care. *Nursing Standard,* [e-journal] 29 (9). Available through: Royal College of Nursing Institute website. [online] Available at: http://journals.rcni.com/doi/full/10.7748/ns.29.9.29.s33 (accessed 22 July 2020).

Pictures to Share (n.d.) Our Books. [online] Available at: https://www.picturestoshare.co.uk/ (accessed 1 February 2021).

Plos Medicine (2018) Impact of Person-Centred Care Training and Person-Centred Activities on Quality of Life, Agitation, and Antipsychotic Use in People with Dementia Living in Nursing Homes: A Cluster-Randomised Controlled Trial. [online] Available at: https://journals.plos.org/plosmedicine/article?id=10.1371/journal.pmed.1002500 (accessed 5 May 2020).

Policy Navigator (2007) Putting People First Was Published by the Department of Health in December 2007. [online] Available at: https://navigator.health.org.uk/content/putting-people-first-was-published-department-health-december-2007 (accessed 9 May 2020).

Poole (2006) *Direct Payments and Older People.* [pdf] London: Kings Fund. Available at: https://www.kingsfund.org.uk/sites/default/files/direct-payments-older-people-wanless-background-paper-teresa-poole2006.pdf (accessed 3 June 2020).

Pratt, R and Wilkinson, H (2001) *TELL ME THE TRUTH the Effect of Being Told the Diagnosis of Dementia from the Perspective of the Person with Dementia.* [pdf] London: The Mental Health Foundation. Available at: https://www.mentalhealth.org.uk/sites/default/files/tell_me_the_truth.pdf (accessed 12 March 2021).

Priestley, M, Finkelstein, V and David, K (1997) The Union of the Physically Impaired against Segregation and the Disability Alliance Discuss Fundamental Principles of Disability. [pdf] Available at: https://disability-studies.leeds.ac.uk/wp-content/uploads/sites/40/library/UPIAS-fundamental-principles.pdf (accessed 22 May 2020).

Prime Minister's Strategy Unit (2005) *Improving the Life Chances of Disabled People Final Report.* [pdf] Department for Work and Pensions, Department of Health, Department for Education and Skills and Office of the Deputy Prime Minister. Available at: https://webarchive.nationalarchives.gov.uk/+/http:/www.cabinetoffice.gov.uk/media/cabinetoffice/strategy/assets/disability.pdf (accessed 15 March 2021).

Public Health England (2015) *Reasons Why People with Dementia Are Admitted to a General Hospital in an Emergency*. [pdf] Public Health England. Available at: https://webarchive.nationalarchives.gov.uk/20170302124526/http://www.yhpho.org.uk/default.aspx?RID=207311 (accessed 4 November 2016).

Realpe, A and Wallace, L M (2010) *What Is Co-production?* [pdf] The Health Foundation. Available at: https://qi.elft.nhs.uk/wp-content/uploads/2017/01/what_is_co-production.pdf (accessed 12 June 2020).

Rogers, C (1951) *Client-Centered Therapy: Its Current Practice, Implications and Theory*. London: Constable.

Routledge, M and Carr, S (2013) *Improving Personal Budgets for Older People A REVIEW.* [pdf] London: Think Local Act Personal and SCIE (Social Care Institute for Excellence). Available at: https://www.adass.org.uk/AdassMedia/stories/Carers/Personal%20BudgetsOlder%20People_FINAL.pdf (accessed 17 January 2021).

Saad, K, Hartman, J, Ballard, C, Kurian, M, Graham, C and Wilcock, G (1995) *Coping by the Carers of Dementia Sufferers.* [pdf] Oxford University Press. Available at: https://www.researchgate

.net/profile/Candida_Graham/publication/14611088_Coping_by_the_Carers_of_Dementia_Sufferers/links/563a510e08ae45b5d284a953.pdf (accessed 3 July 2020).

Saunders (2003) *Miller-Keane Encyclopedia & Dictionary of Medicine, Nursing & Allied Health*. 7th ed. London: Saunders.

Seeds for Change (2020) *Facilitation Tools for Meetings Workshops.* [pdf] Seeds for Change. Available at: https://seedsforchange.org.uk/tools.pdf (accessed 7 August 2020).

Seligman, M E P (1975) *Helplessness: On Depression, Development, and Death*. San Francisco: W. H. Freeman.

Skills for Health and Skills for Care (2018) *Managing Success in Dementia Care.* [pdf] Leeds: Leeds Beckett University. Available at: https://www.hee.nhs.uk/sites/default/files/documents/Managing%20Success%20v3.pdf (accessed 17 May 2020).

Smull, M and Harrison, S B (n.d.) *An Overview of Essential Lifestyle Planning*. [pdf] Annapolis: Support Development Associates. Available at: http://www.allenshea.com/brochure.pdf (accessed 7 August 2020).

Snow, J (2015) *Great Questions: Writings of Judith Snow*. Toronto, ON, Canada: Inclusion Press.

Social Care Institute for Excellence (SCIE) (2011). What Is Personalisation? [online] Available at: https://www.scie.org.uk/personalisation/introduction/what-is (accessed 9 May 2020).

Social Care Institute of Excellence (SCIE) (2012) *Personalisation: A Rough Guide* [pdf] Social Care Institute of Excellence (SCIE). Available at: https://www.scie.org.uk/files/personalisation/introduction/rough-guide/guide47.pdf (accessed 17 June 2020).

Social Care Institute for Excellence (SCIE) (2012) Report 55: People not Processes: The Future of Personalisation and Independent Living. [online] (Last updated March 2012) Available at: https://www.scie.org.uk/publications/reports/report55/barrierstopersonalisation.asp (accessed 5 June 2020).

Social Care Institute for Excellence (SCIE) (2015) Getting a Dementia Diagnosis. [online] Available at: https://www.scie.org.uk/dementia/symptoms/diagnosis/getting-a-diagnosis.asp#:~:text=The%20Alzheimer%27s%20Society%20says%20that,a%20diagnosis%20can%20be%20made (accessed 1 July 2020).

Social Care Institute for Excellence (SCIE) (2017) Using Technology to Support People Living with Dementia. [online] Available at: https://www.scie.org.uk/dementia/support/technology (accessed 3 July 2020).

Social Care Institute for Excellence (SCIE) (2020) Dementia. My Life Is Changing because of Dementia. [online] (Last updated October 2020) Available at: https://www.scie.org.uk/dementia/after-diagnosis/knowing-the-person/life-is-changing.asp (accessed 22 November 2020).

Social Care Institute for Excellence (SCIE) (n.d.) Deprivation of Liberty Safeguards (DoLS). [online] (Last updated December 2011) Available at: https://www.scie.org.uk/mca/dols (accessed 25 September 2020).

Social Care Institute for Excellence (SCIE) (n.d.) Eligibility Outcomes for Carers with Support Needs under the Care Act 2014. [online] Available at: https://www.scie.org.uk/care-act-2014/assessment-and-eligibility/eligibility/outcomes-carer-with-support-needs.asp (accessed 24 June 2020).

Social Care Institute for Excellence (SCIE) (n.d.) News. [online] Available at: https://www.scie.org.uk/news/ (accessed 12 July 2020).

Social Services and Well-Being (Wales) Act 2014. (anaw.4.). Cardiff: National Assembly for Wales.

Stokes, G (2000) *Challenging Behaviour in Dementia : A Person-Centred Approach*. Milton Keynes: Routledge.

The Care and Support (Eligibility Criteria) Regulations 2015 (2015) *SI 2015/313*. London: HMSO.

The Care and Support (Eligibility) (Wales) Regulations 2015. 2015. *SI 2015/1578*. Cardiff: HMSO.

The Health and Social Care Act 2008 (Regulated Activities) Regulations 2014. (2014) *SI 2014/2936*. London: HMSO.

The King's Fund (2018) *Key Challenges Facing the Adult Social Care Sector in England.* [pdf] King's Fund. Available at: https://www.kingsfund.org.uk/sites/default/files/2018-12/Key-challenges-facing-the-adult-social-care-sector-in-England.pdf (accessed 13 June 2020).

The Scottish Government (2017) *Scotland's National Dementia Strategy 2017–2020.* [pdf] Edinburgh: The Scottish Government. Available at: https://www.gov.scot/binaries/content/documents/govscot/publications/strategy-plan/2017/06/scotlands-national-dementia-strategy-2017-2020/documents/00521773-pdf/00521773-pdf/govscot%3Adocument/00521773.pdf (accessed 4 May 2020).

The Scottish Government (2020) Mental Health. [online] Available at: https://www.gov.scot/policies/mental-health/dementia/ (accessed 4 May 2020).

Think Local Act Personal (2011) *Making it Real. Marking Progress towards Personalised, Community Based Support.* [pdf] London: Think Local Act Personal. [online] Available at: https://www.thinklocalactpersonal.org.uk/_assets/Resources/Personalisation/TLAP/MakingItReal.pdf (accessed 25 May 2020).

Think Local Act Personal (2014) *Personalisation Action Plan: Key Activity Underway in Advance of the Care Bill.* [pdf] Think Local Act Personal. Available at: http://www.thinklocalactpersonal.org.uk/_assets/PersonalisationActionPlanFINAL.pdf (accessed 13 May 2020).

Think Local Act Personal (n.d.) Paying for Respite Care - Solutions. [online] Available at: https://www.thinklocalactpersonal.org.uk/Personal-Budgets-Minimum-Process-Framework/Respite-care-provided-through-vouchers/#prc6-solutions (accessed 12 July 2020).

Undercover Care: The Abused Exposed (2011) Panorama, Series 59. [TV Programme]. BBC, BBC1, 31 May 2011, 21.00.

Upton, D, Upton, P, Jones, T, Jutlla, K and Brooker, D (2011) *Evaluation of the Impact of Touch Screen Technology on People with Dementia and Their Carers within Care Home Settings*. [online] (Last updated 17 June 2020) Available at: https://eprints.worc.ac.uk/2162/ (accessed 24 January 2021).

Wells, S (2006) *Developments in Dementia Advocacy: Exploring the Role of Advocates in Supporting People with Dementia*. London: WASSR.

Welsh Government (2018) *Dementia Action Plan for Wales.* [pdf] Welsh Government. Available at: https://gov.wales/sites/default/files/publications/2019-04/dementia-action-plan-for-wales.pdf (accessed 4 May 2020).

West, S and Glover, H (2014) *Best Interest Meeting Guidance*. [pdf] Lincolnshire County Council. Available at: https://www.scie.org.uk/files/mca/directory/best-interests-meetings-guidance.pdf?res=true (accessed 25 September 2020).

Whitehead, H (2020) Over 60% of Community Groups Have Closed or Decreased Services during Covid-19. [online] Available at: https://www.civilsociety.co.uk/news/over-60-of-community-groups-have-closed-or-decreased-services-during-covid-19.html (accessed 29 January 2021).

Whitman, L (2015) *People with Dementia Speak Out: Creative Ways to Achieve Focus and Attention by Building on AD/HD Traits*. London: Jessica Kingsley Publishers.

Williamson, T (2010) *My Name Is not Dementia People with Dementia Discuss Quality of Life Indicators*. [pdf] London: Alzheimer's Society. Available at: https://www.cardi.ie/userfiles/My_name_is_not_dementia_report%5B1%5D.pdf (accessed 25 September 2020).

Wolfensberger, W P, Nirje, B, Olshansky, S, Perske, R and Roos, P (1972) *The Principle of Normalization in Human Services.* [e-book] Toronto: National Institute of Mental Retardation. Available through: University of Nebraska Medical Center website. [online] Available at: https://digitalcommons.unmc.edu/wolf_books/1/ (accessed 24 May 2020).

World Health Organization (WHO) (2011) *World Report on Disability*. [pdf] Geneva: World Health Organization. Available at: https://www.who.int/disabilities/world_report/2011/report.pdf (accessed 23 May 2020).

World Health Organization (WHO) (2012) *Q10: For Carers of People with Dementia, Does Respite Care When Compared to Care as Usual, Produce Benefits/Harm in the Specified Outcomes?* [pdf] World Health Organization (WHO). Available at: https://www.who.int/mental_health/mhgap/evidence/dementia/mh_dementia_q10_respite_en.pdf? (accessed 1 June 2020).

World Health Organization (WHO) (2019) Dementia. [online] Available at: https://www.who.int/news-room/fact-sheets/detail/dementia (accessed 1 July 2020).

Yates, L, Csipke, E, Moniz-Cook, E, Leung, P, Walton, H, Charlesworth, G, Spector, A, Hogervorst, E, Mountain, G and Orell, M (2019) The Development of the Promoting Independence in Dementia (PRIDE) Intervention to Enhance Independence in Dementia. *Clinical Interventions in Aging*, [e-journal] 14: 1615–1630. Abstract only. [online] Available at: https://www.ncbi.nlm.nih.gov/pmc/articles/PMC6748161/ (accessed 17 January 2021).

YouGov (2013) Care Home Concerns. [online] Available at: https://yougov.co.uk/topics/politics/articles-reports/2013/03/06/care-home-concerns (accessed 12 July 2020).

Young Dementia UK (n.d.) Janet & Martin's Story. [online] Available at: https://www.youngdementiauk.org/janet-martins-story (accessed 10 June 2020).

Young Dementia UK (n.d.) Ken H's Story. [online] Available at: https://www.youngdementiauk.org/ken-hs-story (accessed 1 June 2020).

Young Dementia UK (n.d.) Tommy's Story. [online] Available at: www.youngdementiauk.org/tommys-story (accessed 23 May 2020).

Index